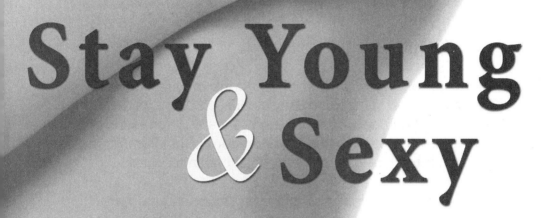

Stay Young
& Sexy

with

Bio-Identical
Hormone Replacement

Jonathan V. Wright, MD

Lane Lenard, PhD

STAY YOUNG & SEXY
WITH
Bio-Identical Hormone Replacement

Jonathan V. Wright, MD & Lane Lenard, PhD

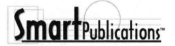

www.smart-publications.com
Petaluma, CA

**Published in the United States of America
Fifth Printing, Second Edition, 2014**

Library of Congress Control Number: 2009934977

ISBN: 1-890572-22-5   978-1-890572-22-8

Warning—Disclaimer

TABLE OF CONTENTS

Take
our
FREE

hormone assessment online at:

www.smart-publications.com/
hormone-self-assessment

JONATHAN V. WRIGHT, MD.,
DEDICATION & ACKNOWLEDGMENTS

For my wife Holly

Lane Lenard, Ph.D., a science writer and researcher with very few equals;

John Morgenthaler, Ed Kinon, and the staff at Smart Publications for waiting so long for this revision and update;

Suzanne Somers for all she's done to bring BHRT and better health to the women (and men) of the world;

Oprah Winfrey, for spreading the word to millions more;

"Anna" (not her real name), who advised me she wasn't a horse and wanted her own human hormones back, and the thousands of women I've worked with who thought for themselves about hormone replacement, from whom I've learned so much;

Ed Thorpe, Pharm.D., of Kripps Pharmacy, Vancouver, British Columbia, for finding the materials for the very first BHRT prescriptions;

Jim Seymour, R.Ph., Bill Corriston, R.Ph., and the staff of Key Pharmacy, Kent, Washington, for filling so many BHRT prescriptions and taking such good care of so many Tahoma Clinic clients;

Joe Grasela, R.Ph., and John Grasela, R.Ph., of University Compounding Pharmacy, San Diego, for organizing and managing the best BHRT seminars in these United States;

The physicians—my colleagues—on the staff of Tahoma Clinic, who continue to research and use better ways to use and monitor BHRT and natural medicine for all those with whom we work.

LANE LENARD, PH.D., ACKNOWLEDGMENTS

For Phyllis, who began using bio-identical hormones long before I ever wrote a word about them (and it shows). Thank you for your encouragement, your creative (and critical) input, and valuable editing help. Most of all, thank you for your patience and understanding.

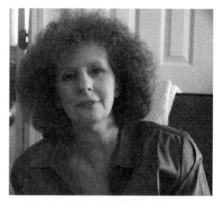

And for Katy. You make it all worthwhile.

I'd also like to acknowledge the critical contribution of Dr. Jennifer Schneider for the chapter on osteoporosis, and the editing advice of Kathryn Pucci and Stan Shaffer.

FOREWORD

YOUR BIO-IDENTICAL HOROMONE REFERENCE BIBLE

By Suzanne Somers

Reading Stay Young and Sexy with Bio-Identical Replacement: The Science Explained is like taking a college course with the premier professors of our time. That would be Drs. Jonathan V. Wright and Lane Lenard. The confusion surrounding menopausal hormone replacement needs to be unraveled, and this book does just that. Replacing lost hormones due to aging or stress is the backbone of anti-aging medicine. Mainstream medicine tends to frown upon anti-aging as though it were a phenomenon that didn't exist, but it is quite clear that human beings are living longer today than ever before. Unfortunately, that longer life may have very little quality left.

At present, people begin to degrade at middle age (which, due to increasing stress, is now becoming younger and younger), and the remedy conventional medicine typically prescribes is one or more pharmaceutical drugs. Can't sleep? Take Ambien®. Depressed? Take Prozac®. High cholesterol? Take Lipitor®. Anxiety or panic attacks? Take Valium®. Then there's blood pressure medicine and pain killers, and soon you have a virtual tackle box of pharmaceuticals and so begins the slow degrade of "you." Your thinking becomes foggy; your joints ache; your libido disappears; the essence of who you are slowly slips away and tends towards disease.

Information Is Power

More than ever before, laypeople need to arm themselves with information that is truly lifesaving. Stay on your present course of pharmaceuticals and chemicals, and you will eventually lose yourself in the fog of drugs and the slow poisoning that is evident in people all around us.

Drs. Wright and Lenard have done the work for us in this informative book. They understand that replacing natural hormones as we age with real, bio-identical hormones, just as we once made in our own bodies, is the backbone of successful aging. In order to take advantage of this new long life that technology has allowed us, we need to keep our bodies' hormone levels in youthful balance.

This book explains the difference between natural hormones and manmade hormones. It is the manmade hormones that have been proven dangerous, but in this book you will see the studies and scientific backup that prove the efficacy and joys of replacing natural hormones with real, bio-identical hormones that have been lost through the aging process or from the stress of today's hectic lifestyles.

It's all here in this book – the ultimate explanation. This is the real science, not encumbered by pharmaceutical agendas. These doctors have gone out on a limb to bring you the truth so that we can all feel better and live the joyous lives we were meant to live.

I recommend that you read this book cover to cover and then use it as your "bio-identical hormone reference bible." Whatever information you are looking for will be here; all the answers lie within. This is a tremendous piece of work that has taken years of intensive study and clinical application to accomplish. Dr. Jonathan V. Wright and Dr. Lane Lenard will one day be known as the doctors who changed medicine against all odds and against violent opposition.

It is a great book.

Suzanne Somers
June 2009

PREFACE

Bringing BHRT into the 21ST Century

By Jonathan V. Wright, MD

Doctors often learn as much from their clients as clients learn from their doctors. One of many times this has happened to me was in the early 1980s, when a woman suffering symptoms of menopause reminded me that she wasn't a horse (*for details, see Chapter 2*), and that she'd prefer to replace her disappearing ovarian hormones with the exact same molecules that menopause had mostly taken away, and not alien-to-human horse hormone molecules. That stimulated me to put together what turned out to be the very first comprehensive "bio-identical hormone replacement therapy" (BHRT) program here in North America. The bio-identical hormones included were estradiol, estriol, estrone (for technical reasons, this third estrogen not used as much any more) along with progesterone, DHEA, testosterone, and thyroid.

The word about BHRT spread first by woman-to-woman communication, reporting to each other how much better they felt. "I feel like my self again" was a very typical comment. Then came articles and books (including the very first book on this topic by Dr. Lenard and me, published in 1997) and many other publications. Since 2004, BHRT has been given enormous publicity by Suzanne Somers' series of books discussing BHRT, and lately by TV superstars Oprah Winfrey (who had Suzanne on one of her shows) in early 2009; "Dr. Phil," and Robin McGraw (Mrs. "Dr. Phil") and the other doctors on the TV show "The Doctors."

Since it's beginning in the early 1980s, comprehensive BHRT has since grown from one woman, one physician, and one compounding pharmacy to hundreds of thousands of women, and (at this time) several thousand physicians and compounding pharmacies. Men have joined the comprehensive BHRT movement, too, of course using the bio-identical pattern for males (*See Chapter 10*).

But even though my comprehensive BHRT prescriptions were the first in North America, I can't really take credit for "inventing" BHRT! The model was there all along, right there in women's (and men's) bodies. I copied — not invented it — as precisely as I could, following the pattern of hormones found naturally, using the exact same molecules, in the same quantities, following the same timing, and using the best ways of getting them into the body. This was all guided by a principle that has always kept my entire medical practice as safe and effective as possible: *Copy Nature!* But I can't even claim to be the first to copy Nature, nor did I do the best job. The first and finest job of copying Nature with BHRT was actually accomplished in China, between the years 1025 and 1833 AD.

Lessons from Ancient China

No, I'm not kidding! The details are discussed at great length in volume 5 of Joseph Needham and GD Lu's classic multivolume series, *Science and Civilization in China.** (For those lacking time to read all 36 densely packed pages on this topic, an excellent 4-page summary can be found in Robert Temple's *The Genius of China.†*) Described in Needham and Lu's book are several methods of preparing complete patterns of human hormones, much more complete than anything available today. These included not only the hormones listed above, but also human growth hormone (HGH), pituitary hormones, such as adrenocorticotropic hormone (ACTH), thyroid-stimulating hormone (TSH), follicle stimulation hormone (FSH), and luteinizing hormone (LH), the thyroid hormones T4, T3, T2, and T1, parathyroid hormone (PTH), calcitonin, cortisol, dehydroepiandrosterone (DHEA), aldosterone, erythropoetin (EPO)... I could go on and on with every hormone mentioned in today's textbooks, but the list still wouldn't be complete, as these preparations also contained every hormone not yet discovered by now, but present in

---

*   Needham J, Lu G-D. Proto-endocrinology: The enchymoma in the test-tube: Medieval preparations of urinary steroid and protein hormones in science and civilization in China, vol. 5: Chemistry and chemical technology, part 5: *Spagyrical Discovery and Invention: Physiological Alchemy.* 1983; Cambridge, UK; Cambridge University Press: 301-337.

†   Temple, Robert. *The genius of China: 3,000 years of science, discovery, and invention.* Part 5, Section 52. *The science of endocrinology.* 1986; New York: Simon and Schuster: 127-130.

the human body all the same. How could this happen, especially in the 11th century, when none of these individual hormones were even identified by scientists until the late 19th and early 20th centuries?

It's all due to the same principle mentioned above: **Copy Nature!** No, these medieval Chinese scientists and chemists had no way of knowing any of the individual hormones, but they correctly guessed that all of the substances that "power" the human body are found in human urine, which has indeed been found by "modern science" to contain every hormone known to be secreted by the human body[*] (and many other things, too, such as sodium, potassium, calcium, magnesium and every other trace element found in our food — but that's a discussion for another time.) Before you go "yuck!" and quit reading, remember that since the late 1960s and up to the present day, millions of American women — and many more overseas — have been prescribed and willingly swallowed pills containing hormones concentrated from **preg**nant **mar**e's **urine** — better known as **Premarin®,** which unfortunately are not bio-identical to humans, and because of that, caused an enormous amount of trouble for decades before "modern medicine" decided to research it thoroughly.

Quite obviously, the urine of young adults is likely to contain the highest quantities of sex steroids (as well as all the others), so for those effects, that's the urine medieval Chinese physicians used, gender-specific for women and men. Needham and Lu provide detailed documentation that from the 11th through the 19th centuries, Chinese physicians — very often famous Taoist physicians — would evaporate or precipitate urine in quantities from a few gallons to hundreds of gallons at a time, thus concentrating every hormone produced by young healthy bodies. These concentrates were then compressed with resins, gums, and spices into pills, and swallowed by various Emperors and Empresses and many others interested in healthy longevity. Needham and Lu report that many of those who took these preparations were observed to appear much younger than their actual ages — even then, this original version of BHRT was known to support healthy aging and help retain a more youthful appearance.

---

[*]   It's very unlikely that modern science has to this day identified all the hormones present in human urine. For example, the hormone hepcidin,an important iron-regulating hormone was unknown it until was discovered in human urine in 2001. (Rossi E. Hepcidin - the iron regulatory hormone. *Clin Biochem Rev.* 2005; 26: 47–49).

For the foreseeable future, "modern" 21st century BHRT will remain far behind medieval Chinese BHRT because of the former's woefully incomplete hormone pattern. The only part of "modern" BHRT that's actually superior are its delivery (into the body) systems, transdermal — or even better, as you'll subsequently read — transmucosal crèmes, which help us "Copy Nature" (there's that phrase again) better than pills. Transmucosal crèmes introduce the hormones they carry directly into the bloodstream, just as our own hormone-secreting glands do. By contrast, pills carry the hormones into the intestines and then to the liver, which is definitely not meant to be the first stop on Nature's route for hormone travel in the body. For many hormones, the liver is actually the most important part of the body's hormone disposal (not use) system. Sending overly large quantities of hormones to be disposed of before they're even used by other body cells leads to potential "side effects," including extra risks of blood clots, heart disease, and cancer.

Catching up with Medieval Chinese Science by 21st Century Recycling

"Modern" BHRT could actually "catch up" — in a decade or less — with comprehensive medieval Chinese BHRT, which included every hormone, major and minor, found in the human body. Ironically, that "catching up" could be done by following a pattern pioneered by a 20th century patent medicine company, by processing urine, *not horse urine,* but human urine. And as "bonus points," if this is done, it could well permanently solve — or greatly lessen — the chronically recurring financial problems of school districts, colleges, and universities across these United States.

"Wait a minute!" you might be thinking. What's he suggesting here? Mixing BHRT with school districts, colleges, and universities? How could public school districts actually hold the key to upgrading 20th century and earlier BHRT to the 21st century, allowing us to equal and surpass Chinese BHRT of the 10th through 19th centuries? I'm sure you've guessed how by now, but just in case not, here it is:

Where are the most healthy and robust adult hormones to be found? In young adults, of course. And where are young adults concentrated regularly in large groups? In high schools, colleges, and universities. By making appropriate use of this presently neglected (literally flushed away) but reliably produced natural resource, which obviously, the young adults don't wish to keep, high schools, colleges, and universities could go a long way toward preventing and even eliminating the financial crises in which they so frequently find themselves.

Yes, that's right. By re-plumbing high school, college, and university restrooms, urine flow could be re-routed to two (one for women, one for men) very high-tech filtration and purification installations, which would totally clean it up and extract only the myriad hormones in ultra-pure concentrated form, discarding or putting to other use all the rest. Working with high-tech processing techniques, this ultra-pure, strongest and best-possible-hormonally-balanced concentrate (as it originated from healthy young women and men) could be divided by compounding pharmacists into individualized daily doses as prescribed by each woman's and man's physician. The compounding pharmacist could also "tweak" the concentrate exactly as prescribed, for example, adding a bit of extra bio-identical progesterone for part of a woman's BHRT cycle, and then put the final individualized result into the most effective and safest delivery form, likely a transmucosal crème or gel. By supplying this system with this most hormonally rich "raw material," participating public school districts, colleges, and universities could achieve total sales of billions of dollars annually, and thereby help solve their financial problems.

Think I'm kidding? You think Americans simply won't "go for" a program in which urine — yuck, urine — is recycled into a "healthy aging" treatment? Think again: Remember Premarin®, concentrated and purified from horse urine? What could be yuckier than that? (Well, yes, but please don't answer that out loud.) (Recall that NASA has overcome the "yuck factor" and developed a way for astronauts on long space voyages or visits to the space station to recycle their own urine for drinking water.) Yet, buoyed by the promise of reversing the symptoms of menopause and slowing many of the normal changes of aging, by 2001 Premarin® sales were over $2 billion annually. A little bit of this would go a long way at your local school district, and at many colleges and universities.

I've discussed this idea at many seminars and public meetings for several years, and many of the physicians and other attendees seem to think it's meant as a joke. It's really not, as it follows many sound principles in health care, including *"First, Do No Harm"* and *"Copy Nature."* It follows sound business principles, too, including "*Sustainable Industry*," "*Recycle 'waste,'*" and on the profit-making side "*Do Well by Doing Good*." The first school districts, colleges, and universities to implement this idea will (if their programs are run well) make the most money. Why not have your educational institution or institutions be among the first? Enough of that. For now, we have the BHRT we have, synthesized from starting material in the Mexican yam and/or soy plants – bio-identical for sure, but incomplete at best. Yet, incomplete as it is, today's BHRT for women is far safer and more effective than horse estrogens and patent-medicine medroxyprogesterone ("Premarin® + Provera® sold for decades as menopausal hormone replacement therapy, or "HRT"). In this book, you'll find more than ample evidence to prove that point, and for your doctor, who may not yet be persuaded that BHRT can safely and significantly reduce your risk of Alzheimer's disease and other cognitive malfunctions; heart attack, stroke, and other cardiovascular and cerebrovascular diseases; osteoporosis; and (for non-tobacco-smoking women) emphysema and COPD; this updated version of our earlier pioneering book includes all the scientific journal support he or she might want.

Just as importantly for many, today's BHRT can noticeably slow the physical *appearance* of aging for any woman who uses it properly and regularly. Nearly any woman who's used BHRT for 5 to 10 years notices herself and hears from others that she "doesn't look her age." After 10 years or more, the difference in appearance between BHRT-using and non-BHRT using women of the same age is obvious to everyone. An example: My wife Holly has been a BHRT user, and lets me show her picture at seminars and print it here along with this question: "How old was she when this picture was taken?"

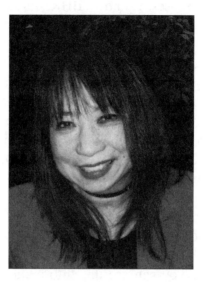

(You can find the answer in the index, under "Holly")

Of course, none of this means that BHRT is perfectly safe! Although BHRT uses exact copies of human hormones and is demonstrably safer than conventional HRT, it still uses hormones. To use BHRT safely, a woman can't expect to get her hormone prescriptions and not see her physician again. Careful follow-up monitoring for both quantities of each hormone used ("not too much, not too little, but just right for you") and for the metabolism of each hormone (does it turn into — ie, metabolize — too many procarcinogens and not enough anticarcinogens?) is very important and can be easily fixed if it is not producing the ideal mix.

Physicians skilled and knowledgeable in BHRT know not only how to order these tests in adjusting quantities of hormones, but also which minerals, vitamins, and botanicals to recommend to restore a safer pattern of metabolism. You'll discover information about how to find such a physician — if you don't know one already — in the book's "Resources" section (*See Chapter 11*).

"Routine" testing is still very important for women using BHRT. Breast check-ups, Pap smears, infrared thermography (as accurate as mammography, but much less uncomfortable and considerably less hazardous) to screen for breast lumps; ultrasound examinations; and even mammograms in some cases. Your own BHRT-knowledgeable physician can, of course, give you the best individual guidance.

But BHRT is only one tool — even though a very important one — for promoting healthy aging. Diet and exercise are, as always, at the top of the list, closely followed by general and individually-specific dietary supplementation. While those are beyond the scope of this book, why not check (*sorry about the shameless plug*) the book *Natural Medicine, Optimal Wellness* (2006) by Alan R. Gaby, MD, and me, for both general guidelines and individual health-problem-specific advice and recommendations?

Dr. Lane Lenard and I hope you enjoy this book, and perhaps learn something about BHRT you might not have known before. More importantly, we hope you can use this information to help you live a long and healthy life!

Jonathan V. Wright, MD
Tahoma Clinic, Renton, Washington
www.tahomaclinic.com
September 2009

PREFACE

THE HANDWRITING ON THE WALL

By Lane Lenard, PhD

It's been more than a decade since we introduced in written form the already over-a-decade-old concept of bio-identical hormone replacement therapy (BHRT) with our book *Natural Hormone Replacement for Women Over 45* (*Wright JVW, Morgenthaler J. Smart Publications, 1997*), at a time when only a handful of clear thinking, knowledgeable doctors had ever heard about bio-identical hormones.[*]

It was also a time when Premarin® and Provera® (combined as Prempro®) were among the best-selling patent medicines in the world, earning their parent company, Wyeth Pharmaceuticals, billions of dollars per year. For women who wanted to alleviate the discomforts of menopause or to protect themselves from the long-term effects of the age-related decline in sex hormones, "hormone replacement therapy" (HRT) – as the patented, horse estrogen + alien-to-the-human body pseudohormone combination was marketed – was virtually the only solution conventional medicine had to offer.

Today, scientific research has proven, even to the FDA, that the combination of Premarin® + Provera® is good for little more than alleviating hot flushes for a couple of years at most. Beyond that limit, and despite the current recommended use of new, but unevaluated lower doses, the risks and uncertainties of conventional HRT make it virtually unusable even for that limited role.

---

[*]   Alert readers will note that our previous book referred to "natural hormone replacement," while now we talk about "bio-identical hormone replacement." While the concepts remain unchanged, the terminology has been altered a bit in order to be more precise as to the source of the hormones and to avoid confusion with other products that may be "natural" but not necessarily *bio-identical* for humans. These include conjugated equine estrogens (eg, Premarin®), which are natural for horses but not for humans, as well as herbal products like black cohosh and dong quai and plant-based estrogens (phytoestrogens) like genistein, which are bio-identical for plants but not for humans.

Our little book pulled back the curtain concealing the true dangers of HRT, and at the same time introduced women and their doctors to the benefits of true *hormone replacement* using bio-identical *human* hormones – estrogens, progesterone, testosterone, and DHEA – that were *molecularly identical to those the human body produces.*

Many women first learned the truth about HRT and BHRT from our book; others later heard about it from TV celebrity Suzanne Somers, who described her personal experiences with a different version of BHRT in the first of a series of best-selling books. But the stampede away from HRT and toward BHRT really began in 2002 with the premature termination of a large, government-funded study – the Women's Health Initiative (WHI) – the results of which confirmed that the risks of conventional HRT unquestionably outweighed its benefits. This study and its aftermath have proven to be a significant threat to Wyeth's profits.

The news of HRT's dangers probably came as no surprise to the millions of women who had started on it but quit after a few months, because they couldn't tolerate its side effects or the "funny" way it made them feel. Then again, what would a woman expect when she puts horse hormones and alien pseudohormones into her body every morning?

By contrast, BHRT is a therapy that sells itself. When women start using it, they soon find how much better they feel (especially if they are experienced with conventional HRT), and they almost invariably stay on it and recommend it to their friends and family.

In the wake of the WHI disclosures, women entering their menopausal years have been flocking to BHRT in record numbers. This trend has not gone unnoticed at Wyeth, which has launched an unprecedented legal, lobbying, and public relations campaign to influence the FDA and the US Congress to – in effect – "eliminate the competition" for them. With the battle moving through the courts and the Congress, it's anybody's guess whether, once the dust settles, BHRT will even be legal in this country.

Surprised? You shouldn't be.

Although HRT has repeatedly been proven to cause unnatural and dangerous changes and reactions in the body, it remains available in every pharmacy in the country. The fact that Premarin® and Provera® are still on the market, despite their proven tendencies to cause cancer, heart disease, and other serious disorders, tells us something about the cozy relationship between Wyeth and the FDA, the federal agency that's supposed to be regulating its products for the good of *all* Americans, not just Wyeth.

The irony of Wyeth's anti-BHRT campaign is that the company purports to be trying to protect women who, it claims, would be exposing themselves to BHRT's alleged "dangers." Yet, the only evidence Wyeth can produce about the BHRT's alleged "dangers" is that drawn from studies of its own admittedly dangerous, FDA-"approved" HRT products, which bear no relation, chemically or molecularly, to bio-identical hormones. Wyeth's argument goes something like this: "If our 'hormone' products are dangerous, so must theirs be," as though HRT and BHRT were the same products.

Conspicuously absent from Wyeth's arguments, though, is even the slightest evidence supporting the alleged "dangers" of BHRT. Along with the FDA, Wyeth refuses to acknowledge the existence or validity of the hundreds of scientific studies that have been published over the years that support the efficacy and safety of bio-identical hormones, not to mention the dangers of conventional HRT. They've recently gone so far as to declare that a benign and long-accepted form of estrogen (estriol), which is produced by every human body (in especially enormous volumes during pregnancy) and is essential to the proper use of BHRT, should be considered an "unapproved drug" and essentially banned from use in the US. This is in spite of the fact that Wyeth has marketed estriol in Europe for years as an "ideal treatment" for menopausal women). Their hypocrisy and dishonesty take the breath away. (*For more about these medicolegal issues, see Chapter 12.*)

Volumes of Research and Years of Clinical Experience

Given all the negative press Wyeth and the FDA have generated about BHRT, combined with the average physician's ignorance or bias about it, it's understandable for women to be a little hesitant about questioning their regular doctor about going on to try bio-identical hormones.

Are you worried about the supposedly unknown risks of BHRT? Certainly concerns about cancer and other serious disorders should always be addressed and the risks carefully monitored. Yet, despite what BHRT critics may allege, literal volumes of scientific research and decades of careful clinical experience vouch for its efficacy and safety. One important purpose of this book is to summarize and bring to light much of this "nonexistent" research and clinical experience.

Over the years, hundreds of comparable, but independent, studies of Premarin® and Provera® and bio-identical estrogens have been conducted – and continue to be conducted – in test tubes, in animals, and in actual human women. They may not always be the large, prospective, double-blind, placebo-controlled trials the FDA likes to hold up as the only kind that can provide valid data. In most cases they are smaller – but usually still well-controlled – studies designed to test some aspect of hormone function, efficacy, or safety, like cholesterol levels, blood clotting, heart function, liver function, propensity for causing cancer, or controlling bone metabolism. Their individual results may not show the "big picture," but, taken together, they offer a remarkable view as to what that big picture is going to look like. Such studies rarely make headlines, but they do make valid scientific points, and they all have one thing in common: when trials are carried out under reasonably comparable conditions, in virtually every case, bio-identical hormones turn out to be clearly safer and more effective than Premarin® and Provera®.

If the devastating results of the Women's Health Initiative came as a shock to the vast majority of conventional medicine practitioners, it's because they had largely ignored these smaller studies – some decades old, but some quite recent – which have served as the handwriting on the wall that clearly predicted the WHI/HRT debacle and the resulting emergence of BHRT. The results and conclusions of most of these smaller studies are as valid today as they were the day they were published, but conventional medicine, controlled as it is by the patent medicine industry and the retrogressive, legalistic FDA, remains wedded to their dangerous but profitable HRT franchise, endlessly repeating the false mantra that there are no valid studies supporting the safety and efficacy of BHRT.

Recently, as the viability of conventional HRT as a big profit-maker has grown lesser and lesser, while the acceptance of BHRT has grown greater and greater, Big Pharma has begun to switch its emphasis to so-called FDA-"approved" bio-identical hormones – primarily commercial versions of the bio-identical estrogen *estradiol*. Individual compounding, they argue, is unnecessary and needlessly risky. This strategy ignores the facts that 1) the one-size-fits-all standard dose of these estradiol products is typically at least 4 times the amount the body can safely metabolize without raising the risk of breast cancer (*See Chapter 9.*); 2) the anticarcinogenic estrogen *estriol* – a mainstay in BHRT – is not only ignored, but is currently being actively and illegally suppressed by the FDA; and 3) no one has ever shown scientifically that carefully compounded hormones or other medications are any more dangerous than mass-produced commercial versions. This last point is a myth supported by a single, decade old, intentionally biased, FDA-sponsored, "limited survey," the lack of scientific validity of which has been acknowledged under oath before a US Senate committee by the "researcher" who ran it. (*See Chapter 12.*)

A Note about Endnotes

As you read this book, you'll no doubt notice a large number of *endnotes* – references to scientific studies that support all the factual statements and arguments we make. Such references, which are listed at the end of each chapter, are standard practice in the scientific literature, but are much less common in "consumer-oriented" books like this one. The conventional thinking is that "nonscientists" probably aren't much interested in exactly how these statements are supported by scientific research; that hardly anyone is going to check back to see what those references actually say; and that they just clutter up the text. If that's the case with you, please feel free to ignore the endnotes. However, at the same time, try to be aware that every time you see something like this[1-3] in the text, it means that that particular statement is supported by 3 scientific studies, which you and/or your doctor are welcome to check out.

On the other hand, given the repeated misstatements by BHRT opponents that, since there is "no scientific support" for its efficacy and safety, it must be considered as dangerous as conventional HRT, we thought it essential to provide that scientific research in as much detail as feasible. That way, those critics, or those inclined to be influenced by them, can see just how wrong they have been. We welcome the opportunity to summarize this research for these critics and hope they will look up every reference listed in this book. If they do that, we would find it difficult to understand how they could stand by their negative position.

If after reading this book, you're still hesitant about the safety of bio-identical hormones, think about this: How could the human species – including all of our ancestors – have survived if normal levels of women's reproductive hormones predisposed them to fatal diseases? If natural or bio-identical human reproductive hormones (administered in physiologic doses (a physiologic dose duplicates the range of amounts naturally produced by human ovaries, neither more nor less), via a sensible route, and on a schedule the body has adapted to over decades of natural ovarian hormone secretion) increased women's risks of heart disease or cancer much at all, as many critics contend today, the human species would likely have gone extinct long, long ago. Beyond such common sense reasoning, in the remainder of this book, we bring to light many examples of "forgotten" or "ignored" scientific studies combined with up-to-date clinical experience that provide solid support for the safety and benefits of BHRT.

Lane Lenard, PhD
Millstone Township, NJ
September 2009

Take
our
FREE

hormone assessment online at:

www.smart-publications.com/

hormone-self-assessment

CHAPTER 1

DON'T LET YOUR DOCTOR GIVE YOU HORSE URINE!

Cancer researchers tend to be quite conservative by nature, typically careful not to use their study results to overstate people's hopes or exaggerate their fears. So it was that in November 2006, something amazing happened at a medical conference in San Antonio, Texas. It was there that medical scientists from Houston's prestigious MD Anderson Cancer Center presented recent study results that left jaws dropping, not only in San Antonio, but all the world over.

The study's senior investigator, Dr. Donald Berry, characterized their results as "astounding." Others called them "fascinating," "provocative," and having "no obvious flaws." Acclaimed another prominent cancer researcher, *"This could well be the study of the year in cancer."*

What was this amazing, astounding, provocative finding that shocked the world of cancer medicine? It was quite simple, really, and not a bit surprising to those of us who have been practicing *natural medicine*, beyond the bounds of the conventional medical wisdom that is strongly biased by the "patent medicine" industry (also known as the "drug" and "pharmaceutical") industry. (See page 435)

What Dr. Berry and his colleagues did was to simply calculate the number of cases of breast cancer that have occurred annually in the United States for about the last 25 years. They then compared those numbers with the number of prescriptions of patented "hormone replacement" therapy (HRT) – daily oral doses of the patent medicines (aka "pharmaceuticals" or "drugs") **Premarin**® (*conjugated equine estrogens, CEEs*) and **Provera**® (*medroxyprogesterone, MPA*) or the combination of the two, **Prempro**®. What they found is summarized in Figure 1-1.

From the mid-1940s until the 1970s, the incidence of breast cancer climbed slowly but steadily. Beginning in the late '70s and early '80s, though, the cancer rate among women *of menopausal age* (45 years and older) began to accelerate, shooting up by more than 300% – with up to 200,000 new cases per year, 40,000 of them fatal – until about 1999, when

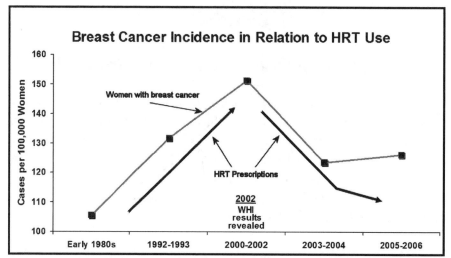

Figure 1-1. The incidence of breast cancer among women aged 45 and older has risen and fallen over the last 3 decades in direct correlation with the number of prescriptions of conventional "hormone" replacement (HRT) therapy (Premarin® + Provera®). Looking at these data, scientists have declared it "the smoking gun" that proves that HRT causes breast cancer.

Adapted from Ravdin PM, et al. *N Engl J Med.* 2007;356:1670-1674 and Glass AG, et al. *J. Natl. Cancer Inst.* 2007;99:1152-1161.

the incidence began to level off. Among women *younger than 45* – ie, premenopausal women – the rate of breast cancer remained essentially unchanged during this period.

Then in 2003 something strange happened that snapped the whole puzzling picture into focus. Compared to the previous year, the rate of *estrogen-positive* breast cancer,[*] the most common form of the disease, fell an astonishing 18%. For the first time since 1945, and for no obvious reason (at the time), the annual incidence of breast cancer had actually declined significantly over the course of a year.

The Smoking Gun

What happened to spark such a sharp rise and fall in breast cancer incidence? The key event occurred in mid-2002, noted Dr. Berry and colleagues. It was the unscheduled, premature termination (after about 5 years) of a huge, placebo-controlled, federally funded clinical trial called

---

[*]   About 70% of breast cancer tumors are fueled by the hormone estrogen. As estrogen levels rise, tumor growth increases and vice versa. Such tumors are termed "estrogen-receptor positive," or "ER+."

the **Women's Health Initiative** (**WHI**). The WHI had been designed to evaluate the efficacy and safety of conventional HRT in women after menopause.*

We'll discuss the pivotal WHI trial in detail in subsequent chapters. Suffice it to say, its results pulled the rug out from under the long-time practice of conventional patented HRT, showing definitively that it was far less useful and far more dangerous than the vast majority of doctors and their menopausal patients had been led to believe.

But the decline in breast cancer was only half the story. Remember that the MD Anderson researchers correlated the rise and fall of breast cancer with the prescribing of HRT. As you can easily see in Figure 1-1, in the 2 decades during which the incidence of breast cancer was "spiking," women were using conventional HRT at an increasing and unprecedented rate, so much so that during that period, Premarin® and Provera® (Prempro®) became among the best-selling patent medicines in the world.

But beginning in July 2002, with the publication of the first of several papers detailing the WHI results, the sales of patentable HRT plummeted. In the 6 months after the WHI results were published, Prempro® prescriptions fell by more than half, from 61 million prescriptions annually in 2001 to 27 million in 2003 to 18 million in 2005. Justifiably frightened by the WHI findings, women were abandoning HRT in droves.

Although the WHI had made it clear that patentable HRT was dangerous, hardly anyone expected that abruptly ceasing use of these pseudohormones would bring about such an immediate and profound benefit for so many women. Yet, the correlation was unmistakable. As many women stopped taking their HRT, their risk of developing breast cancer quickly diminished.[1, 2] The researchers were surprised by both the magnitude and the rapidity of the decline at first. As Dr. Berry later explained, "It makes perfect sense" if you consider that the use of HRT may be an important contributing factor to cancer development.[3]

---

* If you can believe it, despite the fact that Premarin® had been process-patented and approved for use in the 1940s and had been heavily marketed since the '60s, and the combination of Premarin® + Provera® had been in widespread use since the 1970s, no such "gold standard" trial had ever been conducted to evaluate its safety and efficacy. Thus, what doctors *thought* they knew about conventional HRT was based largely on inadequate research, rumor, and myth, topped off with heavy doses of wishful thinking and marketing hype.

Now, just because two events are correlated does not automatically mean that one *causes* the other; the new data do not prove that patented HRT *causes* breast cancer. There could be a third factor – eg, more mammograms – responsible for the increase in breast cancer. Nevertheless, as medical oncologist Peter Ravdin, MD, the lead author on the MD Anderson paper, stated, the somewhat misnamed "hormone hypothesis" seemed to explain the cancer data perfectly, and they could find no other explanation.[2, 4]) "Of course, we're not sure. We never are," said Dr. Berry, "but it fits. *It's a smoking gun.*"[5]

Any doubt about a third factor, like fewer mammograms, as a possible cause for the decrease in breast cancer was recently erased in a major article in the *New England Journal of Medicine* by the WHI researchers themselves. Re-examining their own data, they concluded that "…*the recent reduction in the incidence of breast cancer … is predominantly related to a decrease in the use of combined "estrogen" plus progestin.*"[6]

The Bio-Identical Hormone Option

Although conventional patent medicine HRT was originally developed to relieve hot flushes and other unpleasant symptoms related to the menopausal decline in ovarian estrogen, for decades it has been sold to women and their doctors as a kind of "fountain of youth." The hype began in the 1960s with the publication of the book *Forever Young*, whose physician-author was disclosed decades later to have been financed by the Ayerst Corporation (predecessor of today's Wyeth Pharmaceuticals), the manufacturer of Premarin®, Provera®, and Prempro®. As they came to appreciate the money to be made in the menopausal "hormone replacement" business, Wyeth (along with some other companies) used countless other public relations (PR) gimmicks to tout the alleged benefits of their patented HRT products, all the while downplaying its known risks, even in the absence of convincing scientific evidence.*

At the same time, Wyeth and their compatriots at the FDA have tried to ignore, discredit, and even to eliminate a valuable, identical-to-natural, but generally *unpatentable* alternative known as **bio-identical human hormones.** While studies like the WHI and many others proved that patented HRT had fewer benefits and more risks than previously thought, many other studies – some old and others very recent – have shown **bio-**

---

* For an eye-opening and disturbing review of the early years of HRT, see the book *The Greatest Experiment Ever Performed on Women*, by Barbara Seaman. Hyperion; New York, 2003.

identical hormone replacement therapy (BHRT) to be remarkably safe and effective for eliminating common symptoms of menopause, as well as for warding off such long-term effects of menopausal hormone decline as heart disease, osteoporosis, memory loss, urinary incontinence, and others.

Why Are Human Bio-identical Hormones Superior?

As you've probably heard, conventional patented HRT employs estrogens derived from *horse urine* (more about this later). Nature designed these estrogens to work very well in pregnant female horses, but not so well in female humans (or even in *nonpregnant* mares!). By contrast, bio-identical human hormones are precisely identical biochemically to those the female human body produces on a daily basis; the body cannot distinguish them from those it produces itself.

What a radical idea! Human hormones for human beings!

Not surprisingly, when tested in scientific study after scientific study, bio-identical human hormones virtually always turn out to be safer, more tolerable, and more effective than conventional, FDA-"approved" horse hormone-based HRT regimens.[*]

How could anyone who knows anything about the human female reproductive system presume that horse hormones and pseudohormone patent medicines (like Provera®) could possibly be better and safer for the human body than hormones that are exactly the same as the ones the body produces naturally? It defies reason!

Imagine you're a researcher back at the dawn of the menopausal hormone replacement era and a benevolent company picks you to develop the best hormone replacement product(s) possible. You're given two things: 1) the benefit of all the research and equipment available to any scientist today, and 2) a choice between working with bio-identical *human* hormones or not bio-identical (for humans) *horse* hormones. Which type of hormones would you pick?

---

[*]   A very recent review of 196 studies (Holtorf K. The Bio-identical Hormone Debate: Are Bio-identical Hormones (Estradiol, Estriol, and Progesterone) Safer or More Efficacious than Commonly Used Synthetic Versions in Hormone Replacement Therapy? *Postgraduate Medicine* 2009;129:1-13) makes this point abundantly clear.

It's a safe bet that the average person using common sense, whose sole experience with hormones was limited to secreting them (and perhaps admiring their effects in the opposite sex), would choose human hormones every time. But then, people running patent medicine companies don't use common sense. On the contrary, they choose business sense over common sense almost every time; and for reasons too complex to explain here, the vast majority of practicing physicians tend to go along with the patent medicine approach.

Regrettably, bio-identical hormones step up to the patent medicine (drug) company plate with three strikes already against them. Like air, water, vitamins, blood, mucus, as well as countless other substances, *bio-identical hormones occur in the world naturally*. Consequently, according to law, they are *not readily patentable*. In the world of Big Pharma and conventional medicine, this means that manufacturing and marketing bio-identical hormones would *not be sufficiently profitable*. Like generic drugs that have gone "off patent," anybody can sell them, increasing the competition and forcing down the selling price.

This legal fact of life in the marketing of therapeutic materials, which limits the profits a patent medicine company can make on unpatentable products, has unfortunately paved the way for *patentable but inferior* substances, like Premarin® and Provera®, to become the standard in conventional menopausal hormone replacement therapy. Meanwhile, bio-identical hormones, despite their inherently superior efficacy and safety in the human body, are widely ignored, routinely denigrated, and most recently, illegally suppressed.

You've probably heard lots of things about BHRT in the media or from your doctor in recent years – some good, some bad. If you're confused, we can certainly understand why. Keep in mind that much of the information we encounter about BHRT on TV, radio, magazines, newspapers, and the internet, whether negative or positive, is quite often wrong, or at best, biased. Fortunately, the ever-increasing popularity of books about BHRT— most recently *Breakthrough* — by Suzanne Somers, and earlier this year, two hour-long "Oprah Winfrey" programs and an hour-long "Dr. Phil" program about BHRT, has exposed many more of us to a more balanced view of BHRT.

When it comes to digging up the actual facts about BHRT, media reporters almost always take the easy way out, relying for their information on patent medicine company press releases and/or interviews with company-paid "expert" sources. When an "authoritative" source claims – falsely – that there is no valid scientific support for the safety or efficacy of bio-identical hormones, it is typical for reporters to take such statements at face value and make no serious attempts to verify their accuracy. In fact, if a reporter were to take the trouble to look, he/she could easily find thousands of pro-BHRT papers published in mainstream medical journals. But, who's going to pay for a comparable PR operation for BHRT? And reporters have other stories to write.

BHRT: Doing It the Right Way

Unfortunately, a similar casual relationship with the facts also applies to many who claim to be advocates of BHRT. They may know a good thing when they see it, but they may fail to dig deeply enough into the research and long experience of clinicians educated in BHRT to understand how best to apply its principles. As a result, the advice they give may be misleading or even dangerous and in some cases might wind up doing as much harm as good. Proper application of BHRT means much more than simply substituting estradiol pills for Premarin® pills and progesterone pills for Provera® pills, as some BHRT "experts" advocate.

In this book, we review decades of scientific research and clinical experience related to hormone replacement therapy, using bio-identical hormones as well as patent medicine products. We believe there is no question that the sum total of this research and clinical experience leads to only one conclusion: the practice of medicine is always better served by following Nature, rather than by seeking to maximize patent medicine company profits. If you think this sounds like hyperbole, stay tuned. We know that once you've reviewed this evidence and come to understand how today's patent-based, conventional medicine system actually works, you'll readily agree.

In discussing menopausal hormone replacement, strange as it may seem, we sometimes like to compare doctors with auto mechanics to make a simple but very telling point. Consider this: No auto mechanic in his right mind would substitute crucial parts in a Mercedes with replacement parts made for a Chevy. You don't have to know a whole lot about cars to imagine the consequences of trying to put, say, a Chevy transmission into a Mercedes. It's just common sense.

Yet, many otherwise knowledgeable physicians, who've been prescribing *horse estrogens* and *pseudohormone patent medicines* for women going through menopause, seem to have less common sense than the average auto mechanic.

By the time you've finished reading this book, we have no doubt you'll agree that using bio-identical hormones, the ones Mother Nature *"designed"* for the human body, instead of "the standard" – alien-to-the-human body, but highly profitable substitutes dreamed up in a patent medicine company's labs – offers women a more natural, and hence, safer, healthier, and more worry-free passage through the years of menopause and beyond.

A Little Background on Menopause

From the time she first enters puberty until the end of her last menstrual period, every woman is keenly aware of the monthly cycle of hormonal changes going on inside her body. Except during those months when she might be pregnant, she experiences the complex interplay of her reproductive steroid hormones – estrogens, progesterone, and many others – ebbing and flowing on a regular 26- to 30-day cycle. However, by the time she reaches her late 40s or early 50s, the regularity of her hormonal cycling starts breaking down. This is the beginning of menopause. Just as puberty marked the beginning of her reproductive life, menopause marks the end of it.

In nearly 40 years of medical practice, I (JVW) have helped thousands of women make this transition. Each woman deals with the changes in her body in her own way, with reactions ranging from joy and fulfillment ("It's finally over!") to acceptance, resignation, depression ("I'm not young any more."), to discomfort, and perhaps to chronic illness. There is no "typical" reaction.

Although menopause usually occurs around the time a woman's biologic clock turns 50, its physical discomforts (and some early hormonal changes) might begin as early as age 35. Women "officially" reach menopause once they have missed 12 consecutive menstrual periods. The phase during which their hormonal cycling starts changing rapidly is termed "*perimenopause*" (literally, *around* menopause), while the time after their monthly periods have completely stopped is termed "*postmenopause.*" We generally use the term "*menopause*" to refer to the "official" end of cycling, but sometimes it serves as a kind of shorthand to describe the entire passage from perimenopause to postmenopause.

During the perimenopausal months (or years), the delicate balance of hormonal secretions as evidenced by the regularity of the menstrual cycle – begins to fail. Like a rapidly spinning top that starts to wobble as it slows, the hormonal "wobbling" – which might begin as early as the mid-'30s – becomes more and more erratic with advancing years. By the time most women reach about age 50 to 55, their "menstrual top" probably has stopped spinning altogether.

In terms of physiologic changes, menopause represents the age-related decline in the production and secretion of the steroid hormones *estrogen* and *progesterone* by the ovaries. In most women, menopause is a gradual transition. A fortunate few have no symptoms other than irregular and finally no menstrual periods. However, significant changes in the secretion of such important hormones as estrogens and progesterone are almost always associated with at least some well known signs and symptoms.

Since you're reading this book, you may already be familiar with some of the most common signals that menopause has begun: hot flushes (also called hot flashes); night sweats; vaginal dryness, leading to discomfort or pain during sexual intercourse; depression; mood swings; memory loss ("creeping forgetfulness"); and an acceleration in skin wrinkling. Conventional patent medicine HRT has been, and continues to be, prescribed primarily to prevent these symptoms.

You may have heard about some of the other, longer term changes – and risks – that also greet many women in the years after menopause: heart attacks and strokes; hip, wrist, or spinal fractures (due to osteoporosis, or thinning bones); urinary incontinence (leaking) and sometimes an enhanced vulnerability to urinary tract or bladder infections (cystitis); a progressive loss of "thinking power," including Alzheimer's disease; and cancer, especially breast cancer.

Until recently, *conventional* patent medicine HRT was thought to be a good way to prevent these long-term consequences, but now we know that it can actually make some of them much worse. As we will show, though, scientific studies – *which conventional medicine tries to pretend don't exist* – and clinical experience bear out that BHRT can be more effective and far safer in preventing them.

Yes, *That* Equine!

If menopausal symptoms are related to a decline in certain hormones, the logical, most commonsense way to relieve those symptoms would be simply to restore the missing hormones. Low on estrogen? Take some estrogen. Low on progesterone? Add some progesterone. Same for testosterone. While it's usually best to replace all three hormones (at least), in the interests of keeping our story simple, let's just focus only on estrogens for now. We'll get back to progesterone, testosterone, and the others a little later.

The "estrogen replacement" most doctors have been prescribing for decades is a formerly patented medicine known generically as *conjugated equine estrogens* (*CEEs*). The best known brand of CEEs is Premarin®, which has been available since 1942, but only widely marketed since the 1960s.

So what's the matter with conjugated equine estrogens? Take a close look at the name. Notice the word "*equine*?" Yes, *that* equine! Premarin® is a form of *horse estrogens*. In fact, it is derived from **pre**gnant **mar**e's ur**in**e, hence the brand name.

But, is that so bad, really? Estrogen is estrogen, isn't it? What difference does it make where it comes from? For the most part, that's what most conventional doctors and their patients have been taught to think.

Although much of the willfully blind conventional medical establishment proclaims to see no essential difference between Premarin® and "estrogen" (or between Provera® and progesterone), the critical differences have been spelled out and diagrammed in standard textbooks, scientific journals, and patent applications for over half a century. Other than the obvious differences in spelling, as we'll soon show, the dissimilarities are many, varied, and profoundly important.

Redefining Reality

Part of the confusion has to do with language. People (ie, doctors, drug companies, government regulators, media, and the "average person") all generally refer to the primary female hormone as "estrogen." In fact, though, this is a misleading oversimplification. In fact, there is no single hormone called "estrogen," but rather many different hormones that share a similar molecular structure that places them in the "estrogen class." These hormones, with names like *estriol, estradiol, estrone*, and *equilin*, are correctly referred to *en masse* as *estrogens*, and each can be considered as *an estrogen*. This may seem like a subtle distinction, but it is vital, because it helps explain (along with US patent laws) how horse estrogens have come to be the standard "hormone replacement" therapy for human females during menopause.

This confusion has not come about by accident. By carefully manipulating the language, the drug companies have convinced the vast majority of doctors, medical researchers, government regulators, media, and women themselves of an outright falsehood: that *CEEs are "estrogen"* and that *"estrogen" is CEEs.* Having had the wool (or perhaps the horse hair) pulled over everyone's eyes in this way, when doctors think "estrogen" and reflexively write "Premarin®" on their little blue prescription pads, it becomes a whole lot easier for everyone involved to rationalize that a woman substituting daily doses of estrogens from pregnant horses for her declining ovarian estrogens might not be such a bad idea.

Re-defining terms like "estrogen," "progesterone," "testosterone," and "hormone" has been a cornerstone of patent medicine marketing for the better part of a century, allowing them to sell billions and billions of dollars worth of highly profitable patent medicines to women (and men) who think that what they are taking are actually *human hormones*. To the enormous financial benefit of the industry, their strategy has worked brilliantly. However, for the millions of women (and men) who have taken their so-called "hormones" according to doctors' orders, the consequences have often been less than ideal and sometimes deadly serious.

How Do Women Differ from Horses?

(*Yes, we must admit, it's a rather odd question to be asking in a "medical" book, but please stay with us, there might be doctors reading.*)

Over the last several million years, the reproductive system of female humans (*Homo sapiens*) has evolved to run quite smoothly on at least 15 or more different estrogens and estrogen metabolites.[7, 8] Of these, **estradiol (E$_2$)** is the most potent and most responsible for "secondary sexual development" (eg, breasts, hips) as well as for much of the "female point of view." As shown in Figure 1-2, the other major human estrogens include **estrone (E$_1$)**, **estriol (E$_3$)**, and the major estrogen metabolites **2-methoxyestrone (2-MeOE$_1$)**, and **2-methoxyestradiol (2-MeOE$_2$)**, which is "major" in terms of importance, but not quantity like the others). Table 1-1 lists the best known human estrogens and their metabolites.

On the other hand, the reproductive system of the horse (*Equus caballus*) has evolved to run on an altogether different mix of estrogens. **Estrone** and **estradiol** can be found in both horses and humans, although in very different proportions. However, when a mare becomes pregnant, she secretes at least eight other estrogens, including **equilin, dihydroequilin, equilenin,** and **dihydroequilenin**[9] (Figure 1-2 and Table 1-1). Thus, most of the time the mixture of estrogens we call conjugated equine estrogens are not even suited to a *non*pregnant mare, let alone a menopausal or postmenopausal human female![10]

And even though estradiol and estrone are found in both species, they occur in vastly different proportions. As you can see in Figure 1-2, estrone accounts for about 50% of horse estrogen but only about 33% of human estrogen. Also, human estrogen is comprised of about 44% estradiol and 10% estriol, compared with pregnant horse estrogen, which contains only about 1% estradiol and **nary a drop of estriol, 0%.** Notice also that equilin (22-25%) and other **"equi-"**-type estrogens are nowhere to be found in human estrogen.

We should point out that all the equine hormones, including estrone, equilin, and its metabolites are *extremely potent*. This becomes especially apparent once they enter the human body, which is not accustomed to such potent estrogens, especially in such large quantities. Still, they are estrogens, and as such, can do many things in the human body that estrogens are supposed to do, like suppressing hot flushes and slowing the progression of osteoporosis. Nevertheless, because of their extreme potency and other differences, they also do a lot that's not so good, starting with discomforts like breast tenderness and fluid retention and ranging up to potentially fatal blood clots and cancers in the breast or uterus, all indications of excessive estrogenic activity.

As noted above, significantly missing from horse estrogens is the estrogen *estriol*, which comprises as much as 10% of human estrogen. In addition to its large proportion, estriol is a very "gentle" or *low-potency estrogen*, only about one-quarter as potent as estradiol and only one-eighth as potent as equilin. Research indicates that, due in part to its low potency,

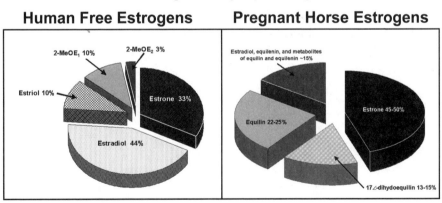

How Women Differ from Pregnant Horses, Estrogenically Speaking

Figure 1-2. Left: The approximate proportions of the major *free* (ie, chemically active) estrogens found in the serum (a portion of blood) of adult, premenopausal women. 2-methoxyestrone (2-MeOE$_1$) and 2 methoxyestradiol (2-MeOE$_2$) are metabolites (chemical transformation products) of estrone and estradiol, respectively. Numerous other metabolites of estrone, estradiol, and estriol are present but at levels too low to be detected by state-of-the-art measuring equipment. (Table 1-1) (*See Xu, et al*[6, 7].)

Right: The approximate proportions of major estrogens found in pregnant mares. Equilin, equilenin, and all their metabolites (Table 1-1) are found only in *pregnant* mares and CEEs.[10, 11] So, not only are they unnatural for the human female, they're also unnatural for *nonpregnant* mares.[9]

estriol may provide invaluable built-in protection against the carcinogenic (cancer-causing) potential of other more potent estrogens. Of course, female horses are built to tolerate all those potent estrogens, but not so female humans.

Looking at Figure 1-2 and Table 1-1, it doesn't take an advanced degree in medicine to conclude that human estrogens and equine estrogens are distant cousins at best. The only estrogens human females and pregnant horses have in common are estrone and estradiol, but in very different proportions.

This difference in reproductive hormones is just one of many differences between horses and humans. You may have also noticed that horses have four hooves, a long tail, a mane, and they're also larger, and can run much faster. We'd never think of transfusing horse blood into a human (or *vice versa*), or transplanting horse organs into humans, and it doesn't make any more sense for humans to be using horse hormones either.

It should come as no surprise then, that the presence of an alien species of estrogens (CEEs) in the human body induces a hormonal imbalance that can cause a woman not only to "feel funny," but also to have significant problems. To most doctors who prescribe Premarin®, this hormonal imbalance has never seemed to carry much weight, at least not until the last couple of years. After all, Premarin® does squelch hot flushes pretty well, doesn't it? And it's FDA-"approved," isn't it? So it must be safe, right?

Table 1-1. Listing of Best Known Estrogens and Metabolites Found in Human Premenopausal Women and in Pregnant Mares

Human Premenopausal Women[a]	Pregnant Mares[b]
Estrone (E_1)	Estrone (E_1)
Estradiol (17β-estradiol, E_2)	17β-estradiol (17β-E_2)
Estriol (E_3)	17α-estradiol (17α-E_2)
16α-hydroxyestrone (16α-OHE_1)	Equilin (Eq)
16-ketoestradiol (16-ketoE_2)	17β-dihydroequilin (17β-Eq)
16-epiestriol (16-epiE_3)	17α-dihydroequilin (17α-Eq)
17-epiestriol (17-epiE_3)	Equilenin (Eqn)
2-hydroxyestrone (2-OHE_1)	17β-dihydroequilenin (17β-Eqn)
2-hydroxyestradiol (2-OHE_2)	17α-dihydroequilenin (17α-Eqn)
4-hydroxyestrone (4-OHE_1)	Δ^8-estrone (Δ^8-E_1)
16-hydroxyestone (16-OHE1)	Δ^8,17β-estradiol (Δ^8,17β-E_2)
2-methoxyestrone (2-$MeOHE_1$)	$\Delta^{8,9}$-dehydroestrone ($\Delta^{8,9}$-DHE_1)
2-methoxyestradiol (2-$MeOHE_2$)	17β-hydroxyequilenin
3-methoxyestrone (3-$MeOHE_1$)	4-hydroxequilenin
4-methoxyestrone (4-$MeOHE_1$)	
4-methoxyestradiol (4-$MeOHE_2$)	

a   Source: Xu, et al[6,7]
b   Source: Woodcock/FDA[11] and Asthana, et al.[12]
Shaded rows (estrone and estradiol) indicate the only estrogens that occur in both human females and mares, although in markedly different proportions as shown in Figure 1-2.

Well, not so fast. One of the primary effects of estrogens is to promote the growth of tissue in the uterine lining and breasts. Normal tissue growth in response to natural ovarian estrogen stimulation is essential for preparing the body for possible pregnancy. However, according to one well-accepted theory, if for some reason, a few cells in the uterus or breast should by chance or genetic predisposition turn precancerous or cancerous, the extra estrogenic boost provided by potent estrogens, like those found in CEEs, could shift that microscopic cancer growth into overdrive.

Using the potent estrogens in Premarin® to treat hot flushes is something like putting out a candle with a fire hose. True, it'll get the job done, but how much power do we really need? As two leading reproductive physiologists pointed out over 20 years ago, "[When women take

Premarin®], ...levels [of equilin] can remain elevated for 13 weeks or more post-treatment due to storage and slow release from adipose [fat] tissue. In addition, metabolism of equilin to equilenin and 17β-hydroxyequilenin may contribute to the estrogen stimulatory effect of therapy."[9] Another metabolite of equilin, 17β-dihydroequilin, has been found to be *8 times more potent than natural endogenous human estrogens* for inducing excess growth of the uterine lining.[13] Of course, none of this can happen with natural or bio-identical *human* hormones, because they do not contain equilin or any of its metabolites (Table 1-1).

Translated into English, this means that Premarin® has tissue-building "estrogenic" activity that is much stronger and longer lasting than that produced by natural, built-in, or bio-identical human estrogens. Under certain conditions, one of these estrogenic overreactions from Premarin® is far more likely to wind up promoting tumor growth in the uterus or breast than human ovarian or bio-identical hormones.

In addition to their secretion, another way to look at hormones is to focus on the antenna-like receptors located on cells throughout the body that receive their stimulation. During the first 50 or so years of her life, the cells in a woman's body bearing estrogen *receptors* "learn to expect" a regular and relatively muted pattern of estrogenic activity caused by the normal activity of human estrogens. From this perspective, it's not hard to see why exposing human estrogen-sensitive tissue to superpotent horse estrogens would be so disruptive and so dangerous.

Strangers in a Strange Land

While CEEs may be quite at home in a pregnant female horse, in a female human they might as well be aliens from another planet, "strangers in a strange land." The female human body has all the enzymes and other chemicals it needs to process (metabolize) estriol, estrone, estradiol and all the other human estrogen metabolites when these hormones occur in their natural human amounts and proportions (Figure 1-2). As a result, the hormones nearly always remain at safe levels and typically do not promote tissue overgrowth or other undesirable effects. On the other hand, humans lack the enzymes they would need to properly metabolize equilin, excess estrone, and the other CEE metabolites.

Is it any wonder, then, why so many women feel "unnatural" on Premarin® and why Premarin® causes so many unpleasant side effects and discomforts (*see box*), many of which are a direct result of estrogen overload? Should it come as any surprise that Premarin® use at the recommended doses (especially in combination with the dangerous progesterone-imposter drug Provera®) has been associated with a significantly increased risk of breast and endometrial cancer[14] – in women, but not in horses?

The patent medicine industry, which has been making billions of dollars selling horse estrogens to women for more than 40 years, has tried to rationalize away the risks and discomforts their products cause by arguing that "estrogen replacement" with Premarin® also cuts the risks of heart disease, strokes, osteoporosis, and perhaps even senility and Alzheimer's disease that often follow menopause: a potentially powerful argument, if only it were true. Unfortunately, the vast majority of *unbiased* scientific evidence, "topped off" by the devastating WHI report in 2002, tells a very different story.

Yet, despite all the well-known shortcomings of Premarin®, purveyors of patent medicine, even in the light of recent findings, remain more than willing to prescribe it without ever asking a ridiculously obvious question: Why use alien species horse hormones in human females? If we have the choice – which we do – wouldn't user-friendly *human estrogens* make a lot more "horse sense?"

Common Side Effects of Premarin® (CEEs)

- Blood clots
- Breast tenderness
- Fluid retention
- Gall stones
- Headaches
- High blood pressure
- Impaired glucose tolerance
- Increased risk of diabetes
- Increased risk of endometrial cancer and breast cancer
- Increased risk of heart attack and stroke
- Leg cramps
- Nausea and vomiting
- Vaginal bleeding
- Worsened uterine fibroids and endometriosis

Which One Is the Woman?

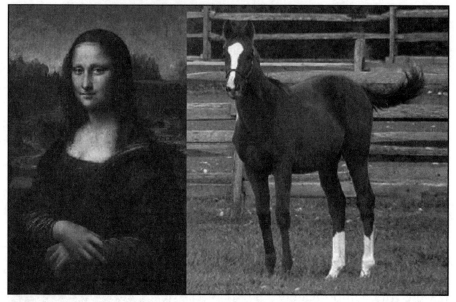

Figure 1-3. Can you tell the difference between a woman and a mare (female horse)? Here's a clue for those of you who might be hampered by a conventional medical school education: the woman is the one with the enigmatic smile.

The Promise of Bio-Identical Hormones

The rise and fall of patented HRT is a vitally important story, but even more important is the promise offered by bio-identical human hormones. We helped introduce the concept of bio-identical hormone replacement in 1997 with the book *Natural Hormone Replacement for Women Over 45*[15], at a time when only a handful of progressive, knowledgeable doctors had ever heard about BHRT. In that book, we summarized much of the evidence then available that demonstrated the promise of BHRT:

- Reducing hot flushes, night sweats, and vaginal dryness and thinning
- Preventing osteoporosis and restoring bone strength
- Maintaining greater muscle mass and strength
- Protecting against heart attacks and strokes
- Maintaining the health and integrity of the urinary system
- Improving blood lipid (cholesterol) levels
- Reducing the risks of uterine and breast cancer
- Reducing the risk of depression
- Improving sleep, mood, concentration, and memory

- Preventing senility and Alzheimer's disease
- Enhancing libido (sex drive)

In the intervening years, much has happened in the world of menopausal hormone replacement. In particular, the evidence supporting the benefits and safety of BHRT has only grown stronger, while the evidence supporting the utility and safety of conventional HRT has been substantially – and unquestionably – diminished. Back in 1997, the risks of conventional patented HRT were becoming increasingly apparent to those who were willing to see them. In 2009, recent research confirms conclusively that patent medicine HRT is both less effective *and* more risky than previously believed. Yet conventional patented HRT remains available by prescription in every pharmacy in the country, while BHRT struggles for its very existence against the combined behemoths of Big Pharma, the FDA, the mainstream media, the US Congress, and the "uneducated" physicians who comprise conventional medicine.

Although it rarely penetrates the world of conventional medicine, the basic principle of bio-identical hormone replacement, copying Nature as closely as possible by replacing declining hormones with *identical-to-human hormone molecules* in identical proportions, with identical timing, and by a route into and around the human body as close to Nature's route as possible, should seem like common sense. However, the sad saga of patented HRT demonstrates what little role common sense plays in the strange world of conventional mainstream medicine, where Big Pharma marketing almost always trumps science, and where safety and efficacy usually get trumped by profits.

Patent Medicine and Patented Medicine: What's the Difference, Really?

In this book, we refer to "patent medicine" quite a bit, and this no doubt makes some people – particularly those associated with the patent medicine industry – uncomfortable, maybe even a little angry. Most people associate the term "patent medicine" with 19th century (and earlier) traveling medicine shows and "snake oil salesmen" selling an endless variety of "nostrums," most of which were probably useless at best and sometimes toxic at worst. They prefer to distinguish this early form of "patent medicine" from today's science-based pharmaceutical industry employing thousands of brilliant and creative scientists using the highest technology to find treatments for our worst diseases.

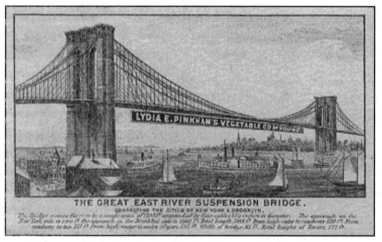

An 1880s advertising card using the newly constructed "high-tech" Brooklyn Bridge to promote Lydia E. Pinkham's Vegetable Compound.

Perhaps the best known of the early patent medicines was "Lydia E. Pinkham's Vegetable Compound." Beginning around 1875, Pinkham's – a therapeutic precursor to today's HRT – was marketed as "a positive cure for all those painful complaints and weaknesses so common to our best female population," including "ovarian troubles" and even uterine tumors, which it was supposedly able to "dissolve and expel…in an early stage of development."

Like most other patent medicines of its day, Lydia Pinkham's was actually *not patented* (as we use the term today). As used then, the term "patent" referred to a centuries-old carryover that once indicated that a product had a royal endorsement. By the 19th century, "patent" had lost all real meaning; the only distinguishing feature of a "*patent*" medicine at that time was its trademark. Anyone could make and sell an identical concoction; they just couldn't call it "Lydia E. Pinkham's Vegetable Compound."

To protect a product from competitors selling cheaper "generic" versions, old patent medicine companies relied on widespread advertising that emphasized its brand name, while asserting that generic substitutes were inferior. In fact, today's advertising industry got its start largely as a vehicle for selling patent medicines.

The old patent medicine industry gave way to the modern patent medicine industry around the turn of the 20th century. As muckraking journalists and government regulators began to expose the wild claims and dangerous and poorly labeled products of the old patent medicine companies, newer companies, working under increasingly tighter regulation, began taking a more scientific approach to drug development.

As the industry matured, and as laws evolved that allowed companies a period of exclusive marketing rights – ie, a *patent* – to their new, *unnatural* drugs – except under extraordinary circumstances, natural substances cannot be patented – the modern *patent medicine* industry came into being. Today's more science-based "pharmaceutical/drug" industry may not like the association, but the description "patent medicine" companies actually fits them better than it did their ancestors, because their products actually are *patented*.

References

1. Ravdin PM, Cronin KA, Howlader N, et al. The decrease in breast-cancer Incidence in 2003 in the United States. *N Engl J Med.* 2007;356:1670-1674.

2. Glass AG, Lacey JV, Jr., Carreon JD, Hoover RN. Breast cancer incidence, 1980-2006: Combined roles of menopausal hormone therapy, screening mammography, and estrogen receptor status. *J. Natl. Cancer Inst.* 2007;99:1152-1161.

3. Decline in breast cancer cases likely linked to reduced use of hormone replacement. *M.D. Anderson News Release.* December 14, 2006; http://www. mdanderson.org/departments/newsroom/ display.cfm?id=A9125328-2686-4886-BA05035B5A3CD6EF&method=displayFull&pn=00c8a30f-c468-11d4-80fb00508b603a14:Accessed August 14, 2007.

4. Kolata G. Reversing trend, big drop is seen in breast cancer. *The New York Times.* December 14, 2006; http://query.nytimes.com/gst/fullpage.html?sec=h ealth&res=9F04E5DA1231F936A25751C1A9609C8B63:Accessed August 8, 2007.

5. Kolata G. Sharp drop in rates of breast cancer holds. *The New York Times.* April 19, 2007; http://query.nytimes.com/gst/fullpage.html?sec=health&res=9A03E6D 91E3FF93AA25757C0A9619C8B63:Accessed August 8, 2007.

6. Chlebowski RT, Kuller LH, Prentice RL, et al. Breast cancer after use of estrogen plus progestin in postmenopausal women. *N Engl J Med.* 2009;360:573-587.

7. Xu X, Duncan AM, Merz-Demlow BE, Phipps WR, Kurzer MS. Menstrual cycle effects on urinary estrogen metabolites. *J Clin Endocrinol Metab.* 1999;84:3914-3918.

8. Xu X, Roman JM, Issaq HJ, Keefer LK, Veenstra TD, Ziegler RG. Quantitative measurement of endogenous estrogens and estrogen metabolites in human serum by liquid chromatography-tandem mass spectrometry. *Anal Chem.* 2007;79:7813-7821.

9. Premarin® (conjugated estrogen tablets). Wyeth Pharmaceuticals, Inc. 2004;Philadelphia, PA 19101:Full Prescribing Information.

10. Evans J. *Horse Breeding and Management*: Elsevier; 1992.

11. Woodcock J. "Bridging what is known and what is not known": FDA perspective and response. *FDA.* http://www.fda.gov/cder/present/ NIHWHI102302/sld018.htm:Slide 18.

12. Asthana S. Alzheimer's Disease: Efficacy of Transdermal 17-ß Estradiol. *http://www.nia.nih.gov/NR /rdonlyres/7DB43991-C46B-40F8-9199-6C282424000F/1982/Asthana.pdf.* University of Wisconsin Medical School.

13. Barnes R, Lobo R. Pharmacology of Estrogens. In: Mishell D, Jr, ed. *Menopause: Physiology and Pharmacology*. Chicago: Year Book Medical Publishers, Inc.; 1987.

14. Heiss G, Wallace R, Anderson GL, et al. Health risks and benefits 3 years after stopping randomized treatment with estrogen and progestin. *JAMA*. 2008;299:1036-1045.

15. Wright J, Morgenthaler J. *Natural Hormone Replacement for Women Over 45*. Petaluma, CA: Smart Publications; 1997.

CHAPTER 2

SHE JUST DIDN'T "FEEL RIGHT"

As a young doctor practicing "natural medicine" in the 1970s, I (JVW) hadn't really given much thought to using bio-identical hormones for women going through menopause. Like just about every other doctor at the time, I was prescribing Premarin®, which, I'd been taught in medical school, was a "natural" hormone, as opposed to a synthetic (laboratory-made) drug. It was derived from actual hormones, albeit hormones that were processed from the urine of female horses (but that seemed like a minor distinction at the time).

Besides, there really weren't any other good options in those days. Bio-identical hormones, as we know them today – pure, safe, inexpensive, easy-to-use, and easily formulated by specially trained compounding pharmacists – were not available. A woman's only real choices were either to use the horse estrogens in CEEs (Premarin®) or to "tough it out" (perhaps with a little help from some traditional herbal preparations) until the symptoms dissipated on their own.

Then, one day in 1982, Anna,* a 48-year-old woman, came to the Tahoma Clinic for her first consultation with me. She described many of her symptoms – infrequent, irregular menstrual periods, hot flushes, night sweats, inability to sleep well, a little memory loss – and told me she'd come to see me because she'd been reading my monthly columns in *Prevention* magazine,† and she wanted to use natural hormones. After we'd talked for nearly an hour, covering her entire health history, discussing the advantages and possible disadvantages of hormone replacement, and reviewing some herbal alternatives, she decided she wanted the hormones. I started to write a prescription for her, but she apparently could read upside-down, and stopped me with several observations and a question.

---

* Not her real name.

† I wrote monthly columns for the original *Prevention* magazine from mid-1976 through mid-1986, monthly columns for *Let's Live* magazine until 1996, and then *Nutrition & Healing* newsletter (published monthly, www.wrightnewsletter.com) with Alan R. Gaby, MD for a few years. From then on, I went on my own with *Nutrition & Healing*, along with a monthly column by Kerry Bone, co-author (with Simon Bone) of *Phytotherapy,* one of the world's leading textbooks of botanical medicine.

"That looks like it'll be a prescription for Premarin®," she said. "I've checked into it, and though I don't know much biochemistry, I've read that horse estrogens are not the same as human estrogens. Do I look like a horse? I want the exact same types of hormones my own body made until a few years ago!" she insisted. Since we'd just met, I skipped answering her question and agreed that some horse estrogens were entirely different from human estrogens, but that my medical school professors had explained that Premarin® (unlike many other molecules also prescribed as "estrogen" at that time, eg, DES) was entirely natural. But the biggest problem was that estrogens in a pattern precisely identical to human just weren't available at that time. Anna smiled. "I'm sure you can take care of that," she said. "I'll be back in 2 or 3 months. Maybe I'll try some of those herbs you mentioned in the meantime.

The textbooks of the time, including those used by medical schools, all emphasized that adult women's bodies naturally produced three primary estrogens: *estriol, estradiol,* and *estrone.* Yet, when it came time to discuss replacement regimens for postmenopausal symptoms, they invariably ignored these human estrogens in favor of horse estrogens.

Reading then-current medical journals wasn't much help either. The vast majority of "hormone replacement" studies published in the foremost peer-reviewed journals (all heavily sponsored by patent medicine company advertising, of course) have long involved the use of CEEs. While the titles of these articles usually cited some action and/or risk of "estrogen," read the text and you find they're almost always reporting on the effects of CEEs and thus, were virtually worthless for helping women like Anna. (*This is an excellent example of how the patent medicine (pharmaceutical/ drug) industry shapes hormone replacement "science" by redefining key terms to suit their marketing agenda; more about this later.*)

Not surprisingly, comparable studies involving bio-identical human hormones, especially at doses that would restore the levels typically found in premenopausal women, have always been far fewer. The main reason is simple and has nothing to do with the relative values of the two options. Such studies cost millions to run. Except for patent medicine companies and government agencies, no one else has the deep pockets to run them. But, patent medicine companies almost never spend a penny to research an unpatentable natural product that could also be marketed by competing companies that might undermine their own already patented products or compete with their own "branded" natural products.

There are exceptions: When patent medicine companies do – under certain conditions – manage to get FDA "approval" for a natural, usually unpatentable substance, they can charge a much higher price than natural food stores or compounding pharmacies for exactly the same item. Moreover, "insurance" will "cover" the high-priced FDA-"approved" version but not the much lower cost product sold without prescription. (Recent examples include ordinary fish oil capsules – renamed Omacor® (and again rebranded Lovaaza®), L-carnitine – renamed Carnitor®," and methylfolate – renamed Deplin®.

What makes this frightening trend even worse, sometimes the FDA, in coordination with the patent medicine company, will attempt to eliminate the "unapproved" – although identical – nonpatented competition. For example, the FDA very recently "ruled" that sales of pyridoxamine (a naturally occurring form of vitamin B6 sold for years in natural food stores) are "illegal." By "coincidence," a patent medicine company is poised to receive FDA "approval" for pyridoxamine – yes, the exact same molecule – renamed Pyridorin®). Of great importance to hundreds of thousands of women (some estimates are as high as 1-2 million) already taking bio-identical hormones, such a battle is currently waging over estriol, an essential form for estrogen in BHRT. (*See Chapter 12 for more detail.*)

Government agencies, like the National Institutes of Health (NIH),* are certainly in a better position to run studies on unpatentable products – and sometimes (rarely) they actually do – but the influence of the patent medicine industry on NIH science and scientists is so pervasive that, for all practical purposes, they all "sing from the same hymnal."

It's no surprise that a large proportion of women taking Premarin® complain about "not feeling right?" Women's brains and bodies have never, ever before been exposed to equilin and other major horse

---

* Many people think the FDA runs such trials, but they do not and could not, even if they were so inclined. By law, the FDA is a regulatory agency, not a research institution. All it can do is review drug studies run by third parties, usually patent medicine companies, which are interested in getting their products "approved".

estrogens! Is it any surprise that as many as half of those who start out down the Premarin® highway soon take the nearest exit ramp,[1,2] reckoning that they'd rather put up with hot flushes and other symptoms than the annoying and dangerous side effects of the patented pseudohormones?

Surely, there had to be a better way, but just as surely, it wasn't going to come from a patent medicine company.

Why Not Simply Copy Nature?

What was so remarkable back in 1982 was not that an alert patient asked me an obvious question: "Why horse hormones for human females?" Rather, it was why hadn't anybody taken the question seriously before?

Remember: the first principle of "natural medicine" is to *copy Nature*! As Anna gently pointed out to me, in the area of hormone replacement, I could have been doing a better job!

Of course, before copying Nature, I first had to determine just what it is I wanted to copy. Specifically, how much of which estrogens circulate through the body of a typical woman at any given time during her premenopausal years? You'd think this kind of information would be readily available, but in the early 1980s, you'd be wrong.

With the focus firmly on horse estrogens, apparently, no one had ever been interested enough to study the question of *human* (not horse) hormone replacement systematically and to publish the results. Certainly, the patent medicine industry, which supports much of the "hormone replacement" research that gets published, could see little profit in finding out. Actually, they assiduously avoided measuring horse hormone levels in women[*]; it might have "blown their cover"! They were more interested in selling equine hormones to humans than in finding out how these compared to bio-identical human hormones.

With so little reliable information to work from, my only option was to find out first hand.

---

[*] If you haven't figured out why, it's because the "normal" level of equilin and other non-human estrogens in the human body is exactly zero!

The Advent of "Triple-Estrogen"

You'd never know it from the mainstream media or most physicians, but there is no single hormone called **estrogen.** It is actually a "group name," describing literally dozens of estrogen subtypes (estrogen metabolites). In recent years (1999-2007), researchers at the NIH, using state-of-the-art assay equipment, published some fairly comprehensive studies about nearly all human estrogen metabolites.[7,8] However, back in the early 1980s there was very little interest in his kind of research. The major estrogens then researched and discussed were estrone, estradiol, and estriol. (These three are now termed "classical estrogens.")

Working with a technician (who coincidentally happened to be having menopausal symptoms herself) at Meridian Valley Laboratories (MVL) (then in Kent, Washington) we asked several large and not-so-large reference laboratories to tell us what the "normal ranges" of these three estrogens (blood levels they usually found in the samples they analyzed). Most of them gave us normal ranges for estrone and estradiol, but told us that estriol was only important during pregnancy, so they would only measure it for a pregnant woman.

Fortunately, though, a few of these reference laboratories had accumulated normal ranges for all three estrogens. We calculated averages from all the lab data, and concluded (at that time) that Nature's estrogen ratios were estriol – approximately 80% – and estradiol and estrone – approximately 10% each. We also sent off blood specimens from healthy nonpregnant women, labeled them "pregnant" (so the labs would test them!) and got back very similar results. That made my decision easy: My estrogen replacement prescriptions should be 80% estriol, 10% estradiol, 10% estrone, just as Nature appeared to intend.

The next problem was where to have these prescriptions filled, since no patent medication company provided these three human estrogens, especially in these proportions. In the early 1980s, nearly all pharmacies and pharmacists had abandoned the centuries-old practice of making up pharmaceuticals from original "bulk" materials right there in the pharmacy. Although more educated than ever in patent medicines and able to guide patients exceptionally well about their benefits and risks, the pharmacists' job in the 1980s (and still the majority of pharmacists' jobs in 2009) involves mostly counting out the correct number of pills at the correct doses. For "estrogen," all they had on their shelves were horse estrogen pills, ethinyl estradiol (usually used in "birth control pills"), and a few other patentable estrogen "take offs." While estradiol was available by injection, pills containing it were hard to find and rarely prescribed.. Pharmacists who actually "put things together" themselves to fill a prescription (now called *compounding pharmacists*) were a rare and endangered species.

I called several compounding pharmacists, but none could help. Finally, though, I found Ed Thorpe of Kripps Pharmacy in Vancouver, British Columbia, Canada, which fortunately was only a 3-hour drive from my "home base" in the Seattle area. Ed formulated capsules (and later a "creme") containing a combination of bio-identical estriol, estradiol, and estrone in what appeared to be Nature's ratio of 8:1:1.

Ed and I named the combination "triple estrogen" or "Tri-Est" (although it was, of course, unpatented). Tri-Est was an "instant hit" with every woman who tried the oral hormone capsules. Over and over, we heard, "My symptoms are gone, and I feel like myself again!"

Later on I noticed (took me awhile sometimes, too) that although we were using Nature's molecules and Nature's ratios, we weren't actually using Nature's ideal route of delivery for these hormones. After all, no woman has her ovaries inside her gastrointestinal (GI) tract, secreting estrogens into her intestines to be absorbed there and delivered first directly to her liver ("first-pass" metabolism). That wouldn't "make physiologic sense," as a woman's liver is her major organ for metabolizing and eliminating estrogens and other steroid hormones from her body. (*See Chapter 9.*)

Nature's pathway for estrogen (as well as progesterone, testosterone, and all other endocrine hormones) delivers these hormones from her ovaries directly into her pelvic veins and from there to her heart, which then pumps them to every part of her body at once (including eventually her liver – "second pass" metabolism), which is the body's natural way of regulating hormone levels.

So Ed and (by then) other compounding pharmacists started putting "triple estrogen" into a "creme" base, designed to be applied to the skin (transdermal application). The hormones easily diffused though the skin and entered the blood stream in a slow, closer-to-natural way. This was in sharp contrast to taking Premarin® (or any other steroid hormone) by mouth, which, in addition to being a highly unnatural way for steroid hormones to enter the body, could open the door to a number of very serious problems.

[Later on, after close monitoring (with lab tests) of many women who used transdermal estrogens, I discovered once more that I wasn't copying Nature as closely as possible, and the recommendation for transdermal application had to be changed again...but that's a topic for Chapter 9.]

In the 1990s, I thought it would be a good idea to re-examine our assumptions about the correct physiologic proportions of estrone, estradiol, and estriol in the body. After all, laboratory techniques had changed considerably since 1982. Many of the women I worked with were now using "Triple Estrogen" (as well as progesterone, testosterone, and DHEA), and MVL was helping me to monitor their blood and urine levels to make sure that the quantities prescribed were correct for each woman. MVL found research volunteers – 26 women between 20 and 40 years of age, healthy, not pregnant, and nonsmokers – and measured their relative plasma levels* of estriol, estradiol, and estrone. The initial results suggested that human estrogen in this population was actually comprised of about 90% estriol, 7% estradiol, and 3% estrone, [Curiously (or perhaps not) no woman we have tested ever showed a trace of horse estrogens!]

As noted above and in Chapter 1, the most recent assays of human estrogens reported by NIH researchers, using much more sensitive (and highly expensive) equipment, have since reported different ratios of these estrogens in urine and in blood.[7, 8] Nevertheless, so many women have done so well by starting with the ratios that I originally derived that the very large majority of bio-identical estrogen prescriptions we write still contain 50% or more estriol. Also, monitoring techniques – especially

---

* **Plasma is the liquid portion of blood, minus all the red and white blood cells, and other solid bodies that normally circulate in the blood stream.**

the multiple-metabolite 24-hour urinary steroid determination – allow prescribing physicians to "tailor" prescriptions to each woman. (*See Chapter 9 for further details of this monitoring technique.*) Since estriol is such a benign and protective (against cancer) estrogen, it appears that its exact proportions may be less important than the fact that estriol levels in replacement prescriptions be far higher than the levels of the more potent – and more carcinogenic – estradiol and estrone.

In the 25+ years since Ed Thorpe and I collaborated on the first batches of Tri-Est, Anna and hundreds of thousands of women like her have used bio-identical estrogen (along with progesterone. DHEA, and testosterone) cremes to restore their hormone levels to approximately the lower end of the range of hormone levels normally found in a premenopausal woman. Their hot flushes vanish, their bones stay strong, their skin improves, they feel good and, for the most part they feel – normal.

What a shocker! Stop the presses!

> "Women Taking Identical Copies of Hormones Their Ovaries Have Been Producing Their Entire Adult Life Feel Normal."

Go figure!

Progesterone, the Hormone the Drug Companies Forgot
(and Why This Was Such a Disaster)

In addition to bio-identical estrogen, doctors who practice BHRT properly always make sure their patients use bio-identical *progesterone* as well. Like estrogen, progesterone is a steroid hormone produced in, and secreted in largest quantities by the *ovaries;* like estrogen, progesterone also declines with menopause, and often before. (The adrenal glands also make considerable amounts of progesterone, much of which is metabolized into other, non-sex steroids.) *For reasons that will soon become apparent, women should never take supplemental estrogen of any kind, no matter what the source, unless they are also taking progesterone.* While this would seem to be obvious to anyone who understands how human reproductive physiology works, the makers of Premarin® chose to ignore it, with devastating consequences.[*]

In the majority of women who are still menstruating, both estrogen and progesterone are normally secreted on an approximate 28-day schedule that is partly responsible for the familiar changes of the menstrual cycle, including ovulation, menstruation (the "period"), and all their associated feelings. In the natural ebb and flow of hormones over the 400 to 500 periods that punctuate a woman's reproductive life, estrogen and progesterone are usually in perfect balance. Until that balance starts to break down during the early days of perimenopause (sometimes as early as a woman's 30s), estrogen never gets secreted without progesterone coming along at just the right time in just the right amounts to modulate its effects.

Over the course of a lifetime, the body's various systems become accustomed to this pattern of rhythmic secretion. (*See Chapter 3 for a more detailed description of what happens hormonally during the menstrual cycle.*) Given the wide range of individual effects that both estrogen and progesterone have, not only in the reproductive organs, but also in many different tissues all over the body, including the breast, brain, bones, urinary tract, and skin, it's not surprising that a woman would feel "strange" or "different" when her estrogen and progesterone go out of balance.

One of estrogen's most important functions is to stimulate the growth of the endometrial lining each month in anticipation of the implantation of a fertilized egg. By contrast, one of progesterone's most important jobs is to "oppose," or limit estrogen-stimulated cell growth in the uterus (and the breast), thus keeping cell growth *in balance*. (*See Chapter 3.*) Unopposed estrogen-stimulated cell growth, due to a prolonged imbalance between estrogen and progesterone, can occasionally lead to cancer, as well as a syndrome named "estrogen dominance," which is associated with certain specific signs and symptoms.

---

[*] At about the same time we were working with early formulations of triple-estrogen, Dr. John R. Lee, a Northern California family physician, was taking a similar approach with bio-identical progesterone. Dr. Lee found that progesterone played many vital roles in the body, including promoting bone growth (preventing osteoporosis), regulating mood, maintaining heart and breast health, and others. At the same time, it also appeared to be extraordinarily safe and well-tolerated. In early 1990s, Dr. Lee began publishing his findings, and in 1996 summed them up in an important book entitled *What Your Doctor May Not Tell You about Menopause* (Grand Central Publishing). For more about Dr. Lee's important work, see Chapter 6.

Progesterone helps prevent endometrial cancer in two ways. First, it reduces the number of estrogen receptors (sites on cells where estrogen molecules normally bind, or attach themselves), such as those in the uterine lining or the breasts; estrogen molecules that are prevented from binding by the action of progesterone cannot then stimulate cell growth. Second, progesterone directly regulates cell division/replication of fully mature endometrial cells, thus inhibiting estrogen-stimulated cellular overgrowth (called *hyperplasia*) and sometimes cancer.[9]

Although patent medicine company researchers must certainly have known about this relationship between estrogen and progesterone from Day 1, they chose to ignore it until, for many women, it was too late. During the early years of "estrogen replacement therapy" (ERT), most women took Premarin® "as directed" without progesterone, during which time thousands went on to develop endometrial cancer (cancer of the uterus). Had drug researchers paid as close attention to the reproductive physiology of *Homo sapiens* as they did to that of *Equus caballus*, they might have had a clue right from the start that something was wrong with their approach, and this tragedy could have been easily averted.

This attitude by patent medicine company researchers indicates that they look at a woman in menopause and see, not someone with her hormonal system out of balance, but as someone with symptoms that need to be suppressed. It's as though she has a headache, so let's give her an aspirin to suppress the pain. From that viewpoint, giving Premarin® "unopposed" by progesterone makes perfect sense ... except for that pesky cancer problem.

The patent medicine companies forgot – or intentionally ignored – a simple physiologic fact: while Premarin® might act like a drug by preventing hot flushes, it was still a potent hormone capable of a wide range of activities that have nothing to do with blood vessel dilation (the cause of hot flushes). They thought of these other activities as *"side effects,"* because they were not really interested in them. Unfortunately, they forgot that they couldn't tell the body to ignore them.

Having finally been forced to face the need to "oppose" estrogen to prevent endometrial cancer, Big Pharma went on to demonstrate its continued cluelessness by offering women, not Nature-proven progesterone, but rather a patented (of course), man-made progesterone-mimicking pseudohormone called *medroxyprogesterone acetate* (MPA), which they marketed under the brand name ***Provera®***. For the sake of convenience – and to prevent women from taking Premarin® without Provera®, which could lead to cancer and *law suits* – they eventually combined Premarin® and Provera® into a single pill they cleverly called ***Prempro®***.

Until women were first asked to swallow it to "oppose" the growth-stimulating effects of Premarin®, the Provera® (MPA) molecule had never seen the insides of a human body. (It actually had never even been found on planet Earth before it appeared in a patent medicine company chemist's test tube! Like most other patent medicines, Provera® was no different than a molecule that might have been brought to earth by a "space alien.") MPA is a synthetic (laboratory-produced) molecule that looks a little like progesterone and, consequently, is capable of doing *a few* of the things that natural/bio-identical progesterone normally does in the human body. Most importantly for the patent medicine industry, Provera® was pretty good at blocking CEE-induced hyperplasia in the uterine lining. When Premarin® is taken with Provera®, the combination can usually be counted on to control hot flushes without significantly increasing the risk of endometrial cancer.

The patent medicine industry liked MPA for two major reasons: 1) It was patentable, *always* the first criterion for any pharmaceutical product; nonpatentable molecules (eg, bio-identical hormones) are routinely passed over, no matter how promising they might be therapeutically*; 2) MPA acts enough like progesterone that it could be used to "oppose" Premarin®-induced endometrial overgrowth, thus minimizing the greatest perceived drawback to Premarin® use at the time, its high risk of uterine cancer.

---

* As noted above, a frightening trend has emerged in the last few years as patent medicine companies see their sales of non-bioidentical, pseudohormones dropping drastically. Adopting the "re-name it, and then get FDA to 'approve' it and then wipe out the competition" strategy, one patent medicine company has re-named estriol Trimesta®, while another has re-named 2-methoxyestradiol as Panzem®. Both companies are racing for FDA "approval" of these natural molecules

Of course, natural (built-in, bio-identical) progesterone accomplishes these same functions and a whole lot more, (*See box.*), but Big Pharma

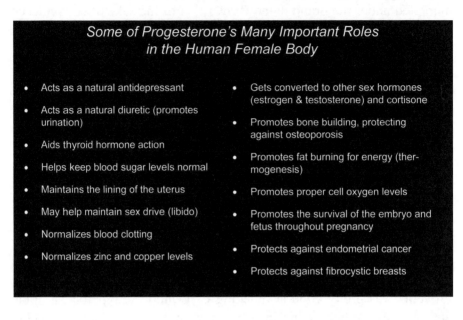

Some of Progesterone's Many Important Roles in the Human Female Body

- Acts as a natural antidepressant
- Acts as a natural diuretic (promotes urination)
- Aids thyroid hormone action
- Helps keep blood sugar levels normal
- Maintains the lining of the uterus
- May help maintain sex drive (libido)
- Normalizes blood clotting
- Normalizes zinc and copper levels
- Gets converted to other sex hormones (estrogen & testosterone) and cortisone
- Promotes bone building, protecting against osteoporosis
- Promotes fat burning for energy (thermogenesis)
- Promotes proper cell oxygen levels
- Promotes the survival of the embryo and fetus throughout pregnancy
- Protects against endometrial cancer
- Protects against fibrocystic breasts

was never really interested in producing an exact analog of progesterone. What they basically wanted was a patentable "one-trick pony" that could oppose estrogen-stimulated hyperplasia. They didn't care much what else it did or didn't do.

So, this is what passes for "hormone replacement therapy" in conventional medical practice in the first decade of the 21st century: a combination of potent estrogens designed for use in a non-human species and a patented synthetic hormone-imposter drug intended not so much to *replace* progesterone as to protect the body from one of Premarin's® potentially fatal side effects. Mission accomplished!

Copy Nature, No More, No Less

The premise of bio-identical hormone replacement therapy is really quite simple: *Copy Nature.* Give the body exactly what it needs to get its systems back in order – no more, no less. Use bio-identical human hormones at doses and on a schedule that restores them to as close to their natural premenopausal levels as possible.

Obviously, you can't do this with patented drugs or pseudohormones. What's the *natural* level of equilin in the human female? What's the *natural* level of MPA? (Just in case you "came in late," it's zero!)

BHRT employs hormones that are chemically identical to those human ovaries have been producing and secreting on a daily basis for millions of years. Biochemists can't tell them apart, and neither can your body. Since the disruption of the normal hormonal environment is responsible for the symptoms of menopause, restoring that environment with exact copies of the missing hormones removes the *cause*, and the symptoms simply vanish as the body returns to its normal hormonal balance.

Restoring a normal hormonal balance has never been particularly high on Big Pharma's agenda. Rather, their principal concern lay in developing patent medicines good for squelching symptoms like hot flushes, etc. Those patent medicines have been among the best selling pharmaceutical products in history. The fact that they focused their efforts on estrogens is merely a matter of convenience. They would have easily used *anything* that worked. In fact, recent studies have touted the possibility of using patent medicines called selective serotonin reuptake inhibitors (SSRIs) – drugs such as Prozac® and Zoloft®, which are commonly used to manage depression and anxiety – to control hot flushes.[10] This is an example of pure symptom suppression that bears no relation to the actual cause of the problem. At least Premarin® and Provera® make an attempt – imperfect as it is – at remedying the cause of the problem.

The Bottom Line, Scientifically Speaking

To this day, nearly everything doctors "know" about hormone replacement in menopausal women comes from studies – often seriously flawed ones – in which human estrogens were "substituted" with pregnant horse estrogens, and human progesterone was "substituted" with Provera®. To use the term "replacement" in this context seems particularly inaccurate.

Signs that the human physiology was never intended to handle these hormonal "bulls in a china shop" have been apparent from Day 1, but conventional medicine has largely dismissed them. The benefits, we've been told over and over again, outweigh the risks. You want to do away with hot flushes? Then you might have to put up with a little breast soreness, fluid retention, and maybe a *slightly* increased risk of cancer. After all, we're reminded, "All drugs have side effects."

Moreover, the use of inexact copies of human hormones has resulted in inexcusably sloppy medical practice. For example, for decades, women were given doses of these powerful pseudohormones with no follow-up testing to determine whether those doses were even safe or effective. Could lower doses have been used with equal (or perhaps greater) benefit and safety? Believe it or not, no one knew, and to this day, no one knows. Since Premarin® and Provera® were first introduced, the "recommended" FDA-"approved" doses have been cut in half twice in the interests of safety, despite the absence of one bit of evidence to support these actions.

Certainly, no matter what their source, hormones and pseudohormones are potent agents, so good medical practice demands that we always stay on the lookout for possible adverse side effects, especially deadly ones like cancer and heart disease. I always tell women I'm working with that

Some of Provera's Many Side Effects*

- Birth defects, if taken during pregnancy
- Breakthrough bleeding or other menstrual irregularities
- Increased risk of breast cancer
- Breast milk production
- Breast tenderness/pain
- Depression and other mental/mood changes
- Memory loss, nervousness
- Sudden severe headache, dizziness
- Changes in vision; ocular inflammation and lesions
- Numbness or tingling in the arms or legs
- Chest pain
- Fluid retention (edema)
- Formation of blood clots, especially in the lungs and brain
- Hair loss, or unwanted facial hair growth (androgenic effects)
- Acne
- Impaired glucose tolerance (pre-diabetic effects)
- Skin rashes
- Weight gain
- Nausea
- Jaundice
- Shortness of breath
- Swelling of the hands or feet
- Pain in the legs

*   Independent of concomitant Premarin® administration

no treatment, not even BHRT, can be considered 100% safe. That's what careful dosing and hormone level monitoring are essential to the proper practice of BHRT, steps that are meaningless and ignored by doctors prescribing patented HRT regimens.

But, let's be sensible about this. Women secrete these hormones for their entire reproductive lives without experiencing most of the problems attributed to Premarin® and Provera®. Moreover, the appropriate use of bio-identical human versions of estrogen and progesterone by hundreds of thousands of women over the last quarter century has yielded not even a hint that they might be causing these serious problems. In fact, the vast majority of the side effects seen with Premarin® (*See box in Chapter 1, page 17*) and Provera® (*See box in Chapter 2, page 38*) are virtually never seen with bio-identical estrogens and progesterone. If anything, the effects of bio-identical hormones are often opposite those seen with Premarin® and Provera®.

If human estrogens and progesterone had anything close to the side effect profiles of their patented pseudohormonal counterparts, few women would survive into adulthood. Based on a number of clinical studies plus the collective experience of thousands of knowledgeable physicians who have been prescribing BHRT, it appears that most of the problems that arise during BHRT are related to the dose – or the metabolism – of the hormone. Reduce the dose or adjust the metabolism and the problems usually go away.

Certainly, it would be a great advantage in terms of acceptance if large-scale clinical trials of bio-identical hormones could be undertaken to convincingly evaluate their benefits and risks, but who's going to run those trials? Independent doctors with busy practices? Don't be silly... no time, no money. A patent medicine company? No way! Where's the profit? The federal government (NIH)? Perhaps, but don't hold your breath.

In the meantime, for those doctors, who are knowledgeable about bio-identical hormones and have been monitoring their use by thousands of women for up to 25 years or more, no further proof is needed.

The WHI and Beyond

HRT proponents have long played up the results of studies demonstrating that long-term treatment with Premarin® + Provera® could reduce the risks of heart disease, osteoporosis, colorectal cancer, dementia, and to improve overall well-being. At the same time, they have downplayed mounting evidence suggesting that the reality of HRT might not quite measure up to its widely cultivated "fountain-of-youth" public image.

The Women's Health Initiative (WHI) was intended to plug some of the major loopholes in the HRT knowledge base. Specifically, "experts" expected the WHI to provide the most definitive answers yet with regard to the role of HRT in cardiovascular disease (heart attacks, strokes, and blood clots) and cancer, clearly expecting that the results would support the use of these products.

The WHI was a large clinical trial of over 161,000 *healthy* menopausal women (aged 50-79 years) conducted by the NIH in 40 different clinics all over the country. Enrollment of participants began in 1993, and the study was scheduled to last 8.5 years. But one day in the middle of summer 2002, after an average of just 5.2 years of treatment, the NIH announced that the primary arm of the study was being terminated ahead of schedule. The reason: a scheduled interim safety monitoring had revealed that the risks of HRT were outrunning its benefits.[3] Almost overnight, the entire HRT house of cards, built up over more than 40 years on myths, promises, and flawed data, suddenly came tumbling down.

Here's what happened. In the primary arm of the study, half the women took Prempro® pills (CEE 0.625 mg + MPA 2.5 mg) and half took identical looking but inactive placebos, or dummy pills. In a secondary arm, women who had had their uterus surgically removed (*hysterectomy*) took either Premarin® pills ("unopposed") or placebos. The study was double-blinded, which meant that neither the participating women nor the investigators knew who was getting which treatment until the study was terminated (or evaluated by an interim safety analysis, as this one was). "Double-blinding" is an important control designed to eliminate the influence of potential investigator or participant bias.

As shown in Table 2-1, most of the supposed benefits of HRT, including protection against heart disease, strokes, cognitive loss, improved mood, and sexual dissatisfaction turned out to be fallacious. After 4 years of treatment, the women who took Prempro® had a 26% *increase* in invasive breast cancer. Moreover, the breast cancers that occurred in these women were slightly larger, more advanced at discovery, and more likely to have spread to nearby lymph nodes, all serious danger signs.

Table 2-1. Key Findings of the WHI Studies[3-6]

Favorable to HRT	Unfavorable to HRT
Prempro® appeared to slow the progression of osteoporosis: 5 fewer cases of hip fracture per 10,000 women.	Prempro® increased the risk of invasive breast cancer by 26% after 4 years; an absolute increase of 8 cases per 10,000 users; risk appeared to be cumulative.
Prempro® was associated with a 37% reduction in the incidence of colon cancer; an overall decline of 6 cases per 10,000 women.	Breast cancers found in women using Prempro® compared to nonusers tended to be slightly larger (1.7 vs. 1.5 cm); to be discovered at more advanced stages; and to spread to nearby lymph nodes more frequently (24.6% vs. 16%).
Premarin® ("unopposed") had no effect (positive or negative) on the risk of heart attack.	Prempro® increased the risk of heart disease in otherwise healthy women: a 29% increase overall and an 81% increase during the first year of use; absolute increase of 7 new cases per 10,000 women per year.
Premarin® ("unopposed") was less likely to cause breast cancer than Prempro®.	Prempro® had no beneficial effects on health-related quality of life (ie, general health, vitality, mental health, depression, sexual satisfaction).
	Prempro® did not improve cognitive function and doubled the risk for developing all types of dementia, including Alzheimer's disease.
	Prempro® doubled the incidence of blood clots in the lungs and legs.
	Prempro® increased the incidence of a stroke by 41%; an increase of 7 new cases per 10,000 users.
	Premarin® ("unopposed") increased the risk of stroke
	Prempro® increased the risk of urinary incontinence

A higher risk of breast cancer was not that big a surprise. The promise of HRT has always been tempered by a risk of cancer, but this risk has been rationalized away by citing the protection supposedly offered against the more common dangers of heart disease, stroke, and perhaps even dementia.

The real revelation of the WHI was that HRT's cardiovascular protection, which had long been assumed and widely promoted, turned out to be an illusion. Many studies prior to the WHI had suggested that HRT was associated with a 30 to 50% reduction in "coronary events."[11-13] However, in the otherwise heart-healthy WHI population at the start of the study, Prempro® actually *increased the risk of heart disease* by 29% overall and by a whopping *81% during the first year of use.* Prempro® also doubled the risk of blood clots in the lungs and legs and increased the risk of stroke by 41%. On the bright side, Prempro® was associated with somewhat fewer hip fractures due to osteoporosis and a slightly reduced risk of colorectal cancer.

If you think this all sounds just a bit too risky merely for snuffing out some hot flushes, you're in good company. That's what the NIH thought also, and it caused them to pull the plug on the Prempro® arm of the study several years ahead of schedule.

Further analyses of the WHI database over the following years continued the theme of promises unkept. HRT was believed to keep women's minds sharper longer, but Prempro® failed to protect cognitive function and actually *doubled the risk* for all types of dementia, including Alzheimer's disease.[5]

And to add insult to injury, not only did HRT not make women healthier, it also failed to make them happier. A sample of the WHI population (about 16,600 women) answered questionnaires designed to assess their health-related quality of life, using a wide range of criteria (including general health, vitality, mental health, depression, sexual satisfaction, sleep, physical functioning, and bodily pain). After 3 years of treatment, though, the results revealed no clinically meaningful differences between the Prempro® and placebo groups on any of the quality-of-life measures.[6]

The other shoe dropped in 2004 with the premature termination (after 7 years) of the "estrogen-only" arm of the WHI. Recall that this study evaluated Premarin® in a variation of the human species called the "woman without a uterus." Although Premarin® did not appear to increase the risk of heart attacks in these women, as Prempro® had done in "women with a uterus," Premarin® did lead to a significant increase in the risk of stroke. On the plus side, there was a decrease in the risk of hip fracture and a questionable reduction in breast cancer risk.[4]

For 40 or more years, Premarin® and Provera® (or Prempro®) had lived comfortably near the top of the drug sales charts, earning billions of dollars for Wyeth Pharmaceuticals, despite a lack of definitive proof that they were either safe or effective, and in the presence of a significant amount of evidence to suggest that they were neither.

In the aftermath of the WHI revelations, conventional medicine was no longer able to convincingly spin the results in its favor. Faced with a tidal wave of negative publicity, women quit HRT in droves. In 2002, before the WHI revelations, 18.5 million women were using HRT, but 2 years later, only 7.6 million women were still using it, a 69% drop. Sales of Prempro® plummeted by 74%.[14]

The FDA's primary response was to alter the official Premarin® and Prempro® labels* – on **all estrogen replacement products**, *not just the CEEs proven by the WHI to cause problems* – to include a "black box" that reiterated the WHI findings, warning of "*increased risks of myocardial infarction [heart attack], stroke, invasive breast cancer, pulmonary emboli [blood clots], and deep vein thrombosis [blood clots again] in postmenopausal women during 5 years of treatment with conjugated equine estrogens (0.625 mg) combined with medroxyprogesterone acetate (2.5 mg) relative to placebo.*"[17]

Despite the dismal history of conventional HRT, of which the WHI is only the most recent reminder, when the forces that control conventional medicine look to the future of menopausal hormone replacement, they still

---

* A drug label, also known as the PI (Product Information or Package Insert) carries all the pertinent information about a drug that the drug company and FDA can agree on. It often comes with each prescription and is usually printed in maddeningly tiny type and folded like a roadmap. Most PIs these days can be found online at the drug company's website, although your pharmacist should be able to supply you with one if you ask.

see only patented pseudoestrogens and synthetic progesterone-mimicking patent medicines. Post-WHI guidelines for treating menopause compiled by such powerful organizations as the American College of Obstetricians and Gynecologists (ACOG),[18] the North American Menopause Society (NAMS),[19] the International Menopause Society (IMS),[20] the United States Preventive Services Task Force,[21] the National Institutes of Health (NIH)[22], and the European Agency for the Evaluation of Medicinal Products (EMEA)[23] barely acknowledge the existence of bio-identical hormones. Where they do mention them, it is in the context of a warning about potential adverse side effects and/or a lack of efficacy in published studies. Nowhere do any of these guidelines offer any evidence of such adverse effects or even suggest the "radical" idea of exploring the therapeutic possibilities of bio-identical human hormones.

Most of the time, when the FDA has strong evidence that a drug causes cancer and has no redeeming life-saving benefits (Nobody ever died from a hot flush.), it pulls that drug off the shelves. In the case of Premarin®/Provera®, however, Wyeth caught a break. Instead of banning the use of Premarin® and Provera®, the FDA "approved" new, lower dosage forms for each drug (Premarin® 0.45 mg and Provera® 1.5 mg; roughly half the previous "approved" dose) under the assumption that the lower dose would be less risky. How did they know the lower doses would be safer? Well, they didn't. No "controlled studies" – or studies of any sort – were done to justify this action. It was just a guess, but the FDA went along with it anyway.[15] In actual fact, a recently published review of "estrogen" replacement research from 1966 to 2003 concluded that low-dose preparations would probably not improve Premarin's® safety profile.[16]

These guidelines recommend some form of conventional HRT only for treating hot flushes and other common menopausal symptoms using the *lowest possible doses for the shortest possible duration*. In other words, once hot flushes go away on their own, HRT should be stopped. Although patented HRT might actually help reduce the risk of bone fractures due to osteoporosis, it is now viewed as a secondary choice for this application, to be used only if patented anti-osteoporosis drugs don't work better. Women who have heart disease should not use HRT, and of course, HRT can no longer be used to prevent heart attacks, strokes, and senility, because the WHI proved that it doesn't work.

Now What? BHRT in the Post-WHI World

While most doctors were "Shocked, shocked!" to learn the truth about the patent medicines they'd been prescribing, for those of us who'd been paying close attention to decades of *pre*-WHI research, the devastating results came as more relief than surprise. In fact, we predicted many of them in our 1997 book.[24]

Many studies – some dating back as far as the 1940s – had suggested that Premarin® treatment was not worth the risks. But these studies almost always had one or more methodologic trap doors that made it easy to dismiss them, or at least minimize the significance of the results if that was your mindset. The WHI avoided most of those loopholes, but it created some enormous new ones of its own. Most notably, the only active treatments tested were *oral* Prempro® and Premarin® alone (in "women without a uterus"). What do the WHI findings – both positive and negative – tell us about the potential benefits and risks of other treatments, especially bio-identical hormones?

The short answer is "virtually nothing." As we have said before, and will continue to reiterate *ad nauseum*, bio-identical hormones and patented pseudohormones are completely different molecularly, and the body responds to them in completely different ways.

Nevertheless, the "official" response to the WHI findings is that, since we don't have large, prospective, double-blind, placebo-controlled studies telling us otherwise, *all options* must be considered equally suspect until proven otherwise in a study comparable to the WHI. While this may represent conservative, lawyerly FDA thinking, it has nothing to do with the realities of medical science and it completely ignores the fundamental differences between alien-to-the-body patent medicines and bio-identical human hormones. Blindly following these dictates would permanently deprive women of what is undeniably a safe and effective resource.

To equate Premarin® + Provera® with bio-identical human estrogens and progesterone is like saying that ordinary 100% natural fruit juice is equivalent to some patented, synthetic chemical drink (eg, Coke or Pepsi). If the latter were discovered to cause a serious health condition in some people (as they have), does that mean we should suddenly start being concerned about the safety of the pure fruit juice we drink too? It's nonsense, of course, but the analogy is valid. It's as clear a demonstration as we've got how the patent medicine industry has "brainwashed" the conventional medical community into believing that Premarin® = estrogen and Provera® = progesterone.

A growing database of scientific research from all over the world, combined with the first-hand experience of hundreds of thousands of women treated by knowledgeable, progressive doctors, who do not limit their practice to what the FDA-Big Pharma axis dictates, is proving the safety and utility of BHRT every day.

Conventional medicine attempts to discredit research favorable to BHRT by arguing that the studies do not meet the FDA's rigid design standards and/or that they may not be published in "reputable" peer-reviewed (ie, drug industry-sponsored) journals. Although large, expensive-to-run, double-blind, placebo-controlled studies are often held up as the ultimate form of scientific "proof," such studies are really only one means of establishing scientific "truth." Close observation of Nature has a long and glorious legacy in the history in medicine. Until relatively recently, most medical research consisted primarily of anecdotes and careful observations.

Not all "uncontrolled" observations need be biased, especially if no money is riding on the findings. Things began to change only with the advent of modern patent-driven, increasingly FDA-regulated medicine in the mid-20th century. The FDA demanded such studies to support claims of drug efficacy and safety, primarily because patent medicine companies had been caught selling dangerous and/or ineffective drugs one too many times. Naturally, the only ones who could afford to run the studies were the big patent medicine companies. By default, then, if the patent medicine industry was not interested in – ie, *can't make a big profit from* – a particular treatment, it doesn't stand much chance of getting the FDA's "approval."

But as we have seen by the raft of recalls and warnings of FDA-"approved" patent medicines over the last few years,* such studies are a long way from being foolproof.† Certainly, they have their place. They offer a high degree of reassurance about the results that rests on a firm statistical foundation. However, such studies usually serve to highlight subtle differences between treatments and/or to confirm (or refute) insights, findings, and observations that originated in less well-powered studies or in careful observations. Moreover, they can be deliberately designed to increase the chance that a desirable result will be found. It's no coincidence that patent medicine-company studies have a much higher likelihood of yielding results favorable to the company's drug than do independent studies.

As noted above, the WHI was not the first study to demonstrate the risks of HRT, only the most definitive. By the same token, many published studies (mostly in European and Asian medical journals) have demonstrated that bio-identical hormones are safe and effective, not only for preventing hot flushes and other common signs of estrogen depletion, but also for protecting against heart disease, osteoporosis, cancer, and cognitive decline, uses for which conventional patented HRT is no longer considered appropriate.[25]

Nevertheless, lacking an FDA "approval," BHRT will remain under attack; actually categorized as potentially the same or worse than Prempro® and the other pseudohormonal treatments; attacked just because they're not "approved" by the FDA – even though Nature has "approved" them for as long as there have been women!

What a shame! But for those who are open to the idea, scientific evidence and clinical experience continues to accumulate in favor of using a balanced combination of bio-identical estrogens plus natural progesterone, and in many cases, other hormones, such as DHEA, pregnenolone, melatonin, and testosterone, to name just a few.

---

* Vioxx, Rezulin, Propulsid, Bextra, Baycol, Fen-Phen, and Redux are just a few of the FDA-"approved" drugs that have been recalled or "voluntarily" withdrawn over the last few years, because in most cases they were killing people or at least making them very, very sick.

† In fact, a very long way from foolproof. A study by the Government Accounting Office of 198 patent medicines "approved" by FDA between 1976 and 1985 found that 102 (51.5%) had serious and often lethal adverse effects.[GAO/PEMD 90-15 *FDA Drug Review: Post" approval" Risks 1976-1985, p.3.*

Like estrogens and progesterone, many of these hormones have also been found to decline with age. And like estrogens and progesterone, restoring many of them to normal levels with bio-identical versions can have a remarkably revitalizing effect on everything from the heart and immune system to mood, cognitive function, bone and muscle strength, energy level, and libido (sexual drive).

References

1. Regan MM, Emond SK, Attardo MJ, Parker RA, Greenspan SL. Why do older women discontinue hormone replacement therapy? *J Womens Health Gend Based Med.* 2001;10:343-350.

2. Vihtamaki T, Savilahti R, Tuimala R. Why do postmenopausal women discontinue hormone replacement therapy? *Maturitas.* 1999;33:99-105.

3. Heiss G, Wallace R, Anderson GL, et al. Health risks and benefits 3 years after stopping randomized treatment with estrogen and progestin. *JAMA.* 2008;299:1036-1045.

4. Anderson GL, Limacher M, Assaf AR, et al. Effects of conjugated equine estrogen in postmenopausal women with hysterectomy: the Women's Health Initiative randomized controlled trial. *JAMA.* 2004;291:1701-1712.

5. Rapp SR, Espeland MA, Shumaker SA, et al. Effect of estrogen plus progestin on global cognitive function in postmenopausal women: the Women's Health Initiative Memory Study: a randomized controlled trial. *JAMA.* 2003;289:2663-2672.

6. Hays J, Ockene JK, Brunner RL, et al. Effects of estrogen plus progestin on health-related quality of life. *N Engl J Med.* 2003;348:1839-1854.

7. Xu X, Duncan AM, Merz-Demlow BE, Phipps WR, Kurzer MS. Menstrual cycle effects on urinary estrogen metabolites. *J Clin Endocrinol Metab.* 1999;84:3914-3918.

8. Xu X, Roman JM, Issaq HJ, Keefer LK, Veenstra TD, Ziegler RG. Quantitative measurement of endogenous estrogens and estrogen metabolites in human serum by liquid chromatography-tandem mass spectrometry. *Anal Chem.* 2007;79:7813-7821.

9. Ferenczy A, Gelfand M. The biologic significance of cytologic atypia in progestogen-treated endometrial hyperplasia. *Am J Obstet Gynecol.* 1989;160:126-131.

10. Amato P, Marcus DM. Review of alternative therapies for treatment of menopausal symptoms. *Climacteric.* 2003;6:278-284.

11. Grady D, Rubin SM, Petitti DB, et al. Hormone therapy to prevent disease and prolong life in postmenopausal women. *Ann Intern Med.* 1992;117:1016-1037.

12. Bush TL, Barrett-Connor E, Cowan LD, et al. Cardiovascular mortality and noncontraceptive use of estrogen in women: results from the Lipid Research Clinics Program Follow-up Study. *Circulation.* 1987;75:1102-1109.

13. Stampfer MJ, Colditz GA. Estrogen replacement therapy and coronary heart disease: a quantitative assessment of the epidemiologic evidence. *Prev Med.* 1991;20:47-63.

14. Berger L. Hormone Therapy: The Dust Is Still Settling. *The New York Times.* June 6, 2004; Available at: query.nytimes.com/gst/health/article-page.html?res=9 E05EFD91E3EF935A35755C0A9629C8B63. Accessed June 21, 2008.

15. FDA. FDA Approves Lower Dose of Prempro, a Combination Estrogen and Progestin Drug for Postmenopausal Women. March 13, 2003; Available at: www.fda.gov/bbs/topics/NEWS/2003/NEW00878.html. Accessed October 14, 2006.

16. Crandall C. Low-dose estrogen therapy for menopausal women: a review of efficacy and safety. *J Womens Health (Larchmt).* 2003;12:723-747.

17. Premarin® (conjugated estrogen tablets). Wyeth Pharmaceuticals, Inc. 2004;Philadelphia, PA 19101:Full Prescribing Information.

18. Task Force Report on Hormone Therapy. Frequently asked questions about hormone therapy. American College of Obstetricians and Gynecologists, 2004: Available at: www.acog.org/from_home/publications/press_releases/nr10-01-04. cfm.Accessed July 5, 2005.

19. North American Menopause Society. Recommendations for estrogen and progestogen use in peri- and postmenopausal women: October 2004 position statement of The North American Menopause Society. *Menopause: The Journal of the North American Menopause Society.* 2004;11:589-600.

20. Naftolin F, Schneider HP, Sturdee DW, et al. Guidelines for hormone treatment of women in the menopausal transition and beyond. *Climacteric.* 2004;7:333-337.

21. U.S. Preventive Services Task Force. Recommendation statement: Hormone therapy for the prevention of chronic conditions in postmenopausal women. Agency for Healthcare Research and Quality: AHRQ Publication No. 05-0576. May 2005. Available at: www.ahrq.gov/clinic/uspstf05/ht/htpostmenrs.htm. Accessed October 14, 2006.

22. National Institutes of Health. Facts About Postmenopausal Hormone Therapy. Bethesda, MD. Available at: www.nhlbi.nih.gov/health/women/pht_facts.pdf. Accessed March 7, 2006.

23. European Agency for the Evaluation of Medicinal Products. Guideline on Clinical Investigation of Medicinal Products for the Treatment of Hormone Replacement Therapy. January 20, 2005.
Available at: www.iss.it/binary/farm/cont/guideline%20treatment%20 hormone%20replacement%20therapy.1109246299.pdf. Accessed June 21, 2008.

24. Wright J, Morgenthaler J. *Natural Hormone Replacement for Women Over 45.* Petaluma, CA: Smart Publications; 1997.

25. Head KA. Estriol: safety and efficacy. *Altern Med Rev.* 1998;3:101-113.

CHAPTER 3

HORMONES AND THE MENSTRUAL CYCLE

(As males, we ask you to please accept our apologies in advance for having the nerve to explain the menstrual cycle to a woman! If you find this chapter unnecessary or boring, please feel free to skip to the next chapter. However, a brief review about hormones may be a help in understanding the logic of BHRT, especially its timing. If you decide to skip this chapter for now, please go right on to Chapter 4. You can always return to review this material later if you feel a need to.)

The female menstrual cycle is an exquisitely calibrated and sensitive system. In fact, it is so complex that medical school professors often speak of it as a symphony, especially when compared to the male reproductive system, which they liken to an on-off faucet. The complexity of this system is one reason why it's so important to mimic the function of the menstrual hormones as precisely as possible. Of course, horse hormones have no place in this system, but BHRT fits in perfectly.

In order to better understand what happens during *perimenopause* (the 2- to 10-year transitional period before *menopause* (complete cessation of menstrual periods), and how hormone replacement works, let's review some basic information about the normal menstrual cycle.

The story of menstruation and menopause is really the story of the relationship and hormonal interactions between the two *ovaries*, the *uterus*, both located in the pelvic region (Fig. 3-1), and the *pituitary*, the master gland located at the base of the brain.

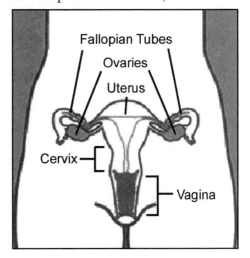

Figure 3-1. Schematic representation showing the major structures of the female reproductive tract.

Within each ovary are thousands of tiny sacs called *follicles*. At the time that a young girl has her first period, her ovaries may contain as many as 500,000 of these follicles, each of which is filled with eggs. Usually, early in each menstrual cycle, just one of these eggs begins to "ripen." (It remains one of Nature's mysteries that only a single egg "knows" when its time has arrived, while the rest "know" to wait their turn until next month.)

Around mid-cycle, a carefully orchestrated interplay of hormones causes the follicle containing the egg to burst open. The ripened egg then passes into the *fallopian tube*, which leads to the uterus. This process is called *ovulation*. If the egg meets sperm, usually somewhere in the fallopian tube, it may be fertilized. The resulting fertilized egg quickly begins to divide and differentiate into multiple cells while continuing its journey to the uterus.

In the meantime, more hormones have been preparing the uterus since the end of the last menstrual period to welcome and nurture the newly fertilized egg. The lining of the uterus (*endometrium*) has become thicker and enriched with blood and nutrients, so when the fertilized egg reaches its destination, it can easily implant itself into the uterine wall and begin to grow into an embryo, a fetus, and eventually an infant.

If the egg is not fertilized, it continues its journey to the uterus. In the absence of a special hormonal signal that fertilization has occurred, though, the uterus halts its preparations for pregnancy and discards the endometrial lining it has built up, as well as the extra blood and nutrients it has amassed.

This familiar event is known by a number of names: menstruation, menstrual bleeding, "the period," "the curse," "the guest/visitor," "that time of month," and many others. In addition to signaling a woman that she is healthy and not pregnant, regular menstruation is a sign that conception could still happen at a future date.

Once menstruation starts to lose its regularity (usually every 26-30 days), it probably means menopause is approaching and that a woman's remaining fertile days are decreasing. One of the first signs of the impending change is a shortening of some menstrual cycles and possibly a lengthening of others. When periods stop altogether – for 12 consecutive months – menopause has "officially" arrived and pregnancy is no longer possible.

The amazing regularity of the menstrual cycle is primarily due to a delicate balance of four primary hormones:

- Estrogen

- Progesterone

- Follicle stimulating hormone (FSH)

- Luteinizing hormone (LH)

Although we often refer to "estrogen" in the singular for the sake of convenience, remember that "estrogen" is really a group of very, very similar molecules with tiny molecular differences. *(Estradiol, estrone,* and *estriol,* are three principal estrogens found in the human body.)* FSH and LH, also known as *pituitary gonadotropins,* are secreted by the pituitary gland. Their purpose is to stimulate the "gonads" (ovaries in women and testicles in men) to secrete their own hormones.

Events of the Menstrual Cycle

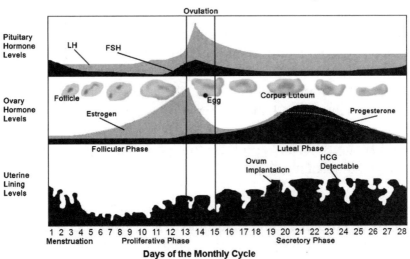

Figure 3-2. Schematic representation of the multiple events that occur simultaneously during each menstrual cycle.

Menstrual cycles blend into each other for approximately 40 years. Although there is no real beginning or end to each cycle, to make things simpler, we typically speak of the first day of menstruation as the end of one cycle and the beginning of the next. Figure 3-2 illustrates in schematic form the multiple events that occur simultaneously during each menstrual cycle.

Days 1-5: During the last few days of the previous cycle, prior to Day 1, the levels of estrogens and progesterone decline, signaling the uterus that pregnancy has not occurred during this cycle. This signal triggers a shedding of the endometrial lining of the uterus. Menstrual bleeding begins on Day 1 of the cycle and lasts approximately 5 days.

Since high levels of estrogen suppress the secretion of FSH, the decline in estrogen secretion now signals the level of FSH secretion from the pituitary to rise. As its name implies, *follicle stimulating hormone* stimulates follicle development. By Day 5 to 7 of the cycle, one of these follicles responds to FSH stimulation more than the others and becomes dominant. As it does so, it begins secreting large amounts of estrogen.

Days 6-14: The large amount of estrogen secreted by the follicle during this phase of the menstrual cycle has several important effects:

- It causes the endometrial lining of the uterus to become thicker and enriched in preparation for implantation of the fertilized egg.
- It suppresses further secretion of FSH by the pituitary gland.
- At about mid-cycle (Day 14), it helps stimulate a large and sudden release of LH from the pituitary. This *LH surge*, which is accompanied by a transient rise in body temperature, is a sign that ovulation is about to occur.
- The LH surge causes the follicle to rupture and expel the ripe egg into the fallopian tube.

Days 14-28: After the follicle ruptures, its walls collapse, and it becomes known as the *corpus luteum*. Immediately after ovulation, the corpus luteum begins secreting large amounts of *progesterone* as well as estrogen, which also helps prepare the endometrial lining for implantation of a fertilized egg. If the egg has been fertilized, a small amount of a hormone called *human chorionic gonadotropin (HCG)* is released. The presence of HCG, which can be detected in urine as early as 7 days after fertilization, is the basis for the early pregnancy tests that have become so popular.

HCG keeps the corpus luteum viable, so it can continue pumping out estrogen and progesterone, which, in turn, keep the endometrial lining intact. By about Week 6 to 8 of gestation, the newly formed placenta takes over the secretion of the very large majority of progesterone.

If the egg is not fertilized, the corpus luteum starts to run out of hormone, causing the levels of estrogen and progesterone to decline. Without these hormones to support it, the uterus soon sheds its lining, and menstruation begins again. In addition, with no estrogen to suppress it, FSH levels again start to rise. Thus, one cycle blends into another.

What Happens During Perimenopause and Menopause?

During the decades that the hormonal top is spinning smoothly, the key to its flawless rotation is balance, specifically the balance among the hormones estrogen, progesterone, FSH, and LH. As a woman enters perimenopause, the hormonal top starts to wobble slightly: estrogen and/or progesterone may begin to cycle at lower than usual levels, while FSH and/or LH levels may rise somewhat higher than before to try to compensate, but cycling still continues. After menopause, the typical hormonal pattern includes continually high levels of FSH combined with continually low levels of estradiol and progesterone.

The follicles remaining in the ovaries of a perimenopausal woman generally lose their sensitivity to FSH stimulation compared to those that preceded them. Increasingly, there are cycles during which no follicle develops fully, and eventually, cycles in which no follicle develops at all. For most of the perimenopause, normal and abnormal cycles tend to intermix. One month a follicle develops normally, and other months, with increasing frequency, it does not.

When a follicle fails to develop properly, it secretes less estrogen. This low level of estrogen cannot fully suppress the secretion of FSH by the pituitary gland. So, as estrogen levels fall, FSH levels rise. If estrogen levels are sufficiently low, they may fail to trigger the LH surge that's supposed to cause the follicle to rupture, and so the egg doesn't get released. This is termed an *anovulatory cycle* (a cycle without ovulation). If the follicle doesn't rupture, the corpus luteum cannot form, and consequently, progesterone is not released at the appropriate time. Irregularities like these can begin as early as a woman's mid- to late 30s, which helps explain why women in their late 30s and early 40s often have difficulty conceiving.

The lack of normal amounts of estrogen and progesterone gives rise to all the familiar discomforts of menopause, from hot flushes and insomnia to depression, mood swings, and palpitations.

The decline of normal estrogen and progesterone secretion by the ovary signals the uterus to shed its endometrial lining prematurely. This results in a general shortening of the length of the cycles. Often, the timing of the estrogen and progesterone secretion decline may vary from month to month, resulting in irregular cycles. Shorter cycles, irregular cycles, or both are often the first signs that the perimenopause has started.

Once ovarian estrogen secretion ceases after menopause, estrogen does not immediately disappear, but its molecular types shift. The primary estrogen circulating before menopause is *estradiol*; after menopause it is *estrone*, which comes from three sources: 1) cells in the adrenal glands (cortex); 2) fat cells, which convert the androgen androstenedione to the estrogen estrone; and 3) the ovaries, which continue producing small quantities of androgens, which are converted to estrogens, primarily estrone.

Levels of testosterone, most of which comes from the ovaries and the adrenals, start declining as far back as a woman's late 20s or 30s, due largely to the age-related decline in the testosterone precursor DHEA. Unlike estrogens and progesterone, testosterone secretion does not take a sudden dive at menopause. More likely, it just continues its steady decline that may have begun 20 to 30 years earlier.

Progesterone Deficiency and Estrogen Dominance Syndrome

As just noted, while menopause doesn't usually occur until around age 50, a woman's "hormonal top" might start going out of balance as early as her mid-30s. The first changes to occur tend to be occasional shortened luteal phases and sporadic anovulatory cycles. Since it is during the luteal phase and ovulation that the corpus luteum secretes the most progesterone, shortened cycles mean a decline in progesterone secretion, even though estrogens remain relatively normal.

This decline in progesterone secretion is far from trivial. As women age into their fourth, fifth, and sixth decade, progesterone levels continue to fall, so that by the time they reach perimenopause, as much as 75% of their youthful progesterone secretion may already be missing as they begin their passage through menopause.

Estrogens and progesterone balance out each other's effects, not just in the uterus, but also in the breast, brain, bones, cardiovascular system, and other locations throughout the body. Thus, when progesterone levels fall while estrogen levels remain normal, the imbalance – even though it may last for just a few days at a time – can cause noticeable and often unpleasant effects.

Because of the absence of progesterone's "growth opposing" effects, menstrual periods during which progesterone is absent or deficient may be characterized by abnormally thick endometrial (uterine) linings – resulting in a "heavy flow." (*In addition, progesterone has a wide range of effects that are largely independent of estrogen. See Chapter 2.*)

Dr. John R. Lee, in his pioneering book, *What Your Doctor May* Not *Tell You About Menopause,*[2] was the first to identify this syndrome as "estrogen dominance." He pointed out that it is not caused by *too much estrogen,* but rather by *too little progesterone* relative to essentially normal amounts of estrogen. (In retrospect, it might have been even more precise – and possibly easier to understand – if this relationship had been named "progesterone insufficiency.")

Little solid research has been done to study estrogen dominance (or "progesterone insufficiency," but according to Dr. Lee and numerous other physicians and clinical researchers, it may be responsible, at least in part, for such common occurrences as premenstrual syndrome (PMS), migraine and other headaches, uterine fibroids, difficulty in conceiving (infertility), fibrocystic breasts, breast tenderness, decreased libido, premenopausal loss of bone mineral density (BMD) leading to a high incidence of osteoporosis after menopause, memory loss, increased blood clotting (raising the risk of stroke), water retention/bloating, anxiety, depression, and many other disorders. Some research even suggests that a relative progesterone deficiency during this time may increase the risk of breast cancer.[3]

In most cases, estrogen dominance can be remedied fairly simply by using supplemental bio-identical progesterone during the portion of the menstrual cycle when progesterone levels would normally be elevated (Days 14-28).

Androgens: Male Hormones in Female Bodies

Androgens, including *testosterone, androstenedione,* and *dehydroepiandrosterone (DHEA),* also decline before, during, and after menopause in most women. A few women are still surprised to learn that their bodies contain "male" hormones, but it is true, albeit at concentrations 20 to 30 times lower than those seen in men. Similarly, men's bodies contain relatively small amounts of estrogens. As we'll see later, even at these relatively low concentrations, male hormones play extremely important roles in female bodies, just as female hormones do in male bodies.

The primary source of androgens in women is their ovaries. Testosterone secretion varies during the menstrual cycle, with peak levels occurring around the middle third of the cycle and remaining moderately elevated into the mid-luteal phase.[4] Unlike estradiol and progesterone, though, the ovaries usually continue secreting testosterone even after menopause.

Other important sources of androgens (as well as progesterone) are the two adrenal glands, which are located atop each of the kidneys. Some of the androgens produced after menopause may be converted into significant amounts of estradiol in sites such as the breast, adipose (fat) tissue, bone, and brain. The ability of these extragonadal tissues to produce estrogens from androgens, especially from DHEA, seems to increase with age. This fact underscores the value of taking supplemental DHEA to replace the inborn hormone, which like all the other sex steroids, declines with age.[5]

Keeping the Hormonal Top Spinning

As we shall see in the chapters that follow, it's possible to keep the hormonal top spinning with a minimum of wobbling even after the ovaries have started shutting down. By taking bio-identical hormones – estriol, estradiol, estrone, progesterone, testosterone, DHEA, and possibly others – at the appropriate times in the appropriate amounts, and by the appropriate routes, it's possible to mimic the natural ebb and flow of the body's own natural hormones, so that the body responds as though the ovaries were still functioning normally (minus ovulation and menstruation, of course), even though they're not.

In addition to estrogens, progesterone, and androgens, even more hormones are involved in the very complex normal menstrual cycle. These include not only FSH and LH, as mentioned above but also "releasing hormones" that trigger the secretion of FSH and LH, and likely others that science hasn't yet discovered or fully described. Not surprisingly, certain "hormones" are totally and conspicuously absent from the human menstrual cycle: *conjugated equine estrogens* (Premarin®), *medroxyprogesterone* (Provera®), and other patented, alien-to-the-human body molecules, which are never a part of any woman's normal menstrual cycling!

References

1.   Hatcher R, Guest F, Stewart F, et al. *Contraceptive Technology 1988-1989*. New York: Irvington Publishers; 1988.

2.   Lee JR. *What Your Doctor May Not Tell You About Menopause*. New York: Warner Books; 1996.

3.   Cowan LD, Gordis L, Tonascia JA, Jones GS. Breast cancer incidence in women with a history of progesterone deficiency. *Am J Epidemiol.* 1981;114:209-217.

4.   Somboonporn W. Testosterone therapy for postmenopausal women: efficacy and safety. *Semin Reprod Med.* 2006;24:115-124.

5.   Schumacher M, Guennoun R, Ghoumari A, et al. Novel perspectives for progesterone in HRT, with special reference to the nervous system. *Endocr Rev.* 2007;28:387-439.

CHAPTER 4

OF HORMONES & DRUGS AND URINE & YAMS

For centuries, humankind has viewed hormones as a kind of "fountain of youth." Long before anyone had the slightest idea what a hormone was, people recognized that some "essence" present in the bodies of young adult men and women defined their health, youth, vitality, and sexuality.

Of course, men being men, early physicians and other *men* who were trying to understand these "essences" and how they might be used to enhance their health, vitality, and longevity, spent most of their efforts searching for the male "essence," which early on was assumed to reside in the testicles. Even primitive "medicine men" could easily see that when the testicles were absent, due to a birth defect, injury, or disease, a man no longer seemed to be a *"man."* The lack of typical masculine qualities, like large muscles, body and facial hair, a deep voice, and working genitalia, was obvious.

The mysterious masculine essence was prized by, among others, certain ancient Chinese emperors, and by the 19th century, it had become the "Holy Grail" of the emerging science of Western medicine. When the "male hormone," a steroid named *testosterone,* was finally isolated in the early 20th century, its two discoverers were awarded a Nobel Prize.[*]

The search for a comparable female "essence" seemed to have had less urgency in the early days (at least from a male perspective). Nevertheless, once estrogens and progesterone (as well as testosterone) were all identified in the 1930s, patent medicine companies quickly saw the marketing possibilities inherent in restoring both men's women's youth, beauty, and sexuality, not to mention the possibilities of contraceptive drugs. But as patent medicine companies always have done and always will do (after all, that's the reason for their existence), instead of trying to use these hormones as Mother Nature had made them, they quickly got to work trying to "improve" on the natural versions to produce something they could patent and thus, earn significantly more money from.

---

[*] But when the first estrogen was isolated, no Nobel Prize was awarded. Some suspect that the gender composition (mostly male) of the relevant Nobel Prize committees may have been part of the reason .

Harvesting Hormones

For decades, the most commonly used "replacement" estrogens in conventional medicine have come from horse urine. If you think that harvesting estrogens from horse urine sounds like a bizarre way to make "replacement" hormones for women, you'd be half right: *horse* urine – yes, certainly bizarre; but urine in general (especially *human* urine) – not so bizarre at all. In fact, the body excretes sex steroid hormones through the urine, so collecting urine has been a long-honored method of harvesting steroid hormones, not to mention for monitoring women's hormone levels (*See Chapter 9*).

From at least the 11th century onward, and possibly starting as early as 1,000 years prior to that date, Taoist physicians in China used preparations of dried human urine solids to promote longevity and restore sexual vigor and potency in people of both sexes. Urine collected from adolescent boys and girls was especially prized because of its extraordinarily high content of what later turned out to be sex hormones[*]. (Apparently teens have been "teens" about as far back as we can go.) The royalty in particular were big users of urine-derived hormones.[1] We don't know for certain if these preparations did anybody any good, but, from what we now know about hormone metabolism, it's very likely that some might have had some beneficial effects.

By the 18th and 19th centuries, scientists in search of a more convenient source of male and female "essences" took to grinding up testicles, ovaries, and other organs from animals – dogs, pigs, guinea pigs, roosters, cows, and bulls – and then processing them. At first, they brewed them into a kind of soup, and in later years, they learned how to chemically extract the active ingredient(s). A few brave people took the resulting products either by mouth or by injection under the skin. Although the thinking behind these crude preparations might have been on the right track, any reported benefits were most likely a result of wishful thinking (better known today as the "placebo effect").[2]

---

[*] Modern analytic techniques prove that urine from men and women in their late teens and early 20s contains not only high levels of sex steroids, but also substantial quantities of adrenal hormones including cortisol, DHEA, and aldosterone, as well as thyroid hormones, human growth hormone (HGH), and every other hormone made by human bodies. Properly collected, concentrated, and purified, urinary hormones from young men and women could be the most potent and comprehensive hormone replacement ever!

By the turn of the 20th century, the patent medicine company Merck, Sharpe & Dohme (known today as Merck) was marketing a product called "*Ovariin*" – made from the desiccated ovaries of cows – for the treatment of symptoms of "climacterica," as menopause was then known. Although Ovariin might have contained traces of bovine estrogen, there are no reliable reports to indicate whether it actually had any estrogenic effects – positive or negative – in the women who took it.[3]*

American researchers during the late 1920s experimented with a derivative of amniotic fluid from pregnant cows, which they tried giving to women with menopausal symptoms.[4] A few years later, Ayerst Labs (an ancestor of today's Wyeth Pharmaceuticals, the maker of Premarin®) introduced "*Emmenin,*" a menopause remedy developed at McGill University in Montreal. Billed as the "first orally effective estrogen," *Emmenin* was a throwback to ancient China, because it was derived from urine – actually *late-pregnancy urine* – collected from pregnant Canadian women. Since the estrogens a woman's body secretes during late pregnancy includes very large amounts of estriol, Emmenin had relatively high concentrations of this form of estrogen. At about the same time, scientists at the German patent medicine company Schering were developing a nearly identical product from "human pregnancy urine" (HPU), which they called "*Progynon.*"[3, 5]

Emmenin and Progynon were certainly steps in the right direction, but they were doomed from the start, and it's not hard to see why. First, imagine the logistical problems inherent in collecting the vast amounts of urine needed from pregnant women in order to extract even small quantity of estrogens. Second, the women who were asked to take these products were understandably reluctant to swallow medications that apparently retained the smell and taste of urine.[3, 4]

Although these products turned out to be marketing dead ends, researchers sensed they were onto something with urine-based estrogens. Regrettably, both the Canadian and German groups soon turned their backs on human

---

* Although ancient physicians recognized that the ovaries and testes served as the respective sources of the female and male "essences," the long-held assumption that these organs also stored these "essences" turned out to be completely wrong. It wasn't until the early 20th century that scientists figured out that most of the hormone produced in the ovaries and testes (as in other endocrine glands) was immediately secreted directly into the blood stream, and very little was actually stored there.

urine to a more abundant source of the hormone – horse urine.* The Canadian group's first choice as an estrogen source was the Percheron *stallion*. Yes, that's right, stallions are male, yet their urine was found to contain the most potent estrogens produced by any animal, male or female. However, stallion-based estrogen was also a nonstarter as a pharmaceutical product due to a nasty little problem with urine collection: evidently the frisky stallions kept kicking over the collection buckets![3]

The scientists soon found that mares, particularly pregnant mares kept in extremely small, restrictive stalls, were much more docile, thus providing a cost-effective means for collecting the huge volumes of urine they needed for large scale production of conjugated equine estrogens (CEEs). Thus was born *pre*gnant *mar*e's ur*ine,* better known today as Premarin®.

The Female Holy Grail

The other major female sex hormone, ***progesterone***, was first isolated around 1930 from the *corpus luteum*, the ruptured follicle from which the ovum (egg) has recently "hatched" *(See Chapter 3)*. Even before they knew it as progesterone, hormone researchers noticed that the luteal extract could be useful for treating certain menstrual disorders as well as for preventing miscarriages.

Toward the end of the decade, scientists found that bio-identical progesterone extracted from corpora lutea could not only help maintain pregnancies, but it could also *prevent* them. This latter role was much more exciting to them, because, if drug companies had a "Female Holy Grail" in those days, it was a pill a woman could take to keep from getting pregnant. By the end of the 1930s, it seemed like progesterone might be their prize oral contraceptive.

However, it quickly became apparent that bio-identical progesterone was not going to make the grade as a birth control pill. First, there was no ready source of progesterone as there was for "estrogen" (horse urine). Even the best sources of progesterone were labor-intensive and extremely uneconomical. For example, one way was to isolate and extract the

---

* Perhaps early hormone researchers may be forgiven for equating equine and human estrogen, because it was not well understood at the time that horse estrogen was both qualitatively and quantitatively different from human estrogen. As far as they were concerned, estrogen was estrogen. The only really important factor at that time seemed to be potency. Today's researchers and doctors should certainly know better.

hormone from the corpora lutea of animals. Sows were a particularly good source, but you still needed 50,000 of the poor pigs' ruptured follicles to yield only about 20 mg of progesterone. That's a lot of pork chops to make barely enough hormone for a couple of human doses.[5] A better option was to manufacture bio-identical progesterone the way the body does it, by starting with cholesterol. As discussed below, cholesterol is the "Mother of All Steroids" (Fig. 4-2). Nevertheless, this was also extremely difficult and costly. Progesterone derived in the lab from cholesterol sold in its day for about $80 per gram, which at the time was nearly 8 times the price of gold![6]

Perhaps the most serious drawback to bio-identical progesterone as a contraceptive agent involved dosing. Because of the way the human metabolism works, if we take progesterone by mouth, most of the hormone gets chewed up (metabolically speaking) in the liver, and very little pure progesterone ever makes it into the general circulation. (*See Chapter 9 for more about the role of the liver in steroid hormone metabolism*) Thus, oral administration would have required very high doses. You could get more hormone into the circulation by injecting the hormone just under the skin, bypassing the digestive system and liver, but this route of administration precluded its use as a convenient, inexpensive birth-control pill.

So, with visions of oral contraceptives still dancing in their heads, patent medicine companies discarded bio-identical progesterone and focused their attention on patented, man-made progesterone-like drugs (which they called "*progestins*") that were designed to remain active and potent after being swallowed.

It was left to a creative, independent-minded chemist from Penn State University, Russell Marker, to discover an easy and inexpensive way to turn out large quantities of bio-identical progesterone.* His method, known as "Marker Degradation," involved the extraction of a steroid precursor chemical (*diosgenin*) from a vegetable called the Mexican yam (*Dioscorea composita*), which grew wild in the state of Veracruz. Once extracted, he found that just a little relatively simple biochemical "alchemy" could turn disogenin into bio-identical progesterone (or, it turned out, into

---

*   In an earlier incarnation, the remarkable Dr. Marker had developed the octane rating system used for gasoline to this day.

virtually any other steroid hormone, bio-identical or not).

In the early 1940s, when Marker was trying to sell his discovery to the patent medicine industry, he could find no takers. The companies were locked onto the idea of *patentable oral* contraceptives, and they had no interest in an unpatentable bio-identical hormone, even if it was cheap to produce. The possibilities of using progesterone as part of menopausal HRT probably never even

Avoid the "Yam Scam"!

The disogenin extracted from Mexican yams is a remarkable substance, because it can be manipulated to produce not only progesterone, but just about any steroid hormone you want, including testosterone, DHEA, all "human estrogens," and glucocorticoids (eg, cortisone), not to mention CEEs and other non-bio-identical steroids (ie, progestins) as well.

However, you can't get a significant amount of these hormones from eating Mexican yams themselves or from using creams based on unprocessed disogenin, because the human body does not possess the chemical cofactors required to convert diosgenin to useful steroid hormones. These can only he found in a properly equipped laboratory.

Unfortunately, this has not stopped some unscrupulous entrepreneurs from marketing yam products as a source of various steroid hormones. Please don't be fooled! If you purchase a cream or other product purporting to contain progesterone, DHEA, or some other steroid hormone, make sure it actually contains that hormone and not just unprocessed disogenin, Dioscorea, or Mexican yam.

crossed their minds, because in those days, they had convinced themselves that "estrogen" (ie, horse estrogens) was all that was needed.

After being turned away by both Merck and Parke-Davis, Marker decided to go it alone. He started his own company – called *Syntex* – based in Mexico and in 1944 began manufacturing vegetable-based bio-identical progesterone. Almost overnight, progesterone went from being one of the rarest "medications" on earth to one of the most readily available and least expensive. Once more precious than gold, progesterone now sold for only about $1 per gram.

But alas, at that price, unpatented progesterone was just not profitable, and Syntex soon abandoned it, and went on to adapt Marker degradation to produce more profitable patentable estrogen and progesterone chemical analogs. In 1960, Syntex became the first company to discover the "Female

Holy Grail," when they introduced the world's first oral contraceptive pill, which consisted of two patented pseudohormones: *ethinyl estradiol* and *norethindrone*, both derived from the same vegetable source.

In the 60+ years since Marker produced the first vegetable-based bio-identical progesterone, the hormone was almost completely forgotten by conventional medicine, which could see little use for it as long as there were lots of patented "progestins" being marketed by the various patent medicine companies.

In the mid-1970s, doctors finally woke up to the fact that the unopposed "estrogen replacement therapy" (ERT) they had been prescribing was giving their patients uterine cancer. But instead of doing the sensible thing and giving them bio-identical progesterone (which had been available for 30 years) to "oppose" CEE-induced overgrowth in the uterine lining, they developed a patented progesterone analog Provera® (medroxyprogesterone, MPA), which has turned out to be an extremely toxic – but still legally prescribable and FDA "approved" – drug.

When Is a Hormone *Not* a Hormone?

Hormones are powerful chemical couriers that make possible an efficient system of precise communication and remote control of vital organ systems throughout the body. Hormone molecules carry "messages" to specific "target cells," often at great distance from the hormone's source. When they encounter target cells presenting special "receptors," the hormone molecules bind, or attach to the receptor, like a key entering a lock. "Turning the key" triggers the target cells to alter their metabolism or behave in some other predetermined way. If a target cell happens to be a muscle cell, it might contract (or relax); a gland cell might secrete (or cease secreting) its hormone; endothelial cells* might accelerate (or decelerate) their replication. As described in Chapter 2, by binding to and then stimulating specific receptors on target cells, estrogens and progesterone can control numerous vital functions all over the body (Fig. 4-1).

---

* Endothelial cells are smooth, delicate cells that line surfaces such as the insides of blood vessels, intestines, urinary tract, and ducts in the breast, as well as the mouth and nasal and respiratory passageways.

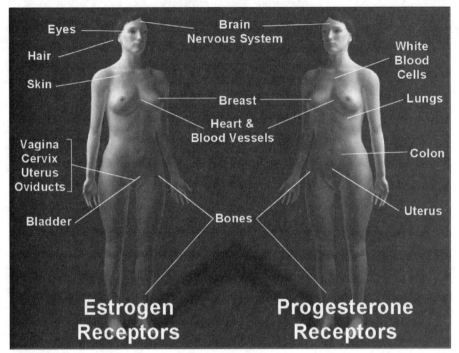

Figure 4-1.

The classic definition of a "hormone," according to *Dorland's Illustrated Medical Dictionary,* is "*a chemical substance **produced in the body** by an organ or cells of a certain organ, which has a specific regulatory effect on the activity of a certain organ.*" (Emphasis added.) For example, as described in Chapter 3, follicle-stimulating hormone (FSH), secreted into the blood stream by the pituitary gland at the base of the brain, travels in the blood until some of it reaches the ovaries, where it triggers the release of estradiol. When estradiol makes the return trip back to the pituitary, it triggers that gland to *suppress* FSH secretion. (This kind of "negative feedback loop" is a common way the body keeps many different hormone systems in balance.)

Dorland's goes on to point out that the definition of "hormone" has been broadened (by some, particularly patent medicine companies) to include the *actions* of hormones as well as their origins. According to this revisionist definition, any molecule – no matter where it comes from, no matter how it was created, or no matter what it looks like chemically – could be said to fall under the hormone umbrella. All it has to do is *act like a hormone* somewhere in the body.

Broadening the definition of "hormone" a little may not seem like a terribly significant event in the history of medicine, but by opening the door to all kinds of substances for use as "hormone replacements" (hormone *"substitutes"* is a more accurate description), it altered the way medicine is practiced today by most doctors. Some of these hormone substitutes (eg, CEEs) are indeed bio-identical hormones, but designed for another species, and consequently, alien to the human body. Others are not hormones at all in the original sense of the word, but rather, patented hormone analogs that were also strangers in a strange land, physiologically speaking.

Why does it matter what a hormone molecule looks like as long as it does what it's supposed to do? It's largely a question of metabolism. The body metabolizes (ie, chemically changes, neutralizes, and/or disposes of) alien hormones or patented pseudohormones differently than it does natural/ endogenous or bio-identical hormones. The metabolism of bio-identical hormones is built into the human body's normal functioning. For every natural hormone, there are enzymes and other chemicals whose sole purpose is help metabolize that hormone safely and efficiently, without producing any toxic by-products. On the other hand, the body lacks the biological "infrastructure" to safely and efficiently metabolize alien and patented pseudohormone, *nonhuman* molecules. Put another way: From hundreds of thousands of years' experience, our bodies "know" exactly what to do with bio-identical hormones, but when presented with patented imitation hormones that are alien to the body, they are relatively "clueless."

Figure 4-2 lays out – in vastly oversimplified fashion – the metabolism of sex steroid hormones, including estrogens, progesterone, testosterone, DHEA, and others as they occur naturally in the human body (male or female). (You don't have to be a biochemist to understand this chart. Just think of it as a kind of genealogic chart that shows which substances "begat" which other substances.) Each listing represents a different hormone in the human steroid family tree. The arrows show the direction of the "begatting." For example, starting at the top, you can see that *cholesterol* (Yes, *that* cholesterol!)* begats *pregnenolone*,

---

* All steroid hormones trace their "ancestry" back to cholesterol. While cholesterol gets a pretty bad (and probably unjustified) rap in the medical press as a "cause" of heart disease, it's a safe bet that doctors who hand out cholesterol-lowering drugs like candy to just about everybody over age 45, never once think about the effects these drugs might be having on their patients' hormone balance. But that's a subject for a whole other book!

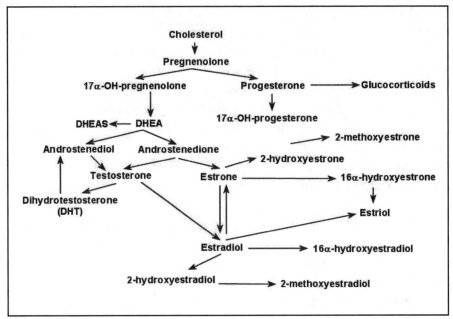

Figure 4-2. Simplified map of the metabolic pathways of human reproductive steroid hormones.

which in turn "begats" two offspring: *progesterone* and *17-hydroxy (OH) pregnenolone*. The right-hand branch essentially ends with *progesterone* and its main metabolite, *17-OH progesterone*. (Actually, the progesterone branch continues on to a whole other family of non-sex steroids, the *glucocorticoids* (which include cortisol and cortisone), but they are beyond the scope of this book.)

The left-hand branch – via the important hormone *DHEA* and two intermediate hormones, *androstenediol* and *androstenedione* – leads to *testosterone*, the primary *androgen,* which in turn leads to three primary human female hormones, the *estrogens: estradiol, estrone,* and ultimately *estriol.* Note that estradiol has two "parents": Some estradiol starts out as *testosterone*, while the rest comes by way of *androstenedione* and *estrone*. As a means of keeping things in balance, *estrone-estradiol* metabolism is a two-way street, with each hormone converting back-and-forth to the other as conditions demand.

One "end of the line" for estrogen metabolism is *estriol*. Both *estradiol* and *estrone* may eventually get metabolized to *estriol: estradiol* directly and *estrone* via the intermediary hormone *16α-hydroxyestrone,* with most *estriol* coming about via the latter route. It is noteworthy that estriol is never converted back to either estradiol or estrone.

So, what would happen if we were to drop some horse estrogens or patented pseudohormones like MPA into this tightly coordinated web of *human* metabolic activity? Lots of things that are not supposed to happen in the human body, including some extremely potent, toxic, and carcinogenic by-products would to be produced.

Figure 4-3 shows the molecular structures of a few of the *steroid* hormones commonly used as replacement "hormones." (Again, please don't panic if you didn't major in biochemistry. Just think of these diagrams as stick-figure pictures of the hormones, which is all they really are.) Three major human estrogens, *estriol, estradiol,* and *estrone,* are shown across the top left of the figure. Just below them are *equilin*, the primary equine estrogen in Premarin®, and *ethinyl estradiol*, an extremely potent, orally active man-made estrogen widely used in contraceptive pills. As shown in the right-hand panel, the molecular structure of Provera® (as well as other progestins, not pictured) is a variation on the theme of endogenous estrogen and progesterone.

In most cases, the differences from one hormone to the other (or from hormone to hormone-like drug) may seem to the untrained eye to be trivial. All possess the basic steroid "skeleton," yet, human physiology can make a very big deal over the slightest variation, like the location of a carbon (C) or oxygen (O) atom, an "OH (hydroxy)-group," or a carbon bond. In fact, apparently minor structural disparities like these can translate into enormous differences in the molecule's hormonal activity, potency, toxicity, and the way the body metabolizes it.

Finally, we come to the molecule called *diethylstilbestrol (DES)*. It's plain to see that DES, which is a man-made molecule, lacks the characteristic steroid skeleton that all the other steroid hormones, including the man-made and equine estrogens and progestins, share. So why is it here?

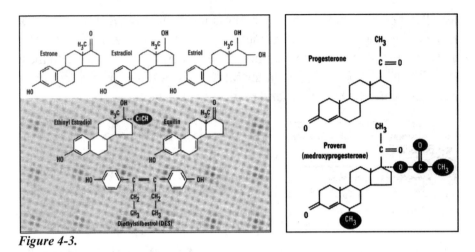

Figure 4-3.

Even though the DES molecule's unusual structure exempts it from the steroid class, it still acts like an estrogen in some ways (eg, it suppresses hot flushes). So, here we have a highly potent, *nonsteroidal* "estrogen" that is readily available (no urine collection needed) and can be easily and inexpensively produced by any laboratory. Back in the early 1940s, when DES was first developed, and the only thing that mattered was function – "if it works like an estrogen, it *is* an estrogen" – it seemed to some like a miracle.

Yet, in all the excitement of the moment, DES's cheerleaders conveniently overlooked unambiguous data showing that it caused cancer in laboratory animals. Doctors following accepted protocols, with the "approval" of just about every relevant medical "authority" including the FDA (*starting to sound like a familiar refrain?*) prescribed DES to millions of women, mostly to prevent miscarriages and other pregnancy complications. (Aside from DES's inherent toxicity, it apparently never occurred to these medical/hormonal "experts" that giving high doses of potent pseudoestrogens to pregnant women could create an extremely unnatural – and potentially hostile – hormonal environment, not only for the mother, but also for the fetus.

After 10 years of giving DES to unsuspecting women, someone finally got around to doing a study to see what the drug was actually doing to their bodies. (Regulation of patent medicines was a lot looser in those days.) What they found wasn't pretty. Despite all its hype, DES turned out to have absolutely *no clinical benefits* for pregnant women.[7] And that wasn't even the really bad news. It took another 20 years – an entire generation of women – before DES's actual toll of toxicity became evident.

By the early 1970s, it became undeniable that millions of women, who had taken DES during their pregnancies, from the 1940s through the '60s, were at increased risk for breast cancer. Even more frightening, though, DES taken by mothers-to-be was found to cause cancer of the breast, vagina, and cervix *in their daughters* and testicular cancer *in their sons* who had been exposed *in utero*. Furthermore, if "DES daughters" tried to become pregnant, they faced hazards like infertility, ectopic (tubal) pregnancy, miscarriage, and premature delivery.

It might be of interest to note that, while DES's molecular structure bears no relation to other members of the steroid family, it does closely resemble another well-known patented compound called *dichlorodiphenyltrichloroethane*. Better known as *DDT*, this pesticide has well-known estrogen-mimicking properties that help make it toxic not only to "pests," but to humans and some animals as well.

One lesson here is that molecular structure is "destiny." Even the tiniest change in molecular structure that varies from what's normally found in our bodies can lead to distinct changes –from relatively small to very large ones – in activity, potency, toxicity, and metabolism. Big differences, like the difference between DES and the steroids, can be devastating.

Hormonal Shell Games

Blurring the lines between hormones and pseudohormonal drugs and between bio-identical hormones and non-bio-identical "hormones" has led to a mind set among doctors (and just about everyone else) that says, "If it *acts* like estrogen (or progesterone), then it must *be* estrogen (or progesterone)." For over 100 years, patent medicine companies have worked very hard to sell us this expanded definition of "hormone," because it gives them a foot in the door to sell enormously profitable patented drugs under a "hormone" label.

How has the patent drug industry pulled off this shell game? Primarily by convincing doctors, via repeated reports of company-sponsored studies, "educational"/promotional programs, advertising copy, PR campaigns, and person-to-person sales calls, that 1) Premarin® = estrogen; 2) Provera® (or other progestins) = progesterone; and 3) it makes perfectly good medical sense to give women daily doses of horse estrogens and progestins. Of course, FDA "approval" to use Premarin and Provera as if they were human hormones was a critical part of the shell game, too.

Thanks to these efforts, the medical literature and consumer media alike are replete with articles and programs that make no distinction between "estrogen" and Premarin® or between progesterone and Provera®. It's ridiculously easy to find countless examples of this. One article, entitled "*Progesterone* Abolishes *Estrogen* and/or Atorvastatin Endothelium Dependent Vasodilatory Effects," describes a clinical study evaluating the effects, not of the hormone *progesterone*, as the title advertises, but *norethisterone acetate*, a *progestin* drug. In the article, norethisterone is described as a "progesterone compound" and a "progesterone derivative," with the implication that there is no need to distinguish it from the real thing.[8] Another article, entitled "The Effect of Low-Dose Continuous *Estrogen* and *Progesterone* Therapy with Calcium and Vitamin D on Bone in Elderly Women," actually describes a study testing the effects of Premarin® and Provera®.[9] A third study entitled, "The Effect of Long-term Use of *Progesterone* Therapy on Proliferation and Apoptosis in Simple Endometrial Hyperplasia without Atypia," claims to describe the effects of "3 months of cyclic *progesterone* treatment," even though bio-identical progesterone was never used. Rather, the researchers used the progestin *noretisterone*.[10] These are but three examples. A casual scan of the medical literature would easily reveal hundreds more.

Provera's® acceptance as a "hormone" equivalent to progesterone has been aided by including it as a member of a *totally fictitious* family of "hormones" known as *progestins* or *progestogens*.* In all of Nature, across all species of animals, one finds classes of sex hormones called "estrogens" and "androgens," but no such hormones as "progestins" or "progestogens." They are total fictions propagated by patent medicine companies, aided and abetted by FDA, to justify the use of drugs like

---

* Although there are no hard, fast rules, "progestins" are usually defined as patented versions of progesterone, while "progestogens" (or "progestagens") may include both progestins and bio-identical progesterone.

Provera® and its chemical cousins. In Nature there is progesterone, and that's all; progesterone has no relatives the way estrogens and androgens do.

Progestins are defined as compounds that share some of molecular attributes of progesterone, but most importantly, that produce at least some of the actions with which progesterone is normally associated – primarily "opposing" Premarin®-induced tissue overgrowth in the uterine lining. Prior to the advent of Provera® and other progestins/ progestogens (eg, norgestrel, norethindrone, norgestimate, levonorgestrel, et al), such a classification was superfluous, because the only molecule that looked like progesterone and also acted like progesterone was, of course, progesterone itself.

This FDA "approved" marketing strategy has been a brilliant success. After generations of indoctrination beginning in medical school, there is hardly a conventional doctor anywhere who has not learned to equate Premarin® with estrogen and Provera® (and other progestins) with progesterone. From the highest echelons of medical research right on down to the "doc down the block," most practitioners of conventional medicine make no distinction between Premarin® and estrogen or between Provera® (or other "progestins") and progesterone. Consider this bit of wisdom courtesy of the prestigious American College of Obstetricians and Gynecologists (ACOG): "Risks [of low-dose Premarin® treatment in perimenopausal women] appear to be relatively low, possibly because your body is still producing its own estrogen and ***progestin***."[11] (Actual word used; emphasis added.) So, to hear ACOG tell it, a woman's ovaries produce *progestin,* not progesterone! Go tell that to Mother Nature!

Here's another example of how woefully clueless "medical experts" can be when trying to distinguish between bio-identical hormones and patented hormone-like drugs. In the aftermath of a large, important National Institutes of Health (NIH)-sponsored clinical study (nicknamed PEPI) on the roles of "estrogen and progestins" (actually Premarin® plus either Provera® or bio-identical "micronized progesterone"*) in women

---

* When bio-identical progesterone is taken orally, the body metabolizes it more efficiently if it is first crushed into extremely small pieces, a process known as *micronizing.* On those rare occasions that conventional medical research has ventured into the world of bio-identical hormones, it has usually opted for the oral route of administration, which is best accomplished by using a micronized formulation. As discussed in Chapter 9, there are good reasons why this is a bad practice.

with heart disease,[12] Dr. Bernadine Healy, then *head of the taxpayer-supported National Institutes of Health ("NIH")*, was frankly amazed at bio-identical progesterone's "surprising" superiority over Provera®. *"We have to find out more about micronized progesterone,"* she remarked during an online roundtable discussion with some of the study's authors that was published on the website of the American Medical Association (AMA). "Why is it so different from Provera? *Physiologically, you wouldn't expect that it should be,"* she said. Duh!

Let's think about what Dr. Healy said here for a moment. She seemed to be viewing bio-identical progesterone as some sort of mysterious substance that science apparently knows little about. Someone should have reminded her that researchers first identified progesterone in the 1930s; that it's been available as a bio-identical hormone since the mid-1940s; and that her very own ovaries had been churning the stuff out for decades. She *"wouldn't expect"* a patented, man-made drug to act any differently from its bio-identical hormone counterpart? *Please!!* At the time she said these things, Dr. Healy was the head of one of the nation's premiere medical research institutions, and yes, she really said those things. Sadly, she shares the pharmaceutically driven mindset of most practitioners of conventional medicine today!

This attitude has given rise to two rather unfortunate misperceptions about Premarin® and estrogen as well as about Provera® and progesterone: 1) Premarin®/Provera® can do anything bio-identical human estrogen/progesterone can do; and 2) any side effects and risks associated with Premarin®/Provera® must also be serious concerns with their bio-identical counterparts. As evidenced by "official" reactions to the WHI, critics attempting to discourage bio-identical hormone use often raise the specter of the proven risks of Premarin® and Provera®, despite the fact that these risks have *never, ever* been documented for properly used bio-identical hormones.

There are signs that some important researchers are beginning to see through the shell game Big Pharma has been playing with them all these years. In a recent comprehensive review of progesterone research, a group of French investigators included the following cautions about terminology:

*"Before discussing the activities of progestagens in the nervous system, it is important to clarify the terminology and to call attention to the fact that not all progestagens behave the same. They do indeed exhibit profound differences according to their structure, and it is certainly not correct to consider them as equivalent compounds, as unfortunately continues to be done. Thus, after the WHI trials, concern has been directed toward progestagens as a single class. Worse, the term progesterone has even been used as a generic one for the different types of natural and synthetic progestagens in recent papers. **'Progesterone' should in fact only be used to designate the natural hormone,** produced in the corpus luteum of the ovary after ovulation, in the placenta during pregnancy, in the adrenal glands and, as shall be discussed later, also in the central and peripheral nervous systems."*[13]

All we can say is, it's about time. But of course this was written in France, where doctors have long been suspicious of conventional HRT and more aware of the benefits of bio-identical hormones. Their thinking seems still not to have penetrated that of "medical authorities" here in the United States.

Cutting Through the Verbal Fog

Even if a "hormone" is "bio-identical" (eg, CEEs for horses), it might still be unnatural for humans; and just because a hormone is "synthetic" doesn't mean it can't be "bio-identical" for humans. Confused? You're in good company. Having played along for decades with the patent medicine industry's language games, most of the medical community, including those who lean toward the "alternative" side, doesn't really understand the differences either.

In 2009, whether a hormone is said to be "natural," "synthetic," "bio-identical," or something else may depend as much on marketing as on science. While everyone will agree that the hormones we're born with are truly "natural," the picture gets cloudier once we start replacing (or substituting) these hormones with versions that originate in a vegetable, a test tube, or a horse's ovaries. However, if we apply informed reason to the subject, the following categories might help cut through the verbal fog:

- **Natural hormones.** There are three major classes of "natural" hormones. The human body produces the familiar natural sex steroids, including *estriol, estradiol, estrone, progesterone, DHEA, pregnenolone,* and *testosterone,* as well as nonsteroids like *luteinizing hormone (LH), follicle-stimulating hormone (FSH), insulin, thyroid hormone,* and many others. This mix of "natural" hormones has been present for millions of years to serve the unique needs of the human physiology. With room for individual variation, all human females produce and secrete roughly the same amounts and proportions of sex steroids, LH, and FSH, and others on about the same schedule, for much of their adult lives.

  A second class of natural hormones includes *equilin* and the other CEEs found in Premarin®. For years, Premarin's® promoters hyped the fact that CEEs were *natural* hormones, which, of course, they are. The catch is that they're natural for horses, not for women. They'd like us to think this is a trivial distinction, but these days, even they know better.

  A third class of natural hormones includes estrogens produced by plants. The best-known natural plant estrogens, or *phytoestrogens,* come from foods like beans, cabbage, soybeans, seeds, berries, fruits, vegetables, grains, and many others. Among the principal phytoestrogens are compounds known as *isoflavones,* especially *genistein* and *daidzein,* which are plentiful in soy-based products (eg, tofu), and *lignins,* which are derived from flax and other sources. Although phytoestrogens can produce estrogenic actions in the human body, these are generally much weaker than those produced by bio-identical (or equine) estrogens (500 to 1000 times less active than estradiol). Phytoestrogens are indeed "natural" estrogens, but like horse estrogens, they are not "bio-identical" for humans. Unlike horse estrogens, though, their low potency makes them much safer as substitutes for human bio-identical hormones.

- **Bio-identical hormones.** "Bio-identical" hormones, sometimes called "isomolecular" hormones, are simply molecules that are structurally identical to the "natural" hormones they are intended to replace. There's no way to tell "bio-identical" and corresponding "natural" hormones apart because *they are exactly the same in terms of molecular structure.* In the body, they are metabolized in precisely the same way that the body's "natural" molecules are metabolized. Paradoxical as it may sound, all bio-identical hormones in use today are derived (ie, synthesized) from a vegetable source, the Mexican yam (*Dioscorea composita*) or soy.[14] Thus, given this terminology, there is nothing wrong in asserting that bio-identical hormones are of *synthetic origin.*

- **Patentable "hormones."** According to the US Patent Office, a molecule can be patented only if it is *not found in nature* (with some important exceptions, which patent medicine companies are increasingly learning to exploit). Thus, molecules that are found in nature, like air, water, vitamins, minerals, and bio-identical hormones, are typically *not patentable.* A common patent medicine company strategy is to take a "natural," unpatentable hormone molecule, such as progesterone or estradiol, and chemically "tweak" it so that it becomes *medroxy*progesterone or *ethinyl* estradiol (or some other similar unnatural molecule), which is patentable (*See Figure 4-3*). If the molecule acts somewhat like progesterone (or estrogen) and doesn't cause too many adverse side effects, compared to an inactive placebo, they give it a brand name (eg, Provera®), run "clinical trials" (which usually are too brief to disclose many serious adverse effects), pay enormous "approval" fees, and then market it, often making no distinction between the patented, alien-to-the-human body molecule and the natural or bio-identical hormone it is supposed to be replacing.

  A company that patents a hormone-like molecule has the exclusive right to sell it for a limited term – usually about 17 years from the time the patent is granted. This means the company can charge for their product as much as the market will bear. A popular product with no direct competition could earn them many billions of dollars. Once the patent expires, though, other companies are free to manufacture and market *generic* versions of the "hormone," which tends to force its price down considerably.

It's certainly understandable, from a *financial* viewpoint, why a patent medicine company would opt for patentable rather than unpatentable products. However, a patent in no way ensures that a product is better or safer than its unpatentable bio-identical counterpart. Quite the contrary, it's a good bet that, since patented molecules are, by definition, alien to human physiology, they are going to be more dangerous.

- **Synthetic hormones.** As hinted above, here's where things really get tricky. The dictionary definition of "synthetic" refers to something that is *artificial, man-made,* or even *fake.* However, when applied to hormones, "synthetic" has come to suggest that the molecule was produced (or *synthesized*) in a laboratory. Thus, Provera® and all other progestins are clearly *synthetic* "hormones," while CEEs, which are collected and extracted from pregnant mare urine, are considered "natural" hormones (at least for horses). On the other hand, patented products called Cenestin® and Enjuvia® are – We kid you not! – *vegetable*-based CEEs made from estrogens that are *synthesized* from Mexican yams. (*See below for more about these bizarre products.*) The big surprise comes when we look at bio-identical human hormones. Because, as noted earlier, since they are *synthesized* from Mexican yams or soy, bio-identical human hormones are, in fact, *synthetic.*

While it's commonplace to use the word "synthetic" to distinguish lab-produced "hormones" from those that are "natural" for humans, in this "age of the yam," this practice has become a distinction without a difference. Aside from Premarin®, which is still made the old-fashioned way – distilled from pregnant mare urine – and some phytoestrogens, which are extracted from plants, virtually all pseudohormones and bio-identical hormones alike in use today are actually *synthetic.*

Readers who want to learn more about bio-identical hormone replacement – and we urge everyone to learn as much as they can – are bound to run into unending language confusion, whether listening to the evening news or reading a medical journal. Please try to be wary of the widespread misuse of terms like "natural," "synthetic," and "bio-identical," not to mention words like "hormone," "estrogen," "progesterone," "progestin," and "progestogen." Whether intentionally misleading, misinformed, or simply careless, misuse of these terms remains the rule rather than the exception in both mass and medical professional media.

As an example, note the sloppy language used in a description of the patented oral "hormone replacement" product FemHRT® (*See box*). If you don't read carefully, you could easily gain the false impression that the "*estrogens*" and "*progesterones*" used in this product are the same as

those produced by the human body. In fact, the "*estrogen*" in FemHRT® is really the highly potent, man-made, patented drug, *ethinyl estradiol*, and the "*progesterone*" is really the man-made, patented drug, *norethindrone acetate*, both of which have long been used in birth control pills.

The blurb also points out that "*progesterones*" are one of the female hormones. That there is more than one "progesterone" is certainly news to us. We presume they meant "progestins" or "progestogens," since that is how norethindrone acetate is usually classified. Whatever the intent of this distortion, though, the result is to suggest – falsely – that ethinyl estradiol is equivalent to "natural" estrogen and that norethindrone acetate is equivalent to "natural" progesterone.

When considering the <u>hormones</u> used in hormone replacement therapy, please remember that the <u>only</u> variable that really matters is whether the molecular structure of the replacement hormone matches exactly that of the "natural" hormone it's intended to replace.

The only hormones that fit this description are bio-identical human hormones. Anything less than an exact match, whether it originates in a Mexican yam, a horse's ovaries, or some other chemical substrate, is almost certainly going to be inferior in terms of safety, tolerability, and efficacy.

A Hormone "Scorecard"

As the saying goes, "You can't tell the players without a scorecard," and that's especially true in the world of hormone replacement, where

Estrogens and "Progesterones"?

"FemHRT® contains two medicinal ingredients: ethinyl estradiol and norethindrone. Ethinyl estradiol belongs to a group of medicines called *estrogens*, while norethindrone acetate belongs to the group of medicines known as *progesterones*. *Estrogens* and *progesterones* are female hormones. They are produced by the body and are necessary for the normal sexual development of the female and for the regulation of the menstrual cycle during the childbearing years."

Source: Medbroadcast.com
http://www.medbroadcast.com/drug_info_details.asp?brand_name_id=1491

there are so many combinations and permutations of hormones and pseudohormones that one's eyes can quickly glaze over when trying to make sense of them. It may help to take a step back from all the confusion to see some of the forest as well as the individual trees. There are several points of interest that become apparent when you look at "hormone replacement" products in this way:

♦ **All bio-identical steroid hormones can be compounded.** As we discuss in detail in Chapter 9, hormones can – and should – be individually prepared for each woman based on her unique physiology and preferences by specially trained "compounding pharmacists." In addition to ensuring that each BHRT prescription is safe and effective, such compounding is essential if unpatented products like bio-identical hormones are to be available, because pharmaceutical companies find them too awkward and unprofitable to market.

Bio-identical steroid hormones are best when compounded into topical creams or gels, designed to be rubbed into the vaginal membranes or the inner surfaces of the labia, or sometimes the skin. Although not the preferred forms, they can also be made into oral pills or capsules to be swallowed, or into sublingual (literally, under the tongue) lozenges designed to be absorbed through the endothelial membranes in the mouth without swallowing. Oral (ie, swallowed) progesterone works best when it is *micronized*, or crushed into extremely small particles, but much higher doses are required.

♦ *A few bio-identical hormones are sold as branded products.* These include *Prometrium*®, a brand name for an oral micronized progesterone product; *Prochieve*®, and *Crinon*®, both progesterone vaginal gels; and *Synapause-E3*®, which is estriol sold as either an oral tablet or a vaginal cream (outside the US only). Recently, an oral form of estriol called Trimesta® has received a European patent for treating multiple sclerosis (MS) and other autoimmune diseases and is undergoing clinical trials in the US. As these examples demonstrate, the presence of a trademark (®) or register mark (®) does not necessarily mean that the product is patented. All it does is protect the product's name from use by anyone else. The hormones used to make them are exactly the same ones used by compounding pharmacists to formulate nonbranded prescriptions.

♦ *The only __human__ estrogen of interest to the major patent drug companies is estradiol.* There are at least 8 trademarked estradiol products on the market, one orally administered estriol product in clinical trials for future "approval" (for MS), no estrone, no "rub-on" estriol, and certainly no estrogen combinations like Tri-Est or Bi-Est. Why estradiol? Probably because it's the estrogen secreted by the ovary and is the most potent of the human estrogens. This choice has nothing to do with replicating human reproductive physiology, but that should come as no surprise by now.

♦ *How can you patent a bio-identical hormone?* The most common way is to incorporate the hormone into some kind of patented patch, cream, gel, or other high-tech "delivery device." Beyond simple creams and gels, there are several hormone-impregnated patches (eg, Estraderm®), which are designed to remain on the skin for several days at a time, while they dispense a constant, measured amount of bio-identical estradiol. Demonstrating an even greater level of scientific muscle-power is the FemRing®, an estradiol-impregnated plastic ring that is placed inside the vagina.

Are such sophisticated delivery devices really necessary? Or better? Not likely. While they have the apparent "advantage" of being FDA-"approved," hormonally they are identical to ordinary unpatented estradiol creams formulated by any compounding pharmacist. Moreover, the unpatented creams usually work better, because they can deliver the hormone on a schedule that more closely approximates the body's natural physiologic rhythm, rather than continuously as the skin patches and vaginal rings do.

Moreover, in addition to higher cost, the added sophistication of the patented devices may have its downside. For example, they are typically sold in only two or three dosage forms at most, which means the dosing may not be appropriate for many women. Also, the adhesives used in hormone patches often cause skin irritation and/or an allergic reactions, which can impede their effective use. Compounded products, by contrast, can be made in any dosage a woman requires and can be incorporated into any suitable base in order to accommodate people with sensitivities or allergies.

♦ *Cenestin® and Enjuvia® are horse estrogens made from the Mexican yam.* These products defy reason, not to mention human physiology. It's one thing if equine hormones are your only choice for treating women's menopausal estrogen deficiencies, as they were in the 1930s and '40s, when Premarin® was developed, especially if you knew as little about steroid hormone physiology as doctors did in those days. But here we are in the 21st century, when – thanks to the Marker degradation process – it's a simple matter to make virtually any steroid hormone you want by merely tweaking a soy or Mexican yam extract in just the right way. Why then, in the name of logic and health, would anyone go to the trouble of creating a *synthetic, vegetable-based, bio-identical horse estrogen* analog, unless you were planning to give it to menopausal horses? In other words, if human hormones are just as accessible as equine hormones, why not use human hormones? It's only common sense. But since when has common sense ever played a role in the world of HRT?

♦ *Climara Pro® and Prefest® are among a growing number of products that combine bio-identical estradiol with a non-bio-identical progestin drug.* Having come to recognize that bio-identical estradiol is better tolerated than horse estrogens, even at the excessively high doses found in these products, many companies have taken to producing such combinations using progestins other than Provera®. It's true that most progestins are better tolerated than Provera®, but if they're going to use a bio-identical form of estrogen (albeit the most potent one), one has to wonder why they didn't also opt for bio-identical progesterone, as well. What's to lose? You guessed it, big profits. A product made from two bio-identical hormones would be unpatentable, so once again, patents and profits trump natural physiology and health.

Is It Ethical for Doctors to Prescribe Premarin®?

It's bad enough that horse estrogens/CEEs/Premarin® can disrupt normal human physiology, but these hormones can cause serious problems for horses, as well. Actually, it's not the hormones themselves that cause problems for the horses, but the way we humans collect them.

Recall that CEEs are derived from the urine of pregnant mares. This may sound innocuous enough, but in order to collect horse urine on a scale that makes production profitable, as many 35,000 pregnant mares are currently confined in tiny stalls not much bigger than the horse under conditions that have raised serious alarms among people concerned with the welfare of these animals.

For 6 months of their 11-month pregnancy, the mares live on restricted fluid intake (so as not to dilute the urine), are allowed little or no exercise, and may not even be allowed to lie down to avoid dislodging their urine collection device. After giving birth, they are allowed only a few months to pasture with their foals before being reimpregnated to begin another round of urine production. In the mean time, most of the foals are sold for slaughter. (Given these hardships, it's easy to understand why estrogens derived from human pregnancy urine never got off the ground in the 1930s and '40s.)

Even if horse estrogens were the only way women could replace their own estrogen, resorting to this kind of cruelty would be questionable. But given the availability of perfectly good bio-identical, or at least vegetable-based, hormone replacement options, there can be no excuse for continuing this barbaric practice.

Perhaps medical doctors are finally getting the message. In an article in the *Journal of Medical Ethics*, Dr. Dennis Cox of Cambridge University Medical School wrote, "I determine that there is *prima facie* evidence to suggest that mares may suffer and that prescription of equine HRT ... would therefore have to be justified in terms of either offering greater benefits to the women or offering greater value for money to the health service. I find that there is no substantial evidence to suggest that equine HRT offers unique advantages over and above estriol."*

Given that incontrovertible evidence has demonstrated that CEEs are carcinogenic, a fact now backed up by the World Health Organization (WHO), it becomes natural to ask, Are doctors who continue to prescribe this product acting ethically?

---

*   Cox ID. Should a doctor prescribe hormone replacement therapy, which has been manufactured from mare's urine? *J Med Ethics*. 1996;22:199-204

References

1. Needham J. *Science and Civilization in China, Vol. 5, Part 5*. Cambridge, UK: Cambridge University Press; 1983.

2. Wright J, Lenard L. *Maximize Your Vitality & Potency*. Petaluma, CA: Smart Publications; 1999.

3. Seaman B. *The Greatest Experiment Ever Performed on Women*. New York: Hyperion; 2003.

4. Jaffe R. Evolution of Estrogen. *http://www.hormone.org/publications/estrogen _timeline/index.html*. 2005;The Hormone Foundation:Chevy Chase, MD 20815.

5. Davis SR, Dinatale I, Rivera-Woll L, Davison S. Postmenopausal hormone therapy: from monkey glands to transdermal patches. *J Endocrinol*. 2005;185:207-222.

6. Redig M. Yams of Fortune: The (Uncontrolled) Birth of Oral Contraceptives. *J Young Investigators*. February 2003:http://www.jyi.org/volumes/volume6/ issue7/features/redig.html.

7. Dieckmann WJ, Davis ME, Rynkiewicz LM, Pottinger RE. Does the administration of diethylstilbestrol during pregnancy have therapeutic value? *Am J Obstet Gynecol*. 1953;66:1062-1081.

8. Faludi AA, Aldrighi JM, Bertolami MC, et al. Progesterone abolishes estrogen and/or atorvastatin endothelium dependent vasodilatory effects. *Atherosclerosis*. 2004;177:89-96.

9. Recker RR, Davies KM, Dowd RM, Heaney RP. The effect of low-dose continuous estrogen and progesterone therapy with calcium and vitamin D on bone in elderly women. A randomized, controlled trial. *Ann Intern Med*. 1999;130:897-904.

10. Bese T, Vural A, Ozturk M, et al. The effect of long-term use of progesterone therapy on proliferation and apoptosis in simple endometrial hyperplasia without atypia. *Int J Gynecol Cancer*. 2006;16: 809-813.

11. Task Force Report on Hormone Therapy. Frequently asked questions about hormone therapy. http://www.acog.org/from_home/publications/press_releases/ nr10-01-04.cfm. 2004; American College of Obstetricians and Gynecologists: Accessed July 5, 2005.

12. The Writing Group for the PEPI Trial. Effects of estrogen or estrogen/progestin regimens on heart disease risk factors in postmenopausal women. The Postmenopausal Estrogen/Progestin Interventions (PEPI) Trial. *JAMA*. 1995;273:199-208.

13. Schumacher M, Guennoun R, Ghoumari A, et al. Novel perspectives for progesterone in HRT, with special reference to the nervous system. *Endocr Rev*. 2007;28:387-439.

14. Taylor M. Unconventional estrogens: estriol, biest, and triest. *Clin Obstet Gynecol.* 2001;44:864-879.

15. Dorgan JF, Baer DJ, Albert PS, et al. Serum hormones and the alcohol-breast cancer association in postmenopausal women. *J Natl Cancer Inst.* 2001;93:710-715.

16. Zumoff B. Does postmenopausal estrogen administration increase the risk of breast cancer? Contributions of animal, biochemical, and clinical investigative studies to a resolution of the controversy. *Proc Soc Exp Biol Med.* 1998;217:30-37.

17. Li CI, Anderson BO, Daling JR, Moe RE. Trends in incidence rates of invasive lobular and ductal breast carcinoma. *JAMA.* 2003;289:1421-1424.

18. Crook D, Cust MP, Gangar KF, et al. Comparison of transdermal and oral estrogen-progestin replacement therapy: effects on serum lipids and lipoproteins. *Am J Obstet Gynecol.* 1992;166: 950-955.

19. Crook D, Stevenson JC. Transdermal hormone replacement therapy, serum lipids and lipoproteins. *Br J Clin Pract Suppl.* 1996;86:17-21.

20. Abbas A, Fadel PJ, Wang Z, Arbique D, Jialal I, Vongpatanasin W. Contrasting effects of oral versus transdermal estrogen on serum amyloid A (SAA) and high-density lipoprotein-SAA in postmenopausal women. *Arterioscler Thromb Vasc Biol.* 2004;24:e164-167.

21. Erenus M, Karakoc B, Gurler A. Comparison of effects of continuous combined transdermal with oral estrogen and oral progestogen replacement therapies on serum lipoproteins and compliance. *Climacteric.* 2001;4:228-234.

22. Koh KK, Mincemoyer R, Bui MN, et al. Effects of hormone-replacement therapy on fibrinolysis in postmenopausal women. *N Engl J Med.* 1997;336:683-690.

23. Scarabin PY, Alhenc-Gelas M, Plu-Bureau G, Taisne P, Agher R, Aiach M. Effects of oral and transdermal estrogen/progesterone regimens on blood coagulation and fibrinolysis in postmenopausal women. A randomized controlled trial. *Arterioscler Thromb Vasc Biol.* 1997;17:3071-3078.

24. Vehkavaara S, Silveira A, Hakala-Ala-Pietila T, et al. Effects of oral and transdermal estrogen replacement therapy on markers of coagulation, fibrinolysis, inflammation and serum lipids and lipoproteins in postmenopausal women. *Thromb Haemost.* 2001;85:619-625.

25. Vongpatanasin W, Tuncel M, Wang Z, Arbique D, Mehrad B, Jialal I. Differential effects of oral versus transdermal estrogen replacement therapy on C-reactive protein in postmenopausal women. *J Am Coll Cardiol.* 2003;41:1358-1363.

26. Stevenson JC, Crook D, Godsland IF, Lees B, Whitehead MI. Oral versus transdermal hormone replacement therapy. *Int J Fertil Menopausal Stud.* 1993;38 Suppl 1:30-35.

CHAPTER 5

RELIEVING THE COMMON SYMPTOMS OF MENOPAUSE

Most women are initially drawn to hormone replacement to help maintain their youthful beauty and to relieve the common symptoms of menopause, Nature's physical signposts that mark the road to ovarian retirement. As you may be all too well aware, these include:

- **Increased skin wrinkling**, because normal estrogen and progesterone levels promote the look and feel of youthful, healthy skin.

- **Hot flushes**, also commonly called hot *flashes*. They are related to changes in the dilation of blood vessels, which is partially under the control of estrogen, and which brings an abundance of warm blood to the skin – at unpredictable moments – leading to a transient warm, often uncomfortable feeling.

- **Night sweats**, which are basically hot flushes that occur while you're sleeping.

- **Vaginal dryness, atrophy, and infection,** which are also due to a lack of estrogen in the genital area; it can cause discomfort and pain, especially during sexual activity.

- **Poor libido (sex drive), unsatisfactory sex,** well known to be associated with low levels of sex steroid hormones, especially testosterone.

- **Sleeping difficulties**, which affect at least half of all women during the menopausal transition.

- **Memory loss, dementia, and mood swings**. No, you're not going crazy! Estrogen, progesterone, and testosterone all help shape mental and cognitive functions, too.

- **Urinary incontinence ("leaking")**, a less well-appreciated, but often very disturbing effect of estrogen decline that becomes more common with age.

- **Urinary tract infection (UTI, bladder infection, "cystitis"),** like incontinence, and for basically the same reason, this risk also increases as estrogen levels decline.

While we often refer to these as *symptoms* of menopause, we should not take this to mean that menopause is a *disease*. On the contrary, while they may be unpleasant and disturbing, these are all *normal* – and *expected* – signs that levels of estrogen, progesterone, testosterone, and other hormone are declining.

Most women find that menopause-related changes like hot flushes, night sweats, sleeping difficulties, and mood swings are transitory. They last only as long as it takes the body to adapt to the new lower hormone levels, a process that can take from a few months to a year or more. However, other changes, such as drying and thinning of skin and vaginal membranes, the loss of urinary tract tone, and waning memory, as well as later developments, such as heart disease, osteoporosis, and cognitive decline, all tend to get worse with age unless hormones are replaced.

The way doctors are advised to prescribe *conventional* HRT today – the lowest possible dose for the shortest possible time – may help minimize hot flushes and the other transitory changes, but that's all. In our post-WHI world, where all bio-identical estrogens and patentable pseudoestrogens are "officially" (but mistakenly) considered equally dangerous, the other menopausal changes must be allowed to run their natural course, or in other words, *to worsen with age*. All mainstream medicine has to offer women for these changes, which are ultimately the most disturbing and the most hazardous, are lots of patented drugs designed to treat the individual symptoms in unnatural and often dangerous ways.

However, this does not mean that the progress of the more degenerative menopausal symptoms cannot be slowed, halted, or even reversed with appropriate bio-identical hormone replacement. In most women, restoring estrogen, progesterone, testosterone, and DHEA to close-to-natural levels on a schedule that copies as closely as possible the way their bodies secreted these hormones prior to menopause slows down all these *natural* degenerative processes. Over the past 25+ years, I have prescribed BHRT for over 2,000 women, and in nearly every case, symptoms have vanished, or at least become less troublesome, with hardly any adverse side effects.

Unfortunately, you'll find no long-term, double-blind, placebo-controlled studies "validating" my experience published in the *New England Journal of Medicine*, the *Journal of the American Medical Association*, or other "bibles" of conventional, pharmaceutical-based medicine. Nevertheless, thousands of other progressive doctors all over the world, who have taken the trouble to learn the facts about BHRT, can verify that BHRT is a safe, tolerable, and effective option for treating menopausal symptoms.

While some may argue that the safety of BHRT has not been proven beyond a reasonable doubt (*A proposition with which we vigorously disagree!*), it's hard to see how anyone could doubt its ability to relieve and prevent menopausal symptoms. If horse estrogens are effective in humans, should human estrogens be any less effective? The thought is laughable, and the evidence, both in the published literature and in the clinical experience of virtually every doctor who has ever prescribed them and every woman who has ever used them, is unassailable.

In the remainder of this chapter, we describe and present scientific evidence supporting the use of bio-identical hormones, especially estriol, to help women safely and effectively relieve the most common and disturbing symptoms of menopausal hormone decline – both transitory and permanent.

Goodbye Hot Flushes and Night Sweats!

Numerous studies published since the late 1970s have confirmed the value of bio-identical estrogens, especially estriol for managing common menopausal symptoms. On the whole, when used properly – at physiologic doses and on a physiologic schedule* – bio-identical estrogen minimizes the occurrence of hot flushes and night sweats, the most common of the menopausal symptoms. Figure 5-1 shows the results of a survey of 78

---

* A physiologic dose (or schedule) is one that approximates what occurs naturally in the body.

women who used compounded BHRT (primarily Tri-Est or Bi-Est). After 6 weeks of treatment, their symptoms occurred far less frequently and on the whole were much milder, compared to before therapy.[3]

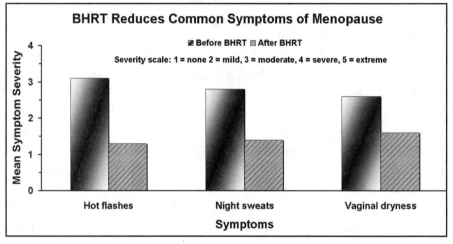

Figure 5-1. BHRT reduces common symptoms of menopause. This graph shows the change in symptom severity in 78 women who used bio-identical hormones for 6 weeks. *Adapted from Vigesaa et al, 2004*

Most importantly, BHRT evinces little or no propensity for promoting abnormal growth in the lining of the uterus, even when taken "unopposed" (without progesterone).[4-9] Recall that such uterine overgrowth is the number one precancerous condition associated with estrogen substitution using Premarin®.

Estriol does not increase blood pressure or other cardiovascular risk factors, and it is effective in women during and after normal menopause as well as in younger women whose menopause occurs literally overnight following surgical removal of their ovaries. Safe and effective doses ranged from 1 to 12 mg per day in these studies, but, like much of the early research, estriol in these studies was given by mouth, which requires doses *20-fold higher* than by topical administration directly to the vaginal epithelial tissue. Subsequent research has shown topical application to be the preferred route of administration of not just estriol, but all sex steroid hormones.[10] (*See Chapter 9 for more about optimal dosing and route of administration of bio-identical hormones.*)

Eliminate Vaginal Dryness, Discomfort, and Pain

Among its many functions, ovarian estrogen supports blood flow to the vaginal lining. With less blood flowing to the genital area, postmenopausal genital tissue loses its sensitivity, leading to reduced arousal and difficulty achieving orgasm.

As estrogen levels decline, vaginal tissue also tends to become dryer and thinner. This atrophy leaves the vaginal walls vulnerable to irritation, making sexual intercourse painful and increasing the risk of infection. Although vaginal dryness and atrophy are common problems, affecting as many as two out of three women after menopause, they are easily treated with estriol and/or estradiol (Fig. 5-1). This effect has been repeatedly confirmed by studies published mostly in European medical journals since the late 1970s.[3, 10-18]

Estriol is far safer for preventing vaginal atrophy than more potent, patented "estrogens." In a study in which 263 menopausal women took oral doses of either bio-identical estriol or the potent, patented, man-made "estrogen" ethinyl estradiol, both the "estrogens" restored vaginal tissue that had begun to atrophy. However, with ethinyl estradiol, the dose that restored healthy vaginal tissue (the therapeutic dose) was nearly the same as the dose that caused uterine overgrowth (hyperplasia), indicating virtually *no safety margin* for this patent medicine; even a normal dose could be dangerous. By contrast, the therapeutic dose of estriol was *3 to 5 times lower* than the dose that caused hyperplasia, a safety margin of 300 to 500%.[17] The next time you hear a BHRT critic claim that there's no data supporting its efficacy and safety, think about this study (and the hundreds of others cited in this book) and also think about who's paying him/her to say it.

Break the Vaginal/Urinary Tract Infection Cycle

Not all women realize that their vaginal fluids are normally slightly acidic, with a pH of about 4 (pH 1 is highly acidic; pH 7 is neutral; and pH higher than 7 is basic, or alkaline). Like everything else in the body, there is a good reason for this degree of vaginal acidity, which comes in part compliments of estrogen. The acidity of the healthy vagina makes it more hospitable to the friendly bacteria, *Lactobacillus acidophilus* (the same bacteria commonly found in yogurt), which thrive in an acidic environment and also contribute to it by secreting lactic acid. The normal acidity also makes the vagina less hospitable to most unfriendly bacteria (and yeasts), which usually find a low pH (about 4 and below) harmful to their health.

The presence of lactic acid-secreting *Lactobacilli* in the vagina thus represents a natural barrier against disease-causing microorganisms. The most common of these pathogenic organisms is the bacteria *Escherichia coli (E. coli)*, which usually originate in the colon and rectum and can easily migrate to the nearby vagina and urinary tract. *Lactobacilli* protect the vagina from colonization by yeasts like *Candida albicans* in a similar way.

After menopause, though, vaginal acidity declines (pH rises) in parallel with the decline in estrogen. This makes the vagina less hospitable to *Lactobacilli* and more hospitable to unfriendly, acid-hating bacteria and yeasts. Once allowed to gain a foothold in the vagina, these "bugs" can cause local infections (called *vaginosis* and *candidiasis*, respectively).[16, 19] About 10 to 15% of women over age 60 have frequent bouts of urinary tract infection (UTI),[20] which are especially common (and potentially serious) when a urinary catheter is inserted into the bladder in a hospital or nursing home.

Conventional treatment of urinary and vaginal infections using antibiotic and/or antifungal drugs can actually make a bad problem even worse. Antibiotic drugs do a great job of killing bacteria. However, their actions are not limited just to the "bugs" causing the infection; they also kill billions of "friendly" microorganisms that live in the vagina (*Lactobacilli*) and in the GI tract, where they perform countless valuable natural functions. Having killed off the infecting organisms, antimicrobial drugs do nothing to help restore the healthy vaginal and urinary tract (or GI tract) epithelial lining, the vagina's normal acidity, or the friendly bacteria that previously lived here. In fact, once the drug is stopped, the microbial "vacuum" that remains actually encourages further infection. (For those who might be interested, there is another safe, effective, and *natural* alternative to antibiotics for women with UTI,* but read on ... BHRT may be preferable for many other reasons.)

Any woman who has ever taken an antibiotic *for any reason* (not just a genitourinary infection) is no doubt quite familiar with the following painful scenario: With the harmless and beneficial *Lactobacilli* wiped out by the drug along with the target infecting organisms, yeasts are free to move in, leading to a vaginal yeast infection, or *candidiasis,* which means it's time for her to start using an antifungal drug (eg, ketoconazole). Once the yeasts are evicted, unless she takes active steps to keep her vagina and urinary tract extraordinarily clean and bacteria free, *E. coli* or some other unfriendly bacteria may return, leading to more antibiotics followed by yet another yeast infection and on and on.

Although a lack of estrogen in the vagina and urinary tract can predispose to a host of problems, in most cases, these can be prevented or reversed by simply replacing the lost estrogen, preferably using topically applied estriol or Tri-Est.

A number of studies have confirmed estriol's ability to maintain a healthful vaginal environment.[15, 16, 21-25] For example, when oral estriol was combined with local application of *L. acidophilus,* postmenopausal women were able to completely restore the epithelial lining of their vagina (and urinary tract) to normal.[26]

In a Swedish study,[25] 41 elderly women (aged 80-90 years) living in a nursing home, took oral estriol (3 mg/day). All the women had been receiving antibiotics for severe, stubborn urinary tract or vaginal infections (the most common "bug" was *E. coli*) but with limited success. Whenever they stopped the drug, the infections kept returning – a familiar story to women who are vulnerable to UTI. However, after 4 to 5 weeks on estriol (plus an antibiotic), all the women became virtually infection-free. Furthermore, protective *Lactobacilli* started to return spontaneously to the vaginas of about one-third of the women. During up to 1,219 patient-weeks of estriol treatment, the women required antibiotics during only 9 patient-weeks (0.7% of the time). Overall, when the women were using

---

* Approximately 90% of all urinary tract infections can be eliminated by using a safe, natural sugar called **D-mannose.** For details, see *D-Mannose and Bladder Infection, the Natural Alternative to Antibiotics,* by Jonathan Wright, MD and Lane Lenard, PhD. 2001; Dragon Art, 36646 32nd Avenue South, Auburn, Washington, 98001.

estriol, antibiotic use plummeted 16-fold. Noted the authors, "From our experience it will be clear that the therapeutic and prophylactic effect [of estriol] in urogenital infections is striking."

Perhaps the most impressive illustration of estriol's ability to prevent UTI was reported in the prestigious *New England Journal of Medicine.*[23] (Remember, according to the FDA, *"There's no data supporting the safety or efficacy of bio-identical hormones, especially estriol."*) In this double-blind, placebo-controlled study, 93 postmenopausal women with a history of recurrent UTI (about 5 infections per year on average) were randomly assigned to use either a vaginal estriol cream (0.5 mg) or an inactive placebo cream. Over the course of 8 months, the researchers found the following results:

- The annual rate of infection was 0.5 for the estriol group and 6.0 for the placebo group. This amounts to more than a 10-fold or 1000% decline in the incidence of UTI in women treated with estriol (Table 5-1, Fig. 5-2).

- Eight (8) of 50 women (16%) in the estriol group had a total of 12 episodes of infection, compared with 27 of 43 women (63%) in the placebo group, who had 10 times more episodes of infection – 111.

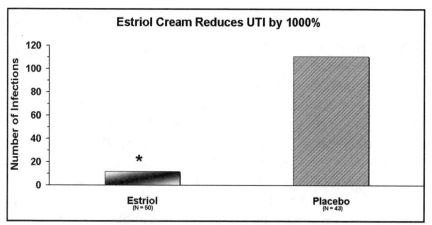

Figure 5-2. In postmenopausal women with a history of UTI, vaginal application of estriol cream significantly reduced the occurrence of bacterial infections in the urinary tract by a factor of 10 (1000%) over an 8-month period, compared with an inactive placebo cream.

* $P = 0.001$ Source: Raz & Stamm, 1993

- Over the 8-months of the study, the estriol-treated women used antibiotics for an average of 7 days vs. 32 days for the placebo-treated women.

- Estriol replacement also resulted in a significant increase in vaginal acidity. As shown in Figure 5-3, for the estriol-treated group, vaginal pH declined from a bacteria-friendly pH 6 to a normally acidic, bactericidal pH of 3.8 after 1 month and to 3.6 after 8 months.

Table 5-1. Estriol Reduces Urinary Tract Infections and Antibiotic Use

	Estriol	Placebo
UTI rate (infections/year)	0.5*	5.9
Number (%) of women with UTI	8 (16%)*	27 (63%)
Total UTI episodes	12*	111
Antibiotics (mean number of days of use)	6.9*	32.0

* $P \leq 0.001$ *Source: Raz & Stamm, 1993*
UTI = *urinary tract infection*

- At the start of the study, both groups of women had no friendly *Lactobacilli* in their vaginas. However, after 1 month of treatment, *Lactobacilli* returned spontaneously in 61% of the estriol-treated women but *never returned* in women in the placebo group.

You don't find too many clinical study results much clearer than these. Positive results in preventing UTI have also been reported in women using a patented estradiol-impregnated silicone ring that is left in the vagina,[27] but since estradiol is so much more potent than estriol, even low doses are likely to cause more unwanted side effects.

Unfortunately, the same is true about conventional HRT. Even if you could use HRT on an extended basis – which current treatment guidelines strongly discourage – the effects of Premarin® alone or in combination with Provera® on genitourinary infections have been equivocal at best. Three studies found little or no change in risk,[28-30] while one found that postmenopausal women taking oral "estrogen" for at least a year actually had an *increased risk of UTI*.[31] Perhaps the results would have been better

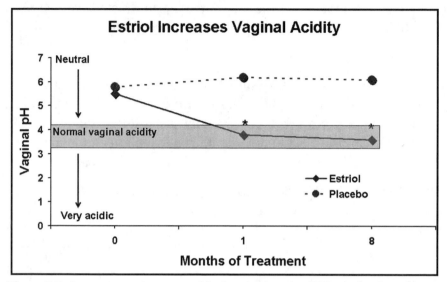

Figure 5-3. In menopausal women with chronic recurring UTI, application of
a vaginal estriol cream resulted in a significant reduction in vaginal pH, from a
bacteria-friendly 6 (near neutral) before treatment to a normal, antibacterial pH of 3.8
after 1 month of treatment and 3.6 after 8 months. Use of a placebo cream caused no
change in vaginal acidity. * P <0.001

Source: Raz & Stamm, 1993

if Premarin® had been studied for its ability to prevent UTIs in aging
mares! These studies show, once again, why human estrogens are far
preferable for humans!

Avoid "Leakage" and Other Urinary Problems

For many of the same reasons that low estrogen levels predispose to
vaginal atrophy and genitourinary infections in the years after menopause,
they also increase the likelihood of urinary incontinence ("leaky bladder")
and pain or difficulty in urinating (*dysuria*). Urinary incontinence affects
20 to 40% of older women.[32] Because they help restore normal blood flow
to urinary tissues and muscles that support and control the structures of
the urinary system, estriol and BHRT can be very effective for preventing
and treating these common urinary tract problems.[33, 34]

Most commonly, leakage occurs during coughing, laughing, exercising,
or other actions that increase abdominal pressure. This is called "stress
incontinence." Leakage may also occur following a strong urge to void,

whether the bladder is full or not. Known as "urge incontinence" (and also as "overactive," "unstable," or "spastic bladder"), it may happen spontaneously during sleep or be triggered by drinking water or even by merely touching water or hearing water running in a sink or shower.

However it manifests, urinary incontinence (UI) is usually due to weakened muscles in and around the bladder and urethra, the tube that transmits urine out of the body. The tone and strength of these muscles depends in large part on the presence of estrogen. In some premenopausal women, the natural decline in estrogen during the week before menstruation is enough to cause the muscles surrounding their urethra to weaken and temporarily lose their grip. The permanent decline in estrogen after menopause often means a permanent state of intermittent incontinence.

Not surprisingly, the prevalence of UI increases with age. Recent research revealed a prevalence of 28% in younger women (aged 30-39 years) and more than 50% in women in their 60s and older.[35, 36] Depression also rises as the severity of UI increases.[37]

Mainstream medicine has had little to offer women with postmenopausal stress incontinence besides patent medication, diapers, absorbent pads, and in extreme cases, surgery. Perhaps for this we should be grateful. Patent medicines that merely increase urethral muscle tone are widely advertised (*"Gotta go, gotta go, gotta go right now!!"*), minimally effective, and can have many disturbing side effects, including blurred vision, nausea, constipation, dizziness, and headache.[38]

At the same time, medical science has known for a long time that the best treatment for both types of incontinence is estrogen replacement. However, until recently, it was widely assumed that the horse estrogens in conventional HRT could help women with UI. Then, in the harsh light of well-controlled research — the Women's Health Initiative (WHI), the large, double-blind, placebo-controlled clinical trial conducted by the National Institutes of Health (NIH) — another myth evaporated. At the start of the study, more than 23,000 participants had some form of UI. They were randomly selected to receive Premarin® + Provera®, Premarin® alone ("women without a uterus"), or placebo.

After 1 year of treatment, women who had been continent at baseline (the start of the study) and received conventional HRT, had just about *doubled their incidence of urinary incontinence.* In women who were already incontinent at baseline, horse hormone (Premarin®) replacement significantly increased the risk of leakage. The authors concluded unequivocally, *"Conjugated equine estrogen with or without progestin should not be prescribed for the prevention or relief of UI."*[39] Moreover, even if HRT had been shown to be effective, the elevated risks of heart disease and cancer demonstrated in the WHI would now preclude its long-term use, so any relief obtained from the treatment would have been short-lived.

Similar results came out of the Heart Estrogen/Progestin Replacement Study (HERS), in which 1,208 women took Premarin® + Provera®. Shockingly, within just 4 months, both stress and urge incontinence began to appear in the horse hormone-treated women, and after more than 4 years of treatment, nearly two-thirds of the women (64%) were adversely affected, compared with about half (49%) of the women in the placebo group.[40, 41]

Unlike horse estrogens, *unpatentable* bio-identical human estriol actually works in women with urinary incontinence. A group of 48 postmenopausal Swedish women with urinary incontinence took estriol orally for up to 10 years, during which 75% of the women reported subjective improvement. Objective measures confirmed that estriol improved the health of the women's urinary tract tissue and muscle; intraurethral pressure increased and leakage stopped.[42]

In another study, a group of 135 German women with postmenopausal UI used estriol intravaginally. After 3 months, leakage had slowed in 63% of the women. At the start of the study, 14 women were reporting pain or difficulty in urinating (*dysuria*). By the end of the study, it was completely gone. Frequency, associated with "overactive bladder," also subsided significantly.[43]

It would never occur to conventional medicine to use what appears to be an ideal treatment for urinary incontinence – bio-identical *estriol*. Despite the ready availability of many relevant studies, the most recent guidelines for the management of urinary incontinence put out by the American College of Obstetricians and Gynecologists (ACOG) don't mention the use of topical estriol or even patented estradiol vaginal rings.[38, 44, 45]

Keep Your Skin Looking and Feeling Youthful

One of the surest ways many women have of telling that menopause is upon them (other than the obvious cessation of their menstrual periods) is simply to look in the mirror. Within a few months after the onset of menopause, the skin – the body's largest organ – may start to noticeably age.[46] It becomes thinner, drier, less elastic, and more easily bruised. Over time it may start to sag; wrinkles may deepen; and wounds may heal more slowly. These skin effects are the first real outward sign of menopause, and for many women, looking in the mirror can become an aversive experience, a daily reminder of the loss of their youthful beauty.

All these skin changes are due at least in part to the loss of estrogen, which in turn leads to a loss in collagen, hyaluronic acid, and other important substances.[47]* Young skin's elasticity and resiliency comes from youthful levels of *collagen,* an important protein that helps give skin, bone, tendons, and cartilage their *great tensile strength.*

Collagen levels seem to be particularly sensitive to estrogen levels, because women begin to lose collagen in their early 40s, the very earliest days of the perimenopause. At the same time, the rate at which new skin cells form and old ones die off slows down. As the old cells hang on long past their useful life, the skin becomes leathery, dull, and more likely to wrinkle.[48]

One small but interesting study, conducted by a German physician, dramatically illustrates the influence that estrogen levels can have on a woman's appearance of youthfulness.[49] Within the first minute that new women patients entered their outpatient clinic, the physician and his staff estimated (and recorded) their estimates of the women's age – ie, before they knew anything about them. During subsequent standard procedures, they measured the women's serum estradiol levels (and, of

---

* The health of the skin depends on a wide variety of life-long factors in addition to estrogen, including sun exposure, cigarette smoking, moisture content, and nutrition.

course, recorded their actual age). Some of the women, who ranged in actual age from 35 to 55 years, were premenopausal, and others were postmenopausal.

After collecting data from 100 women, they compared their initial estimates of the women's ages with their actual ages and plotted these against their levels of estradiol. As shown in Figure 5-4, regardless of their actual age, women with higher levels of serum estradiol were judged at their initial appearance to be significantly younger looking. As the researchers noted, "…Women with high estrogen concentrations looked younger, women with low estradiol concentrations older than they really were. The discrepancy between estimated and real age could be as high as 8 years in either direction."

While skin health has long been linked to estrogen levels, research has begun to explain exactly how estrogen keeps skin from aging and how replacement estrogens can even erase some of the years from aging skin. For example, skin cells are covered with estrogen receptors, special protein configurations that attract estrogen molecules and bind them to the cell, where they trigger vital cell functions. When estrogen binds to

Estrogen Makes Your Skin Appear Younger

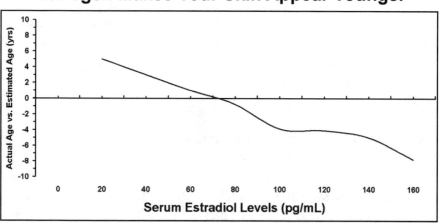

Figure 5-4. The results of this study showed that estimates of a woman's age by a physician and his staff depended to a large degree on the women's levels of estrogen (estradiol). Those with higher levels of estradiol were judged to be significantly younger than those with lower levels, regardless of their actual chronological age.

Adapted from Wildt & Sir-Peterman. The Lancet. 1999;354:224.

these receptors, it improves the structure of elastic fibers[50, 51] and also promotes the growth of new blood vessels in skin, helping keep the influx of nutrients and outflux of waste flowing smoothly.[52] By stimulating the growth of special cells called *fibroblasts* and *keratinocytes* and encouraging the release of substances, such as mucopolysaccharides and hyaluronic acid, bio-identical estrogens increases skin thickness and water content.[46, 53, 54]

One study by Austrian researchers[55] evaluated the effects of bio-identical estrogen replacement using creams made from 0.01% estradiol or 0.3% estriol in 59 postmenopausal women (mean age, ~54 years), who were showing signs of aging skin. The women applied the estrogen creams directly to their neck and face. Wrinkles, hydration, and other skin parameters were measured objectively before and after treatment began. After 7 weeks in the estriol group and 9 weeks in the estradiol group, nearly every woman saw clear improvement in the firmness and elasticity, enhanced moisture content, and vascularization (new blood vessels) of her skin, as well as a 61 to 100% decrease in wrinkle depth and pore size. Both estrogens were equally effective, but not surprisingly, the much more potent estradiol caused more dose-related side effects.

Enhance Your Sexuality

It is quite common for women to experience sexual "problems" during their perimenopausal, menopausal, and postmenopausal years. These include vaginal dryness and thinning, sensitivity and pain during intercourse (*dyspareunia*), declining libido/sexual desire/sexual interest, and decreased frequency and enjoyment of intercourse. In many women, these symptoms may be associated with depression, persistent fatigue, and an impaired sense of general well-being.

As we all know, the link between sex hormones and sex begins in adolescence, and it never really ends. As the hormones decline with age, sexuality also tends to fade away with them, unless replaced by bio-identical replacement versions.

In men, the hormone we typically associate with sexuality is *testosterone*, sometimes hyped as the "hormone of desire." (*See Chapter 10.*) Well, it turns out that, while estrogens and progesterone are important for keeping women's sexual organs normal and healthy, testosterone and other androgens are largely responsible for women's feelings of sexual desire and their enjoyment of sexual activity, too, serving much the same functions they do in men. Of course, men's bodies produce at least 20 times more testosterone than women's bodies, an important point for women to keep in mind when it comes time to replace this hormone.

The relationship between estrogens, androgens, and sexuality in women is quite complex. We have described earlier how estrogens, whether produced by the ovaries or replaced by bio-identical supplements, support vaginal tissue by keeping it thick, moist, and free of bacterial and yeast infections, thus eliminating significant sources of pain and discomfort during intercourse, which can discourage sexual enjoyment all by themselves. However, estrogens have little direct effect on libido.[56]

But it is the androgens, including *testosterone, androstenedione, DHEA, and DHEA-S,* which are primarily responsible for subtler feelings, such as arousability, sexual desire, and fantasy, as well as frequency of sexual activity, orgasm, and satisfaction and pleasure from the sexual act.[57]

In women, androgens originate primarily in the ovaries and the adrenal glands, with each directly contributing about 25% of the total. In premenopausal women, ovarian secretion of testosterone increases by about 10% to 15% around the time of ovulation, with the obvious "purpose" of encouraging mating, leading to fertilization. The remaining 50% of androgen production arises from the conversion in peripheral tissues of androgen "precursor" hormones, such as androstenedione, DHEA, and DHEA-S, to testosterone. Keep in mind that the androgens, testosterone and androstenedione, can also serve as precursors for the formation of estradiol and estrone, which is especially important in postmenopausal women, because their ovaries have ceased the production of estradiol. (*For a reminder of how all these hormones are related to each other metabolically, see Figure 4-2 on page 74.*)

Like most hormones, androgen levels decline with age, but unlike estrogens and progesterone, the decrease in androgens has little to do with the events surrounding menopause. First, adrenal secretion of DHEA and DHEA-S, the most abundant steroid hormones in the body, declines steadily as a function of age, beginning as early as a woman's late 20s.[58]

Partly as a result of the decline in DHEA and DHEA-S, androgen levels in premenopausal women in their 40s may already be 50% lower than those in women in their 20s.[59] During and after menopause, as the ovaries shrivel up and cease secreting estradiol and progesterone, their secretion of testosterone nevertheless continues pretty much unabated.

One of the most important factors in keeping testosterone flowing after menopause is a decline in steroid hormone binding globulin (SHBG), which as noted above, normally gobbles up circulating testosterone and permanently inactivates it. The menopause-related decline in SHBG concentrations leaves more testosterone to circulate as *free testosterone.* One reason SHBG levels fall after menopause is the absence of estrogens, which are normally responsible for triggering their rise. As estradiol secretion declines, SHBG levels fall right along with them. This is fine in as much as it leads to androgen elevation, but it can become a problem in women taking high *oral* doses of potent "replacement estrogens," such as Premarin® or estradiol, which elevate SHBG levels and thus, indirectly lower their androgen levels. Topical application of bio-identical estrogens has no effect on SHBG levels.[60] (*In case you needed another reason to avoid oral, non-bio-identical hormones, how about loss of sexuality?*)

To summarize, women who go through *natural* menopause lose a significant portion of their androgen concentrations due to the normal age-related decline in the secretion of the testosterone precursors, DHEA, DHEA-S, and androstenedione from the adrenals. Still, the ovaries generally continue to secrete testosterone throughout a woman's lifespan, long after they've lost the ability to secrete estradiol. Moreover, the postmenopausal decline in SHBG also helps free up testosterone that would have been removed "from the game" in the presence of normal concentrations of ovarian estradiol, thus helping to boost testosterone concentrations.

Research shows that the steepest decline in women's testosterone levels occurs during their early *reproductive* years. This is followed by a leveling off around menopause and then a slight increase.[61] In one study, women in their 60s were found to have testosterone levels equal to those in premenopausal women.[62] (*We warned you this was complex!*)

Testosterone, Free and Not So Free

As testosterone circulates in the blood stream, about 80% of it is tightly bound to a glycoprotein called sex hormone binding globulin (SHBG); about 18 to 19% is loosely bound to albumin, and the remaining 1 to 2% is unbound and termed free testosterone. SHBG-bound testosterone is permanently inactivated, while albumin-bound testosterone, although also inactivated, can be freed up under certain conditions. Thus, at any given time, only free testosterone is physiologically active, which means only about 1 to 2% of circulating testosterone is available to modulate androgenic activity.

Unfortunately, many doctors who order blood tests to measure testosterone levels (in women or men) do not take this distinction seriously. The only measurement that has any real clinical meaning is free testosterone, yet it is common for doctors to ignore this and measure only total testosterone, which includes testosterone bound to SHBG and albumin, as well as free testosterone. Because as much as 99% of total testosterone may be inactive, such a measurement tells doctors almost nothing about the state of a person's androgens.

Thus, when having your androgen levels tested, it is always a good practice to make sure your doctor is testing for free testosterone and not just total testosterone. Doctors who are skilled and knowledgeable about bio-identical hormone replacement are likely to be well aware of these differences.

Up to now we've been talking about women who go through *natural* menopause, but women who have had their ovaries surgically removed – *overnight surgical menopause* – are a whole different story. Since postmenopausal ovaries continue secreting testosterone and androstenedione – a fact that many doctors overlook – women who've had their ovaries surgically removed lose one of their two primary sources of androgens, which means that their levels decline by about half. (Their adrenals continue to supply the remaining half.)

Not surprisingly, women who've gone through overnight surgical menopause are especially susceptible to the physical, psychological, and sexual effects of androgen depletion. Even if they use estrogen replacement (or partly because of it, if they use potent, patentable *oral* "estrogens," such as SHBG-boosting Premarin®), their sex lives tend to go rapidly downhill, including a loss of sexual desire, diminished sexual pleasure and satisfaction, not to mention depression and insomnia.[59]

What's the Best Testosterone Replacement for Women?

Testosterone and other androgen replacements have been available for treating men's sexual and other "male menopausal/andropausal" disorders for 60 or 70 years. However, the FDA has never "approved" an androgen replacement regimen for postmenopausal women, who have low sex drive and other androgen-related sexual problems. As far as the FDA is concerned, these women are essentially on their own. Women in Europe are indeed more fortunate, since female-sized doses of testosterone are legal and widely available.

Another problem is that, because of the high doses of androgen products developed and marketed for men, women cannot even use them "off label." Women's bodies need (and can tolerate) only a tiny fraction (3 - 5%) of the testosterone and other androgens that men need. Even half a normal male dose of testosterone would cause disturbing or serious side effects. At present, the only way for women to obtain a testosterone replacement product suitable is to have it specially prepared by a compounding pharmacist, an option that the powers behind conventional medicine would prefer not be exercised, regardless of the consequences.

The sole "androgen" currently FDA-"approved" for use by women is an oral pill called Estratest®, which consists of a combination of two patented pseudohormone drugs: 1) *esterified estrogens* (*EEs*), and 2) *methyltestosterone*. This dangerous drug has been around for decades and is officially "indicated" for treating recalcitrant cases of hot flushes, despite the fact that the evidence supporting its effectiveness for this condition is marginal at best. Conventional doctors who wish to prescribe Estratest® for women with sexual problems must do so "off-label." While methyltestosterone may have a few positive sexual effects in some women, it is generally deemed too risky for long-term use.

The problems with Estratest® have less to do with the estrogen side of the pill (Overall, EEs seem to be less risky than Premarin®.), and more to do with the pseudotestosterone side. Methyltestosterone is a patented derivative of natural testosterone, whose primary claim to fame is that, unlike bio-identical testosterone and most other bio-identical steroid hormones, when taken by mouth, the liver does not rapidly and completely neutralize it.

Originally developed in the 1940s as a patented substitute for natural testosterone for treating "menopausal/andropausal" *men*, methyltestosterone is the "granddaddy" of all the oral *anabolic steroid drugs* (the ones used by athletes to help them "bulk up"). Methyltestosterone use by men turned out to be an unmitigated disaster, causing untold cases of liver failure, liver cancer, blood clots, heart attacks, strokes, and other disorders, many of them fatal. It also helped to "poison the well" for research on safer androgen replacements for decades to come. Ironically, though, the drug is still around, continuing to be used by muscle-hungry athletes and body builders. More importantly, methyltestosterone remains the only "testosterone" product officially "approved" by the FDA for use in *women,* but not for sexual problems.* (*Really! We're not making this up.*)

Apparently, though, the bio-identical-hormone message has been getting through at some level to practitioners of conventional medicine. Virtually all new patented testosterone replacement products employ *bio-identical testosterone* in formulations designed for topical application. The best known of these are bio-identical testosterone skin patches, gels, and creams, but these are being marketed only in male-size doses by a few large patent medicine companies. Even though these products have been FDA-"approved" for use by men, comparable products have never been "approved" in doses suitable for use by women (although several are under development).

In recent years, patented testosterone patches, creams, gels, and vaginal rings have been tested and found to be generally safe and effective for treating women diagnosed with "*hypoactive sexual desire disorder"(HSDD)* after having had their ovaries surgically removed. In one pair of placebo-controlled clinical trials, over 1,000 women with surgically induced menopause were randomly assigned to use either the testosterone patch (applied to the abdomen twice a week) or a placebo

---

* The methyltestosterone catastrophe in men beginning in the 1940s was a harbinger of disasters to come once female "hormone replacement" therapy took hold a couple of decades later. Our walk down Hormone Memory Lane brings back such fond reminiscences as DES-linked cancers in women and their offspring; Premarin-induced uterine cancer (before Provera® and other "progestins" were recruited to "oppose" Premarin's inherent carcinogenicity); increases in breast cancer, heart disease, and dementia, as recently confirmed by the WHI and other studies (paradoxically caused at least in part by Provera®). Oddly, each time one of these disasters is revealed, conventional doctors are invariably "shocked."

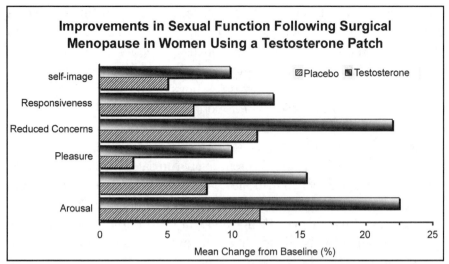

Figure 5-5. Surgically postmenopausal women (aged 20-70 years) also taking "estrogen" replacement (oral or topical patch) were randomly placed in either a *testosterone* patch group or *placebo* patch group for 24-weeks. Sexual function, as measured by a series of validated questionnaires, was significantly improved in the testosterone-treated women on every variable measured, compared to placebo.

Adapted from Kingsberg, S., 2007

patch for 24 weeks. The women were all also using some form of oral or topical estrogen replacement (the precise type of estrogen was not specified).[63]

As shown in Figure 5-5, testosterone replacement in these women led to significant improvement in a wide range of self-assessed variables related to sexual function. In addition, the testosterone-treated women had significant increases in satisfying sexual activity, number of orgasms, and sexual desire, as well as a significant decrease in "personal distress."[63, 64]

The most common adverse side effect in these studies was a skin reaction at the site of the patch, which occurred in 30 to 40% of the users. This side effect is quite common in women using patented, standardized topical patches, regardless of the medication or hormone they deliver. It underlines an important advantage of compounded hormone products, which pharmacists can formulate in a variety of topical base creams or gels to suit any individual sensitivities or allergies.

When the manufacturer of the testosterone patch used in the studies described above applied to the FDA for approval for use in women with HSDD due to surgically induced menopause, a "gun-shy" advisory panel made up of 17 outside "experts" turned them down by a unanimous vote, despite the clear benefits and low risks shown by these and other studies of topical testosterone products for women.

Having been "burned" by the WHI findings a couple of years earlier and still failing to understand the difference between patented pseudohormone drugs and bio-identical hormones, the panel demanded more long-term safety data before recommending FDA approval. They feared that prolonged use of topical bio-identical testosterone (more than the 12 months already tested) might somehow increase women's risk of breast cancer or cardiovascular disease, as Premarin®, Provera®, and methyltestosterone had been shown to do. They were also afraid that the patch might be prescribed "off-label" to naturally menopausal women or even, Heaven forbid, premenopausal women. The precise basis for these fears is unclear, since bio-identical testosterone in the physiologic doses supplied by these patches (or by Mother Nature!) has never been associated with any of these risks in women at any age.

The FDA's misguided "guidance" leaves women with natural or surgical menopause-related sexual disorder with only two options: 1) oral Estratest® prescribed "off-label"; and 2) topical bio-identical testosterone in customized creams or gels prepared by compounding pharmacists. Unbelievable as it sounds, since the FDA seems to be opposed on principle to any bio-identical hormone product coming from a compounding pharmacy, we can only assume that they would prefer that women take the demonstrably dangerous and only marginally effective – but nevertheless FDA-"approved" – Estratest®.

Other experts, including the usually very conservative North American Menopause Society (NAMS)[65] as well as the more progressive International Hormone Society (IHS),[66] actually agree that menopausal women – whether of the natural or surgically induced variety – are better off using bio-identical testosterone replacement if they have signs and symptoms suggesting a testosterone deficiency that is confirmed by laboratory tests. Since the only sources of bio-identical testosterone in female-suitable doses in the US at present are compounding pharmacies, this puts NAMS in the rather awkward position of having to grudgingly present this as the only realistic option, despite their habitually strong misgivings about anything that doesn't have an FDA-"approved" label on it.

The IHS, which points out that "all women who live long enough may expect to be in need of testosterone supplementation," has no reservations about compounded topical testosterone formulations.[66] They recommend doses that restore testosterone levels to those typically found in women in their 20s or 30s. They prefer that women also use adequate doses of topical bio-identical estrogens and progesterone, not just for the normal hormone replacement benefits, but also to prevent signs of virilization (eg, facial or body hair, deepening voice, and acne), which might occur with testosterone replacement in the absence of the "female" hormones. (NAMS also recommends female hormone replacement, although they're basically satisfied with one of the patented versions of HRT.)

Nonsexual Benefits of Testosterone Replacement
In men, testosterone replacement has well-documented benefits not only for libido and sexuality, but also for such nonsexual factors as a general sense of well-being, mood, energy level, bone and muscle mass, cardiovascular health, and cognitive function. Although good strong clinical evidence has not shown similar nonsexual benefits in women, a limited number of small studies,[57, 67] as well as clinical experience by the many doctors who have been prescribing it, suggest that, as long as women use topical, physiologic doses of *bio-identical testosterone*, they may indeed benefit in terms of the following:

- Enhanced sense of well-being
- Reduced fatigue
- Less depression
- Lower risk of osteoporosis
- Increased lean body mass and reduced fat tissue mass
- Improved cognition, lower risk of dementia
- Reduced risk of breast cancer

Use of oral methyltestosterone (Estratest®) would no doubt negate all these benefits and also increase the risks of breast cancer and cardiovascular disease; on the bright side, though, it's FDA-"approved".

Keeping Your Mind and Memory Sharp

One of the complaints women voice most frequently during and after menopause is that they're suddenly becoming more forgetful. Loss of memory and other aspects of "mental sharpness" are common in women (and men) as they grow older, with symptoms ranging from the occasional "senior moment" to full blown Alzheimer's disease. Studies show that at least 10% of men and women already have some form of cognitive impairment by age 65; by age 85, the incidence rises to 50%.[68]

Since cognitive symptoms tend to increase with the advent of perimenopause and menopause, it's been widely hypothesized that the decline in mental function is at least partially a result of falling levels of estrogen and progesterone (as well as testosterone, although, as noted above, the decline in testosterone is independent of menopause). This connection is bolstered by numerous lab studies showing that all three hormones act directly on neurons (nerve cells) in the brain, providing a variety of plausible biologic mechanisms, including:

- Facilitating neurotransmission
- Protecting neurons from attack by neurotoxins and free radicals
- Enhancing cerebral vasodilation and blood flow.

Through these and other actions, the hormones could protect against loss of memory and cognition and the progression of dementia.[69, 70]

HRT's Effects on Cognitive Function: The WHI Strikes Again

Early clinical studies using conventional patented HRT in naturally menopausal women offered a muddy picture on the whole, at best failing to confirm or refute any benefits of "hormone replacement" on cognitive function or protection against cognitive loss and dementia.[69, 71, 72] Some studies suggested improvement related to HRT, but others not. Moreover, the positive findings were usually difficult to trust due to serious weaknesses in study methodology, including the so-called "healthy woman effect." According to this effect, which also seems to have biased early studies of HRT's effects on cardiovascular disease (See Chapter 8.), women who choose (and possibly ask their doctors for) HRT tend to be generally healthier, better educated, and of a higher socioeconomic status, compared with those not opting for HRT. Thus, any apparent improvements in cognitive function in the HRT group may have been due, at least in part, not necessarily to HRT treatment, but to the women's superior health, education, and socioeconomic status prior to treatment.

While HRT may or may not have prevented cognitive impairment in these studies, hardly anyone expected that it would actually make things worse. Then along came the Women's Health Initiative again. This time it was an adjunct of the WHI, the ***Women's Health Initiative Memory***

The Unkindest – *and Least Necessary* – Cut of All

It has unfortunately become common practice for women undergoing pelvic surgery, especially removal of the uterus (hysterectomy), to also have their otherwise healthy ovaries removed (*oophorectomy*), regardless of their risk of ovarian cancer or the consequences for their subsequent sexual life and general well-being.

The reasoning goes something like this: With menopause either already at hand or imminent, women no longer need their ovaries anyway, so why hold onto them and risk the possibility – remote as it may be – of developing ovarian cancer?

This attitude and practice can be traced to the early 1980s after a Swedish survey predicted a 10% reduction in ovarian cancer incidence if all women over age 40 would just have their ovaries out prophylactically as long as the surgeons were already "in there" removing their uterus, or some other organ. Wrote the male authors, "*Not to perform prophylactic oophorectomy during pelvic surgery after the menopause seems to us to be an unreasonable practice.*"[1]

Aside from the fact that healthy postmenopausal ovaries continue secreting testosterone and androstenedione, perhaps for the rest of a woman's life, a series of studies from the Mayo Clinic[2] have shown that premenopausal ovarian removal (especially if both ovaries are removed) is linked – in an age-dependent fashion – with significantly higher risks of cardiovascular disease, osteoporosis, cognitive impairment and dementia, Parkinson's disease, a decline in sexual function and psychological well-being, as well as premature death from all causes.

We can only wonder whether similar reasoning would ever be applied to men to encourage them to have their testes removed once they were no longer considering fathering children, just to reduce the remote risk of prostate cancer.

Study (WHIMS), which was designed to be the last word on conventional HRT's effects on the menopause-related risks of cognitive impairment and dementia, just as the WHI itself had been for heart disease, stroke, and breast cancer. WHIMS was by far the largest randomized, double-blind, placebo-controlled, prospective clinical trial to date comparing the effects of conventional HRT – Prempro® (or Premarin® only in "women without a uterus") with placebo – on the incidence of dementia, mild cognitive impairment (MCI), or global cognitive function. HRT was started long past menopause in these women, who were aged 65 to 79.[73-75]

To just about everyone's surprise, WHIMS convincingly showed that both Prempro® and Premarin® alone actually *doubled the risk of probable dementia*, compared to placebo. (In absolute numbers, the differences amounted to an annual increase of 23 newly diagnosed cases of probable dementia per 10,000 women treated.) The increased risk was evident as early as 1 year into the study, and it persisted through 5 years of follow-up.

The WHIMS results also showed that, in women who had early signs of cognitive loss *even before starting on HRT*, "hormone" replacement using *horse estrogens,* rather than slowing the progression to dementia, actually accelerated it.[75] This finding led the study authors to caution that such women using conventional HRT could be putting themselves at a particularly high risk for severe dementia.

A later examination of the WHIMS data suggested a possible reason for the increased dementia in HRT users. Using MRI scans of the brains of 1,403 women, aged 71 to 89, who had participated in WHIMS, the researchers found that approximately 3 years after the Prempro® arm ended and 1.4 years after the Premarin®-only arm ended, Premarin® use was associated with a significant increase in brain atrophy compared to placebo, especially in such crucial areas for cognition as the frontal lobes and hippocampus.[76]

Endogenous Estrogens and Cognitive Function: A Stronger Connection?
Another way of looking at the connection between hormones and mental function is to compare women with and without cognitive loss in terms of the total exposure to their own *endogenous natural estrogens* over the course of their lives, from menarche (first menstrual period) to

menopause. If estrogens (and other hormones) were truly protective, women who had experienced greater total hormone exposure (eg, more years between menarche and menopause) would be expected to manifest a lower incidence of cognitive loss as they aged. Unfortunately, such studies are extremely difficult to conduct, and only a few have tried to examine this relationship. Not surprisingly, their results have been conflicting and inconclusive.[71, 77, 78]

Perhaps the most unambiguous illustration of a connection between endogenous estrogen and cognitive function can be found in women undergoing surgically induced menopause – the sudden, complete withdrawal of all ovarian hormones. In a study from the Mayo Clinic in Rochester, Minnesota, women who had had either one or both ovaries surgically removed prior to natural menopause were found to have a *46% higher risk of developing cognitive impairment or dementia*, compared to women who retained their ovaries. This effect was age-dependent: the younger the women were at the time of surgery, the greater was their risk of developing cognitive impairment or dementia,[79] (not to mention increased risks of cardiovascular disease, osteoporosis, Parkinson's disease, impaired sexual function and psychological well-being, and premature death from any cause).[80, 81] (*See box: The Unkindest – and Least Necessary – Cut of All, on page 119.*)

Is there a "Window of Opportunity" for Improving Cognitive Function?

Are we confused yet? No one will deny that the relationship between estrogen (and other sex steroids), cognitive function, and the risk of dementia is extremely complex and not very well understood. There is no easy answer at this point as to whether high ovarian hormone exposure or HRT is beneficial or detrimental in the long run.

Nevertheless, recent findings have suggested a way out of the dilemma. One possible reason for much of the uncertainty may lie in the timing of the hormone replacement. Most studies that have found "estrogen" replacement to be ineffective in preventing loss of cognitive function, including the WHIMS, which initiated HRT at least 10 years after menopause. On the other hand, studies showing a benefit generally began HRT right around the time that menstrual periods ceased. These data suggest the existence of an optimal *"window of opportunity"* during which hormone replacement must be initiated in order to protect crucial brain structures from age-related damage.[82]

The best clinical evidence so far for such a critical therapeutic window comes from the Cache County Study, which examined the risk of Alzheimer's disease in 1,889 women (mean age, 74.5 years) who lived in Cache County, Utah between 1995 and 2000.[83] Among those women who had used HRT (most likely Premarin® + Provera®) at some time after menopause, there was an overall 59% reduction in Alzheimer's incidence. Most importantly, though, those women who had initiated HRT shortly after menopause and continued it for at least 10 years had a 2.5-fold lower incidence of Alzheimer's disease, compared with nonusers of HRT. On the other hand, HRT offered little, if any, protection when started 10 or more years after menopause and therefore, closer to the onset of Alzheimer's symptoms.

These results make sense in light of the fact that overt mental symptoms of Alzheimer's disease (eg, memory loss, confusion) don't typically become apparent until brain damage is already very far advanced. In other words, if HRT (or BHRT) is initiated early on in the Alzheimer's pathogenic process, before much damage has occurred, it is likely to be much more effective in slowing or even halting disease progression.
In this regard, the Cache County investigators found a lower risk even among women who had started HRT early but had quit after a few years, compared with users who started HRT many years after menopause, and were still using it at the time of the study.

These findings were echoed in small, placebo-controlled trial (343 women), in which the women received HRT for just 2 to 3 years beginning shortly after menopause and then stopped, but they were monitored 5, 11, and 15 years later. As long as 15 years later, the risk of cognitive impairment was 64% lower in the HRT-treated women than in those in the placebo group.[84] In fact, a close look at the results of the WHIMS trial revealed a similar effect: a reduced risk of dementia was seen only in women who had started and quit HRT, shortly after menopause, but prior to enrolling in the study, rather than 10 to 15 years afterwards.[75]

Bio-identical Hormones vs. Conventional HRT: Do They Differ in Cognitive Protection?

There is little hard evidence to answer this question, since the vast majority of relevant studies have employed Premarin® + Provera® or Premarin® alone. However, a few studies have employed bio-identical estradiol, and their results are telling. One meta-analysis (an analysis of the results of several similar studies) found that 5 of 7 studies that employed estradiol showed cognitive protection, compared to 0 of 3 studies that used Premarin®.[85]

In single study of postmenopausal women, 10 women taking Premarin® (+ a progestin) and 4 taking estradiol (+ a progestin) underwent a functional MRI (ƒMRI), a neuroimaging procedure that measures blood flow (hence, mental activity) in specific regions of the brain in real time. During the ƒMRI procedure, each woman completed a series of cognitive tests. The results showed that the women taking Premarin® had poorer memory performance overall than did those taking estradiol or those taking no "hormone replacement" at all.[86]

Another study evaluated the combined effects of endogenous and exogenous hormone exposure on cognitive function in Swedish twins, aged 65 to 84.[87] The estrogen replacement in this study consisted primarily of a transdermal, topical, or oral preparation of either estriol, estrone, or the, highly potent, patented "estrogen," ethinyl estradiol (Premarin® + Provera® is used very rarely in Sweden and the rest of Europe). At the conclusion, the women who had had the greatest total estrogen exposure (endogenous + exogenous estrogens) showed the least cognitive impairment. Moreover, those who used hormone replacement (primarily estradiol) had an average 40% reduction in the risk of cognitive impairment.

Not only do bio-identical estrogens provide important neuroprotection in the brain, so also do progesterone and testosterone. Studies in lab animals have demonstrated that progesterone (but not patented progestin drugs) has a variety of neuroprotective effects, including antioxidant activity, promyelinating effects (preserving and restoring the myelin sheaths that surround, insulate, and protect neurons), and neuroregenerating effects. By contrast, medroxyprogesterone (Provera®) antagonizes estrogen's neuroprotective and memory-promoting effects.[70]

In summary, based on extensive laboratory evidence, but limited clinical evidence, it seems likely that menopausal hormone replacement may enhance cognitive function and reduce the risks of dementia and Alzheimer's disease in postmenopausal women, but only under certain conditions. Hormone replacement (preferably BHRT) should take advantage of an apparent "window of opportunity," beginning as soon after menopause as possible (or during perimenopause), and it should be continued for as long as possible.

Clinical studies suggest that bio-identical hormones (ie, estradiol and progesterone) are superior to horse estrogens and patented progestin drugs (eg, Provera®) due to the former's inherent, well-documented ability to protect brain neurons and cognitive function and the latter's often destructive effects. Moreover, to the degree that conventional HRT might be effective for protecting cognitive function, prohibitions against its extended use due to its proven risks (eg, heart disease, strokes, breast cancer) make it impractical for this purpose anyway. Since no such risks have been associated with properly used BHRT, long-term use is possible and may well provide important protection against cognitive loss.

Get a Good Night's Sleep, with a Little Help from Progesterone

It is quite common for peri- and postmenopausal women to experience sleep problems, most commonly difficulty falling asleep, waking up frequently, and difficulty falling back to sleep. As many as 60% of postmenopausal women have been reported to suffer from insomnia.[88, 89] Such disturbances, which appear to have many causes, including hormonal changes, vasomotor symptoms (hot flushes/night sweats), anxiety, depression, and stress,[90] can lead to daytime fatigue, loss of concentration, mood changes, and a deterioration in sensorimotor coordination.

Conventional HRT has been reported to improve sleep in some women, but not so in others. Recent research suggests that a key factor in improving sleep in menopausal women may be *bio-identical progesterone.*

A small study (21 women) from France compared sleep patterns in women taking either conventional HRT (Premarin® + Provera®) or Premarin® + oral micronized progesterone.[91] It is worth noting that the women were not selected for the study on the basis of having a sleep problem, and none reported any sleep problems at the start of the study. The women spent 2 nights in a sleep lab at the start of the study (baseline) before starting "hormone replacement" and 2 more nights in the lab after 6 months of treatment. While in the sleep lab, the researchers were able to closely monitor the women's sleeping patterns.

The results showed that the women in the progesterone group had a significant improvement in sleep efficiency – faster sleep onset, fewer awakenings, and more than 40 minutes more total time sleeping throughout the night – compared with those in the Provera® group.

While taking a typical patented "sleeping pill" (hypnotic drug) might be expected to produce similar results, the sleep-inducing effects of progesterone are superior, because the hormone does not alter normal sleep "architecture" (the various regular stages of sleep) as most such drugs do, nor is progesterone associated with daytime sleepiness.

Progesterone's sedative effects are well known. In fact, its only noteworthy side effect from too high a dose (especially oral formulations) is daytime sleepiness. While oral micronized progesterone was used in this study, applying the hormone as a vaginal cream has been shown to be superior for promoting the length and quality of sleep (as well as other progestogenic effects), because it improves absorption and bioavailability.[92] (*See Chapter 9 for more on preferred dosing strategies.*)

Relieving Depression

Depression occurs with greater frequency in women during times of hormonal fluctuation, such as during the days prior to menstruation (*premenstrual syndrome, PMS*), during the months after giving birth (*postpartum depression*), and during the years immediately preceding menopause (*perimenopause*). In fact, women who tended to get depressed as part of PMS when they were younger are at higher risk for depression during the perimenopause, especially the late perimenopause.[93] However, once women complete the transition to menopause, the frequency of depression is likely to decrease. Indeed, it is not uncommon for women with long-standing depression to find their dark clouds lift once they stop menstruating.

Although a variety of psychosocial, physiological, genetic, and other factors can predispose a woman to depression, when it occurs at these particular times, sex steroid hormones, particularly estrogen, testosterone, and DHEA, may well be involved. The rationale for this effect is quite clear. Many studies in lab animals have shown that sex steroids affect neurologic events in the areas of the brain known to be involved in mood control.[94]

Does hormone replacement relieve depression? Generally, "estrogen" replacement (using either oral Premarin® or topical estradiol) has been shown to have a significant antidepressant or "mood-elevating" effect in women suffering from depression during the 2 to 3 years before menopause, but after menopause, it doesn't help much at all.

In one typical double-blind, placebo-controlled study, 50 perimenopausal women with depression used estradiol or placebo skin patches for 12 weeks. Among the estradiol-treated women, 68% (17/25) experienced a remission of their depression, compared with 20% (5/25) of those in the

Repeat after Me: *Provera® Is Not Progesterone*

As these studies on cognition and sleep once again remind us, contrary to the conventional medical wisdom, Provera® is not progesterone!

While they both "oppose" Premarin®-induced overgrowth of the uterine lining, progesterone has many more beneficial effects throughout the body. Helping to protect against dementia and to induce and maintain sleep are just a couple of such actions. (See Chapter 2.)

In light of these results and many, many others, to maintain that progesterone is needed only in "women with a uterus" in order to prevent Premarin®-induced uterine cancer is beyond absurd. This may be true for Provera® and other progestins, which, in fact, don't have many other benefits, but it makes absolutely no sense for progesterone.

placebo group.[95] In another small, double-blind, placebo-controlled study in 34 women with perimenopause-related depression, estradiol treatment resulted in complete or partial improvement in 80% after just 3 weeks, compared to 22% in the placebo group.[96]

Don't Forget Your Androgens!

In addition to estrogen, both testosterone and DHEA replacement have also been shown to significantly enhance mood and/or relieve depression in women whose levels of these hormones have declined significantly.[97-101]

Preventing Estrogen-Related Blood Clots

Abnormal blood clotting (venous thromboembolism, VTE) due to "estrogen" has been a concern ever since the early days of oral contraceptive pills. These pills, which are typically composed of a patented, potent "estrogen" (eg, ethinyl estradiol) and a patented progestin, have always been associated with a relatively high risk of *thrombophlebitis* (clotting in inflamed veins, usually in the legs), especially in women who smoke. Thrombophlebitis can also occur during pregnancy, when estrogen (primarily estriol) levels are also unusually high. Blood clots in the legs are troublesome and painful enough, but if they should break away and travel to the heart, lungs, or brain, as they are prone to do, the consequences can be devastating.

Over the years, patented "estrogen" levels in oral contraceptives have been reduced, which has diminished the risk of VTEs. In women on conventional HRT, which employs doses of patented "estrogen" that are generally far lower than those used in the "pill," the risk is relatively low (about 1.5 cases in 10,000 women per year[102]). Nevertheless, the risk is significantly higher than it is in women not using conventional HRT. Recent epidemiologic and retrospective analyses of postmenopausal women find that those who used oral Premarin® had about a 2- to 3-fold higher risk of VTE than those who did not. The risk appears to be higher during the first year of HRT use (when it is about 3- to 4-fold higher).[102-105]

The route of estrogen administration is also a very important factor. No surprise here! In studies comparing oral and topical administration, oral Premarin® significantly activated various blood clotting factors and increased the risk of thromboembolism by a factor of 3.5, while the topically applied bio-identical estrogen (eg, estradiol or estriol creams) had no detrimental effects.[106, 107]

Does estriol increase the risk of thromboembolism? At high levels, such as those occurring during pregnancy, it's possible, since pregnant women, who have very high levels of estriol are at increased risk. However, the risk of abnormal blood clotting from the estriol in topically applied BHRT is extremely small (*For more on this topic, see Chapter 9*).

Nevertheless, there are safe, natural measures women can take to reduce their risk even further. Over the years, I've (JVW) observed that combinations of cod liver oil (1 - 1½ tablespoons daily) and vitamin E (400 - 800 IU of "mixed tocopherols" daily) help enormously in preventing phlebitis. When taken regularly, these items are nearly 100% effective for preventing abnormal blood clotting, even during pregnancy.

Acceptance & Tolerability of BHRT

Unlike conventional HRT, which has so many unpleasant side effects (not to mention increased risks of cancer, heart disease, blood clots, etc) that at least half the women who start on it quit within a few months, women tend to be very happy with bio-identical hormones. For example, Japanese women using oral estriol replacement following natural or surgically induced menopause, had high (about 75%) satisfaction scores right from the start of treatment and improved steadily over the next 12 months to 85% and 93%, respectively (Fig. 5-4).[9]

Another survey of 78 menopausal women in the US using bio-identical hormones from compounding pharmacies asked the women to report any side effects they might have experienced.[5] Of these women, 55 had previously used conventional HRT. Figure 5-5 shows that earlier treatment with conventional HRT consistently produced more adverse side effects than subsequent BHRT. Overall, 58% of the women reported fewer adverse side effects with BHRT.

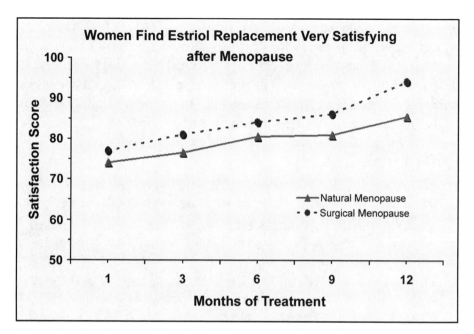

Figure 5-4. Satisfaction with oral estriol replacement therapy increases over 12 months of treatment in women following natural or surgically induced menopause.
Adapted from Takahashi et al, 2000

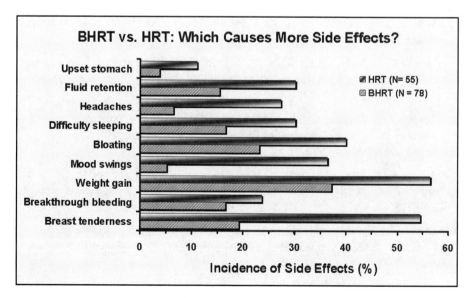

Figure 5-5. Postmenopausal women taking bio-identical hormones reported far lower incidence of side effects compared with their previous experience using conventional HRT.
Adapted from Lauritzen, 2000

Admittedly, this study has a built-in bias in favor of BHRT, since many of the women switched to BHRT precisely because of HRT's side effects. Nevertheless, it illustrates what doctors who prescribe BHRT know quite well: that women generally tolerate bio-identical hormones far better than the patented "hormones" used in conventional HRT. The very few side effects associated with BHRT can usually be reduced or eliminated by adjusting the dose or the metabolism of the hormones.

References

1. Grundsell H, Ekman G, Gullberg B, et al. Some aspects of prophylactic oophorectomy and ovarian carcinoma. *Ann Chir Gynaecol.* 1981;70:36-42.

2. Shuster LT, Gostout BS, Grossardt BR, Rocca WA. Prophylactic oophorectomy in premenopausal women and long-term health. *Menopause Int.* 2008;14:111-116.

3. Vigesaa K, Downhour N, Chui M, Cappellini L, Musil J, McCallian D. Efficacy and tolerability of compounded bioidentical hormone replacement therapy. *Int J Pharmaceutical Compounding.* 2004;8:313-319.

4. Tzingounis VA, Aksu MF, Greenblatt RB. Estriol in the management of the menopause. *Jama.* 1978;239:1638-1641.

5. Lauritzen C. Results of a 5-year prospective study of estriol succinate treatment in patients with climacteric complaints. *Horm Metabol Res.* 1987;19:579-584.

6. Perovic D, Kopajtic B, Stankovic T. Treatment of climacteric complaints with oestriol. *Arzneimittelforschung.* 1975;25:962-964.

7. Yang TS, Tsan SH, Chang SP, Ng HT. Efficacy and safety of estriol replacement therapy for climacteric women. *Zhonghua Yi Xue Za Zhi (Taipei).* 1995;55:386-391.

8. Takahashi K, Manabe A, Okada M, Kurioka H, Kanasaki H, Miyazaki K. Efficacy and safety of oral estriol for managing postmenopausal symptoms. *Maturitas.* 2000;34:169-177.

9. Takahashi K, Okada M, Ozaki T, et al. Safety and efficacy of oestriol for symptoms of natural or surgically induced menopause. *Hum Reprod.* 2000;15:1028-1036.

10. Mattsson LA, Cullberg G. Vaginal absorption of two estriol preparations. A comparative study in postmenopausal women. *Acta Obstet Gynecol Scand.* 1983;62:393-396.

11. Mattsson LA, Cullberg G. A clinical evaluation of treatment with estriol vaginal cream versus suppository in postmenopausal women. *Acta Obstet Gynecol Scand.* 1983;62:397-401.

12. Mattsson LA, Cullberg G, Eriksson O, Knutsson F. Vaginal administration of low-dose oestradiol--effects on the endometrium and vaginal cytology. *Maturitas.* 1989;11:217-222.

13. Luisi M, Franchi F, Kicovic PM. A group-comparative study of effects of Ovestin cream versus Premarin cream in post-menopausal women with vaginal atrophy. *Maturitas.* 1980;2:311-319.

14. Kicovic PM, Cortes-Prieto J, Milojevic S, Haspels AA, Aljinovic A. The treatment of postmenopausal vaginal atrophy with Ovestin vaginal cream or suppositories: clinical, endocrinological and safety aspects. *Maturitas.* 1980;2:275-282.

15. Heimer GM, Englund DE. Effects of vaginally-administered oestriol on post-menopausal urogenital disorders: a cytohormonal study. *Maturitas.* 1992;14:171-179.

16. Molander U, Milsom I, Ekelund P, Mellstrom D, Eriksson O. Effect of oral oestriol on vaginal flora and cytology and urogenital symptoms in the post-menopause. *Maturitas.* 1990;12:113-120.

17. Hustin J, Van den Eynde JP. Cytologic evaluation of the effect of various estrogens given in postmenopause. *Acta Cytol.* 1977;21:225-228.

18. Willhite LA, O'Connell MB. Urogenital atrophy: prevention and treatment. *Pharmacotherapy.* 2001;21:464-480.

19. Yoshimura T, Okamura H. Short term oral estriol treatment restores normal premenopausal vaginal flora to elderly women. *Maturitas.* 2001;39:253-257.

20. Romano JM, Kaye D. UTI in the elderly: common yet atypical. *Geriatrics.* 1981;36:113-115, 120.

21. Kirkengen AL, Andersen P, Gjersoe E, Johannessen GR, Johnsen N, Bodd E. Oestriol in the prophylactic treatment of recurrent urinary tract infections in postmenopausal women. *Scand J Prim Health Care.* 1992;10:139-142.

22. Parsons CL, Schmidt JD. Control of recurrent lower urinary tract infection in the postmenopausal woman. *J Urol.* 1982;128:1224-1226.

23. Raz R, Stamm WE. A controlled trial of intravaginal estriol in postmenopausal women with recurrent urinary tract infections. *N Engl J Med.* 1993;329:753-756.

24. Raz R, Colodner R, Rohana Y, et al. Effectiveness of estriol-containing vaginal pessaries and nitrofurantoin macrocrystal therapy in the prevention of recurrent urinary tract infection in postmenopausal women. *Clin Infect Dis.* 2003;36:1362-1368.

25. Brandberg A, Mellstrom D, Samsioe G. Low dose oral estriol treatment in elderly women with urogenital infections. *Acta Obstet Gynecol Scand Suppl.* 1987;140:33-38.

26. Kanne B, Jenny J. [Local administration of low-dose estriol and vital

Lactobacillus acidophilus in postmenopause]. *Gynakol Rundsch.* 1991;31:7-13.

27. Eriksen B. A randomized, open, parallel-group study on the preventive effect of an estradiol-releasing vaginal ring (Estring) on recurrent urinary tract infections in postmenopausal women. *Am J Obstet Gynecol.* 1999;180:1072-1079.

28. Oliveria SA, Klein RA, Reed JI, Cirillo PA, Christos PJ, Walker AM. Estrogen replacement therapy and urinary tract infections in postmenopausal women aged 45-89. *Menopause.* 1998;5:
4-8.

29. Ouslander JG, Greendale GA, Uman G, Lee C, Paul W, Schnelle J. Effects of oral estrogen and progestin on the lower urinary tract among female nursing home residents. *J Am Geriatr Soc.* 2001;49:803-807.

30. Brown JS, Vittinghoff E, Kanaya AM, Agarwal SK, Hulley S, Foxman B. Urinary tract infections in postmenopausal women: effect of hormone therapy and risk factors. *Obstet Gynecol.* 2001;98:1045-1052.

31. Orlander JD, Jick SS, Dean AD, Jick H. Urinary tract infections and estrogen use in older women. *J Am Geriatr Soc.* 1992;40:817-820.

32. Hunskaar S, Burgio K, Diokno A, Herzog AR, Hjalmas K, Lapitan MC. Epidemiology and natural history of urinary incontinence in women. *Urology.* 2003;62:16-23.

33. Klutke JJ, Bergman A. Hormonal influence on the urinary tract. *Urol Clin North Am.* 1995;22:629-639.

34. Tsai E, Yang C, Chen H, Wu C, Lee J. Bladder neck circulation by Doppler ultrasonography in postmenopausal women with urinary stress incontinence. *Obstet Gynecol.* 2001;98:52-56.

35. Melville JL, Katon W, Delaney K, Newton K. Urinary incontinence in US women: a population-based study. *Arch Intern Med.* 2005;165:537-542.

36. Brown JS, Grady D, Ouslander JG, Herzog AR, Varner RE, Posner SF. Prevalence of urinary incontinence and associated risk factors in postmenopausal women. Heart & Estrogen/Progestin Replacement Study (HERS) Research Group. *Obstet Gynecol.* 1999;94:66-70.

37. Melville JL, Delaney K, Newton K, Katon W. Incontinence severity and major depression in incontinent women. *Obstet Gynecol.* 2005;106:585-592.

38. Urinary incontinence in women. *Obstet Gynecol.* 2005;105:1533-1545.

39. Hendrix SL, Cochrane BB, Nygaard IE, et al. Effects of estrogen with and without progestin on urinary incontinence. *JAMA.* 2005;293:935-948.

40. Steinauer JE, Waetjen LE, Vittinghoff E, et al. Postmenopausal hormone therapy: does it cause incontinence? *Obstet Gynecol.* 2005;106:940-945.

41. Grady D, Brown JS, Vittinghoff E, Applegate W, Varner E, Snyder T. Postmenopausal hormones and incontinence: the Heart and Estrogen/Progestin

Replacement Study. *Obstet Gynecol.* 2001;97:116-120.

42. Iosif CS. Effects of protracted administration of estriol on the lower genito urinary tract in postmenopausal women. *Arch Gynecol Obstet.* 1992;251:115-120.

43. Schar G, Kochli OR, Fritz M, Haller U. [Effect of vaginal estrogen therapy on urinary incontinence in postmenopause]. *Zentralbl Gynakol.* 1995;117:77-80.

44. Ballagh SA. Vaginal rings for menopausal symptom relief. *Drugs Aging.* 2004;21:757-766.

45. Ballagh SA. Vaginal hormone therapy for urogenital and menopausal symptoms. *Semin Reprod Med.* 2005;23:126-140.

46. Schmidt J. Perspectives of estrogen treatment in skin aging. *Exp Dermatol.* 2005;14:156.

47. Sator PG, Schmidt JB, Rabe T, Zouboulis CC. Skin aging and sex hormones in women -- clinical perspectives for intervention by hormone replacement therapy. *Exp Dermatol.* 2004;13 Suppl 4:36-40.

48. Hudson T. Women's health update: women and skin conditions. *Townsend Letter for Doctors & Patients.* May 2003.

49. Wildt L, Sir-Petermann T. Oestrogen and age estimations of perimenopausal women. *Lancet.* 1999;354:224.

50. Punnonen R, Soderstrom KO. The effect of oral estriol succinate therapy on the endometrial morphology in postmenopausal women: the significance of fractionation of the dose. *Eur J Obstet Gynecol Reprod Biol.* 1983;14:217-224.

51. Punnonen R, Vaajalahti P, Teisala K. Local oestriol treatment improves the structure of elastic fibers in the skin of postmenopausal women. *Ann Chir Gynaecol Suppl.* 1987;202:39-41.

52. Schmidt JB, Lindmaier A, Spona J. Hormone receptors in pubic skin of premenopausal and postmenopausal females. *Gynecol Obstet Invest.* 1990;30:97-100.

53. Grosman N. Study on the hyaluronic acid-protein complex, the molecular size of hyaluronic acid and the exchangeability of chloride in skin of mice before and after oestrogen treatment. *Acta Pharmacol Toxicol (Copenh).* 1973;33:201-208.

54. Grosman N, Hvidberg E, Schou J. The effect of oestrogenic treatment on the acid mucopolysaccharide pattern in skin of mice. *Acta Pharmacol Toxicol (Copenh).* 1971;30:458-464.

55. Schmidt JB, Binder M, Demschik G, Bieglmayer C, Reiner A. Treatment of skin aging with topical estrogens. *Int J Dermatol.* 1996;35:669-674.

56. Utian WH. Effect of hysterectomy, oophorectomy and estrogen therapy on libido. *Int J Gynaecol Obstet.* 1975;13:97-100.

57. Simon JA, Abdallah RT. Testosterone therapy in women: its role in the management of hypoactive sexual desire disorder. *Int J Impot Res.* 2007;19:458-463.

58. Nair KS, Rizza RA, O'Brien P, et al. DHEA in elderly women and DHEA or testosterone in elderly men. *N Engl J Med.* 2006;355:1647-1659.

59. Basaria S, Dobs AS. Clinical review: Controversies regarding transdermal androgen therapy in postmenopausal women. *J Clin Endocrinol Metab.* 2006;91:4743-4752.

60. Serin IS, Ozcelik B, Basbug M, Aygen E, Kula M, Erez R. Long-term effects of continuous oral and transdermal estrogen replacement therapy on sex hormone binding globulin and free testosterone levels. *Eur J Obstet Gynecol Reprod Biol.* 2001;99:222-225.

61. Davison SL, Bell R, Donath S, Montalto JG, Davis SR. Androgen levels in adult females: changes with age, menopause, and oophorectomy. *J Clin Endocrinol Metab.* 2005;90:3847-3853.

62. Laughlin GA, Barrett-Connor E, Kritz-Silverstein D, von Muhlen D. Hysterectomy, oophorectomy, and endogenous sex hormone levels in older women: the Rancho Bernardo Study. *J Clin Endocrinol Metab.* 2000;85:645-651.

63. Kingsberg S. Testosterone treatment for hypoactive sexual desire disorder in postmenopausal women. *J Sex Med.* 2007;4 Suppl 3:227-234.

64. Simon J, Braunstein G, Nachtigall L, et al. Testosterone patch increases sexual activity and desire in surgically menopausal women with hypoactive sexual desire disorder. *J Clin Endocrinol Metab.* 2005;90:5226-5233.

65. The role of testosterone therapy in postmenopausal women: position statement of The North American Menopause Society. *Menopause.* 2005;12:497-511.

66. The International Hormone Society. Physician Consensus: Testosterone Therapy of Testosterone Deficiency in Women. December 5, 2005; http:// intlhormonesociety.org/index.php?option =com_content&task=view&id=37&Ite mid=71&tomHack_idp=8:Accessed September 20, 2007.

67. Somboonporn W. Testosterone therapy for postmenopausal women: efficacy and safety. *Semin Reprod Med.* 2006;24:115-124.

68. Yaffe K. Estrogens, selective estrogen receptor modulators, and dementia: what is the evidence? *Ann N Y Acad Sci.* 2001;949:215-222.

69. Yaffe K, Sawaya G, Lieberburg I, Grady D. Estrogen therapy in postmenopausal women: effects on cognitive function and dementia. *Jama.* 1998;279:688-695.

70. Schumacher M, Guennoun R, Ghoumari A, et al. Novel perspectives for progesterone in HRT, with special reference to the nervous system. *Endocr Rev.* 2007;28:387-439.

71. Geerlings MI, Ruitenberg A, Witteman JCM, et al. Reproductive period and risk of dementia in postmenopausal women. *JAMA.* 2001;285:1475-1481.

72. LeBlanc ES, Janowsky J, Chan BKS, Nelson HD. Hormone replacement therapy and cognition: Systematic review and meta-analysis. *JAMA.* 2001;285:1489-1499.

73. Espeland MA, Rapp SR, Shumaker SA, et al. Conjugated equine estrogens and global cognitive function in postmenopausal women: Women's Health Initiative Memory Study. *JAMA.* 2004;291:2959-2968.

74. Shumaker SA, Legault C, Kuller L, et al. Conjugated equine estrogens and incidence of probable dementia and mild cognitive impairment in postmenopausal women: Women's Health Initiative Memory Study. *JAMA.* 2004;291:2947-2958.

75. Shumaker SA, Legault C, Rapp SR, et al. Estrogen plus progestin and the incidence of dementia and mild cognitive impairment in postmenopausal women: the Women's Health Initiative Memory Study: a randomized controlled trial. *Jama.* 2003;289:2651-2662.

76. Resnick SM, Espeland MA, Jaramillo SA, et al. Postmenopausal hormone therapy and regional brain volumes: the WHIMS-MRI Study. *Neurology.* 2009;72:135-142.

77. Yaffe K, Haan M, Byers A, Tangen C, Kuller L. Estrogen use, APOE, and cognitive decline: evidence of gene-environment interaction. *Neurology.* 2000;54:1949-1954.

78. Yaffe K, Lui LY, Grady D, Cauley J, Kramer J, Cummings SR. Cognitive decline in women in relation to non-protein-bound oestradiol concentrations. *Lancet.* 2000;356:708-712.

79. Rocca WA, Bower JH, Maraganore DM, et al. Increased risk of cognitive impairment or dementia in women who underwent oophorectomy before menopause. *Neurology.* 2007;69:1074-1083.

80. Rocca WA, Bower JH, Maraganore DM, et al. Increased risk of parkinsonism in women who underwent oophorectomy before menopause. *Neurology.* 2007.

81. Rocca WA, Grossardt BR, de Andrade M, Malkasian GD, Melton LJ, 3rd. Survival patterns after oophorectomy in premenopausal women: a population-based cohort study. *Lancet Oncol.* 2006;7:821-828.

82. Genazzani AR, Pluchino N, Luisi S, Luisi M. Estrogen, cognition and female ageing. *Hum Reprod Update.* 2007;13:175-187.

83. Zandi PP, Carlson MC, Plassman BL, et al. Hormone replacement therapy and incidence of Alzheimer disease in older women: the Cache County Study. *Jama.* 2002;288:2123-2129.

84. Bagger YZ, Tanko LB, Alexandersen P, Qin G, Christiansen C. Early

postmenopausal hormone therapy may prevent cognitive impairment later in life. *Menopause.* 2005;12:12-17.

85. Hogervorst E, Williams J, Budge M, Riedel W, Jolles J. The nature of the effect of female gonadal hormone replacement therapy on cognitive function in post-menopausal women: a meta-analysis. *Neuroscience.* 2000;101:485-512.

86. Gleason CE, Schmitz TW, Hess T, et al. Hormone effects on fMRI and cognitive measures of encoding: importance of hormone preparation. *Neurology.* 2006;67:2039-2041.

87. Rasgon NL, Magnusson C, Johansson AL, Pedersen NL, Elman S, Gatz M. Endogenous and exogenous hormone exposure and risk of cognitive impairment in Swedish twins: a preliminary study. *Psychoneuroendocrinology.* 2005;30:558-567.

88. Kuh DL, Hardy R, Wadsworth M. Women's health in midlife: the influence of the menopause, social factors and health in earlier life. *Br J Obstet Gynaecol.* 1997;104:1419.

89. von Muhlen DG, Kritz-Silverstein D, Barrett-Connor E. A community-based study of menopause symptoms and estrogen replacement in older women. *Maturitas.* 1995;22:71-78.

90. Owens JF, Matthews KA. Sleep disturbance in healthy middle-aged women. *Maturitas.* 1998;30:41-50.

91. Montplaisir J, Lorrain J, Denesle R, Petit D. Sleep in menopause: differential effects of two forms of hormone replacement therapy. *Menopause.* 2001;8:10-16.

92. Gruber CJ, Huber JC. Differential effects of progestins on the brain. *Maturitas.* 2003;46 Suppl 1:S71-75.

93. Callegari C, Buttarelli M, Cromi A, Diurni M, Salvaggio F, Bolis PF. Female psychopathologic profile during menopausal transition: a preliminary study. *Maturitas.* 2007;56:447-451.

94. Schmidt PJ. Depression, the perimenopause, and estrogen therapy. *Ann N Y Acad Sci.* 2005;1052:27-40.

95. Soares CN, Cohen LS. The perimenopause, depressive disorders, and hormonal variability. *Sao Paulo Med J.* 2001;119:78-83.

96. Schmidt PJ, Nieman L, Danaceau MA, et al. Estrogen replacement in perimenopause-related depression: a preliminary report. *Am J Obstet Gynecol.* 2000;183:414-420.

97. Arlt W, Callies F, Allolio B. DHEA replacement in women with adrenal insufficiency--pharmacokinetics, bioconversion and clinical effects on well-being, sexuality and cognition. *Endocr Res.* 2000;26:505-511.

98. Davis SR, Goldstat R, Papalia MA, et al. Effects of aromatase inhibition

on sexual function and well-being in postmenopausal women treated with testosterone: a randomized, placebo-controlled trial. *Menopause.* 2006;13:37-45.

99. Goldstat R, Briganti E, Tran J, Wolfe R, Davis SR. Transdermal testosterone therapy improves well-being, mood, and sexual function in premenopausal women. *Menopause.* 2003;10:390-398.

100. Schmidt PJ, Daly RC, Bloch M, et al. Dehydroepiandrosterone monotherapy in midlife-onset major and minor depression. *Arch Gen Psychiatry.* 2005;62:154-162.

101. Shifren JL, Braunstein GD, Simon JA, et al. Transdermal testosterone treatment in women with impaired sexual function after oophorectomy. *N Engl J Med.* 2000;343:682-688.

102. Miller J, Chan BK, Nelson HD. Postmenopausal estrogen replacement and risk for venous thromboembolism: a systematic review and meta-analysis for the U.S. Preventive Services Task Force. *Ann Intern Med.* 2002;136:680-690.

103. Castellsague J, Perez Gutthann S, Garcia Rodriguez LA. Recent epidemiological studies of the association between hormone replacement therapy and venous thromboembolism. A review. *Drug Saf.* 1998;18:117-123.

104. Daly E, Vessey MP, Hawkins MM, Carson JL, Gough P, Marsh S. Risk of venous thromboembolism in users of hormone replacement therapy. *Lancet.* 1996;348:977-980.

105. Perez Gutthann S, Garcia Rodriguez LA, Castellsague J, Duque Oliart A. Hormone replacement therapy and risk of venous thromboembolism: population based case-control study. *BMJ.* 1997;314:796-800.

106. Scarabin PY, Alhenc-Gelas M, Plu-Bureau G, Taisne P, Agher R, Aiach M. Effects of oral and transdermal estrogen/progesterone regimens on blood coagulation and fibrinolysis in postmenopausal women. A randomized controlled trial. *Arterioscler Thromb Vasc Biol.* 1997;17:3071-3078.

107. Scarabin PY, Oger E, Plu-Bureau G. Differential association of oral and transdermal oestrogen-replacement therapy with venous thromboembolism risk. *Lancet.* 2003;362:428-432.

CHAPTER 6

PREVENTING AND REVERSING OSTEOPOROSIS

As women get older, especially into their 70s and beyond, one of the most devastating long-term consequences of menopause becomes more and more common. Who hasn't had an elderly mother or grandmother chronically hunched over with a "dowager's hump"? Or an aunt who falls and breaks her hip, and then spends her final months immobile and bedridden in a nursing home?

Because of a progressive disease called ***osteoporosis*** (literally, *porous bones*), as the years after menopause add up, bones can use up their stores of calcium and other minerals, leaving them increasingly fragile. Coupled with weakening muscles and impaired vision and balance, and complicated by the use of patent medicines that might make them sleepy or dizzy, the risk of a fall leading to a broken hip, spine, wrist, or rib grows with each passing year.

Osteoporosis threatens 50% of American women (and 25% of men) aged 50 or older with debilitating fractures. According to the National Osteoporosis Foundation, 8 million women already have the disease, while an additional 27 million have an early stage called *osteopenia*, in which the bones have begun to thin but are not in immediate danger of breaking. A Canadian study of more than 10,000 *randomly selected women* aged 50 or older found that 16% had osteoporosis in their spine or hip.[1]

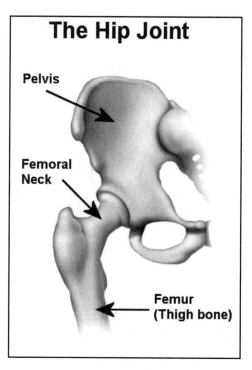

The Hip Joint

Pelvis

Femoral
Neck

Femur
(Thigh bone)

Figure 6-1. Artist's rendering of the right hip joint. Most hip fractures occur at the femoral neck.

The risk of hip fracture increases as more bone is lost, doubling with every decade of age.[5] Each year in the US, osteoporosis is directly responsible for more than 300,000 broken hips,[6] a risk greater – statistically speaking – than that of breast, uterine, and cervical cancer combined.[6]

For many women, an osteoporotic hip fracture signals the beginning of the end: one in five such fractures results in an extended – and often permanent – nursing home stay, and one in four leads to death inside of a year.[7]

The "Dowager's Hump" and Spinal Osteoporosis

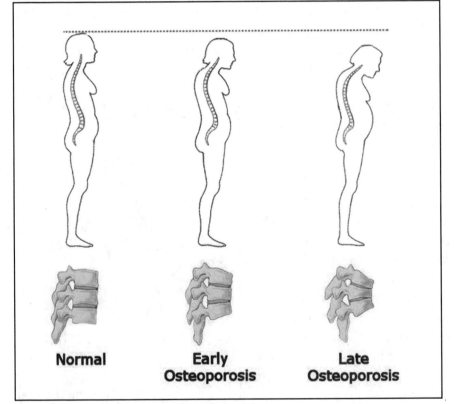

Normal   **Early Osteoporosis**   **Late Osteoporosis**

Figure 6-2. The "dowager's hump" is an abnormal outward curvature of the vertebrae of upper back caused by osteoporosis. As the disease progresses, compression fractures of the front (anterior) portion of the involved vertebrae cause the spine to bend forward (*kyphosis*). The vertebral collapse leads to the formation of a hump in the upper back combined with pain and a loss of up to several inches in height.

Osteoporosis is sometimes called a "silent disease," because bone tissue usually dissipates slowly over many years with no symptoms. Unless she undergoes special diagnostic tests to measure her bone density, the day a woman falls and breaks her hip may well be the day she discovers she has osteoporosis. For some women, it's a fall that causes their fracture. But for many others, whose bones are extremely fragile, a bone may fracture spontaneously, due to no particular event or stressor, and cause them to fall.

In addition to the *femoral neck of the hip* (Fig. 6-1) and the *vertebrae* of the spine (Fig. 6-2), the bones most vulnerable to osteoporotic fracture include those in the wrist, shoulder, and ribs. Osteoporotic vertebrae are subject to being crushed largely by the force of gravity, and they collapse due to the accumulation of many small compression fractures. As osteoporosis progresses, back pain increases, along with a loss of height and, after many years, a characteristic curvature of the spine, popularly known as a "dowager's hump," slowly evolves.

What the hip, spine, and other vulnerable bones have in common is a high proportion of sponge-like *cancellous* (or *trabecular*) bone beneath their thin, smooth surfaces (Fig. 6-3). Cancellous bone is found at the ends of long bones of the arms and legs (eg, hip (femoral neck), shoulder, and wrist) and the inner parts of flat bones (eg, ribs). By contrast, the main body of long bones like the *femur* (thigh bone)

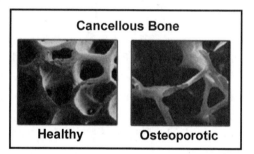

Figure 6-3. Close-up photos of sections of healthy and osteoporotic cancellous bone, as might be found in the femoral neck of the hip, vertebrae, wrists, and ribs.

are composed primarily of harder, denser *cortical* bone, which makes them much more resistant (but not invulnerable) to osteoporotic wasting and fracture.[8]

The major advantage of softer cancellous bone is its ability to be rapidly reshaped or *remodeled* in response to the body's physical and metabolic needs. The idea of skeletal remodeling, or *turnover*, may sound strange, because people sometimes forget that, for all bones' rigidity and strength, they are living tissue that is constantly renewing and reshaping itself, albeit at a much slower rate than soft tissues, such as muscle and skin. That is, after all, how fractures heal.

Although adult bones have long stopped growing in length, they continue to remodel themselves under the influence of such factors as exercise and weight distribution, as well as the actions of various hormones, vitamins, minerals, and other natural biochemicals.

The Road to Osteoporosis

Bone remodeling begins when bone gets broken down – as a normal aspect of body function – by "PacMan"-like cells called *osteoclasts*, which travel through bone tissue in search of older bone cells. When they encounter such old bone cells, osteoclasts dissolve them, releasing the bone's calcium and other minerals into the circulation, a process known as *bone resorption*. Following in the osteoclasts' wake are *tissue building* cells called *osteoblasts*. Like road crews filling in potholes, osteoblasts fill the pits left by osteoclasts by drawing calcium and other minerals out of the circulation and using it to build fresh, new bone tissue.

In addition to performing the normal skeletal functions we're all quite familiar with, bones also serve as a reservoir for minerals – especially calcium – that may be needed by other parts of the body. When we consume a healthy diet that supplies enough calcium (and other nutrients) to meet the body's regular daily needs, which can be substantial, we do not need to dip into our bone storage "vaults."

Under most conditions, osteoclasts and osteoblasts live in perfect harmony in the adult skeleton, helping to keep bones hard and strong. However, on the road to osteoporosis, the osteoclasts start to outpace the osteoblasts. To the extent that the diet is deficient in calcium and other nutrients, the body may be forced to raid its bone mineral stores to make up the deficit. Over time, if these minerals are not replaced, bone mass declines, the bones begin to thin out, and their structure degrades progressively.

Figure 6-3 shows close-up views of dense, healthy cancellous bone and osteoporotic bone. Looking at these side-by-side, it's easy to see why diseased bones break so easily. With the bulk of their superstructure gone, what's left is thin, weak, and fragile. When bone quality is so poor, bone not only fractures easily, but fractures may also heal poorly or not at all.

Why Estrogen Is Not Enough

Dietary calcium, the mineral primarily responsible for bone strength, can't form new bone tissue all by itself. Building and maintaining new bone requires a host of other factors to help incorporate calcium and other minerals. These include the major sex steroid hormones (*estrogen, progesterone, testosterone,* and *DHEA*), as well as parathyroid hormone, vitamin D, prostaglandins, growth factors, and many others.[8]

Estrogen helps maintain the remodeling balance, primarily by reining in "bone-eating" osteoclast activity. Before menopause, as long as you engage in weight-bearing exercise (exercising your bones as well as your muscles) and maintain an adequate diet, your bones will remain strong. However, once you approach menopause, with your estrogen levels in decline, osteoclasts begin to run roughshod over your bones, leading to a corresponding increase in *bone resorption.* It's not surprising, therefore, that when estrogen is nearly completely absent, as occurs following surgical removal of the ovaries, the risk of hip fracture grows by 7-fold.[9]

But estrogen is not the only hormone active in bone metabolism. Just as estrogen and progesterone are the Yin and Yang of the menstrual cycle (*See Chapter 3.*), so the two steroid hormones are also inextricably linked in the life cycle of bone tissue. *Progesterone is a key – but widely overlooked – factor needed by osteoblasts to build new bone*. While estrogen is linked to the function of osteoclasts, the decline in progesterone in the years before, during, and after menopause deprives your bone-building osteoblasts of a growth factor that is essential to their efficient activity.

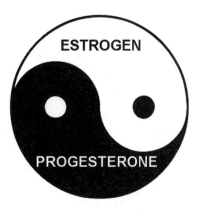

To reprise a now familiar theme, bone health and strength depend on a favorable balance between these two hormones. If estrogen is deficient, unrestrained bone resorption strips bones of vital calcium and other minerals. If progesterone is deficient, new bone cannot form to replace that which is lost to normal or accelerated postmenopausal resorption. When the two deficits are combined – as is typical in menopause – the effects are additive, possibly causing bone to waste away at an alarming rate, especially if important nutrients like calcium and vitamin D are deficient, as well.

The approach to the prevention and treatment of osteoporosis most favored by conventional medicine and aggressively promoted and promulgated by the patent medicine industry, is a one-dimensional focus on the resorption (estrogen) side of the equation. Until the Women's Health Initiative (WHI) results came out in 2002, Premarin® (with or without Provera®) was generally deemed the best available protection against menopause-related osteoporosis. The WHI did indeed demonstrate that conjugated equine estrogens (CEEs), despite their generally negative cardiovascular and carcinogenic profile, appeared to offer a small but statistically significant degree of protection against osteoporosis – a reduction of 5 to 7 hip fractures per 10,000 women, compared to placebo.[10, 11]

It's true. Estrogen replacement, using virtually any type of "estrogen," including Premarin®, can help put the brakes on menopausal bone loss. Estrogen slows osteoclast activity while, at the same time, enhancing calcium retention and absorption. The effects are dose- and time-dependent: the higher your estrogen levels, and the longer those levels remain elevated, the stronger your bones.[13]

But while estrogen helps slow bone loss, it is of virtually no help in rebuilding new bone to replace that which has already been lost.[12] Thus, "estrogen" replacement, primarily using Premarin® slows the rate of bone loss by *only about one-third* overall and decreases the fracture risk by only about 50%.[13] For the rebuilding task, you also need *progesterone*. In addition, parathyroid hormone, the androgens ("male" hormones) – *testosterone* and *DHEA* – are important, as are foods and supplements containing *calcium, magnesium, strontium, vitamin D*, and other nutrients, along with regular and frequent *weight-bearing exercise*.

In the years immediately after menopause, bone loss can be considerable, but for most women, osteoporosis doesn't usually become an important factor in fractures for another 20 or 30 years. The stronger your bones are before menopause, the longer it takes for them to thin out. Women don't usually become highly vulnerable to osteoporotic fractures until their 70s and 80s, decades after they've stopped menstruating and probably many years after most have stopped taking their patented HRT pills.

To improve her bone strength – usually measured by *bone mineral density* (*BMD*) – a woman needs to stay on "estrogen" for up to *10 or more years.*[5] Ideally, it would be nice if you could put some bone "in the bank" during these years, so you could have stronger bones when you're much older. Unfortunately though, "banking" bone using HRT doesn't really work. As soon as you stop taking "estrogen," your bones start resorbing again, and at an even more rapid rate. After only 5 years without "estrogen," all the fracture protection you may have built up during your years on HRT is likely to be completely spent, at which point you'd be no better off than if you'd never even started taking patented HRT.[12, 14]

In recent years, it has become evident that conventional HRT, with all its inherent risks and side effects, was never particularly well suited to treating a progressive disease like osteoporosis. Recall that the initial purpose of patented HRT was to relieve hot flashes, a function for which it works pretty well, just as long as you don't count its many adverse effects and long-term risks.

Unfortunately, most women hoping to improve their bones with conventional patented HRT have it all backwards: they start taking their "hormones" in their early 50s, while their bones are still relatively strong. But by the time they reach their 70s and 80s, with their bones growing thinner and weaker by the day, and just when they need their hormones most, nearly all have long since stopped taking them.[5]

Advocates of conventional HRT, desperately trying to find something positive to say about their ailing billion-dollar cash cow, continue to point out that Premarin® reduced the rate of hip fracture by about 33% in the WHI study.[15] True enough, but because it increases the risk of cancer, heart disease, and stroke, patented HRT is prescribed today at the lowest possible dose for the shortest possible time. Obviously, such a regimen is useless for preventing or treating osteoporosis, which requires continuous treatment after menopause, or else your bones will quickly begin resorbing.

While this realization may have taken a bite out of Prempro® sales, fear not for the global patent medicine industry; they've got lots of patented high-tech, anti-osteoporosis medicines they'd love to sell you. After the WHI study, when "estrogen" fell out of favor as a menopause and osteoporosis treatment, conventional medicine shifted its focus, not to other natural hormonal and nutritional approaches, but to a series of patented medications. These drugs are designed to preserve bone, but they do so in a decidedly *unnatural* – and potentially harmful – way that is discussed in detail below.

Suffice it to say, natural bone preservation and rebuilding, using *unpatented* BHRT and other important nutrients, is more effective and far safer. What follows now is a review of some of the evidence that BHRT is effective and safe in keeping bones strong and healthy, evidence that medical "experts" have been trying to convince us does not exist.

Progesterone: Forgotten *Again*!

Conventional medicine has yet to come to grips with natural progesterone, which has been "in use" in the human body for hundreds of thousands, perhaps millions of years. Only grudgingly did medical "authorities" come to recognize the importance of progesterone in the menstrual cycle as a counterbalance to Premarin-stimulated growth of the uterine lining. And then, as is typical in conventional medicine, instead of opting for the bio-identical (Nature's original) version of the hormone, they turned to patented *progestin* drugs – chemical cousins of progesterone that originated in the mind of a drug biochemist, but have no place in the natural biochemistry of the human body. The best known, most commonly used, and most dangerous of the progestins is Provera® (medroxyprogesterone).

Historically, Big Pharma has placed most of its osteoporosis money on the estrogen side of the equation. Makes sense; they already had a patented medicine – Premarin® – that can slow bone resorption. As far as they were concerned, preventing osteoporosis was estrogen's job; the *only* reason they added progestins to the mix was to keep Premarin-stimulated growth of the endometrial (uterine lining) from overheating and possibly causing cancer. Any positive effect Provera® might have had on bone growth was purely incidental.

We can't make this point strongly enough, or often enough: ***Progestins are not progesterone***.

Most doctors have been taught to make no distinction between progesterone and progestin, which makes the people who sell patent medicines very happy. (*As we noted in Chapter 4, they've been going to a lot of trouble for a lot of years to blur the lines.*) Skeptics are quick to cite the lack of strong clinical evidence supporting progesterone's role in bone metabolism, and yes, it's true, there aren't any large, long-term, double-blind, placebo-controlled WHI-like studies evaluating progesterone in people at risk for osteoporosis. Such studies would be great to have, but they are simply too expensive for anyone but Uncle Sam or Big Pharma to sponsor, and neither of them is interested in researching a nonpatentable hormone.

The publication deck is also stacked against progesterone (and other unpatentable agents). Medical journals, most of which depend on Big Pharma's big bucks to stay afloat, publish primarily progestin-based studies, the vast majority of which are sponsored directly or indirectly by patent medicine companies. By contrast, published studies of bio-identical progesterone – lacking the financial backing of patented progestins – tend to be older, fewer, smaller, sometimes less well-controlled, and often originating in other countries (where English is not the primary language). This makes it much easier for mainstream medicine to ignore or dismiss them. Nor does progesterone have a multimillion dollar advertising and public relations structure, as progestins do, to bring it to the attention of doctors and patients alike.

The Case for Progesterone

"Bullet-proof," FDA-style clinical studies of progesterone's role in osteoporosis prevention and treatment are certainly lacking at the present date. However, a considerable body of evidence, both from laboratory research and studies in actual menopausal women, as well as years of close clinical observation by physicians who prescribe BHRT, all point to the same conclusion: progesterone may be just as important as estrogen – and maybe even more important – for bone health (*not to mention dozens of other normal functions; see Chapter 2.*) throughout a woman's lifetime.

Progesterone Loss Starts Early

Healthy young women's ovaries secrete estrogen for most days of their cycles. On the other hand, most progesterone is produced and secreted by the ovaries primarily after the estrogen-ripened *follicle* ruptures each month to form the hormone-secreting *corpus luteum*. (This is in addition to a normal "baseline" amount of progesterone produced and secreted every day by the adrenal glands.) Since follicle rupture (ie, ovulation) occurs around mid-cycle – typically Day 14 to 16 – progesterone secreted by the ovaries peaks *only* during the final 10 to 16 days of the cycle, a period known as the *luteal phase.** In other words, the first half of the menstrual cycle is dominated by relatively high estrogen levels with little progesterone of ovarian origin, while the latter portion is dominated by relatively high progesterone levels along with moderate levels of estrogen.

In studies in surgically castrated (ovaries removed) laboratory rats, administration of either bio-identical *progesterone*[16] or a patented *progestin/progestogen* drug[18-20] slowed the loss of bone minerals (eg, calcium) and increased the rats' rate of bone formation. Human studies of progesterone's role in bone metabolism, where they exist at all, have tended to be small and to use Provera® or some other patented progestin rather than bio-identical progesterone itself. Nevertheless, they have generally shown an increase in new bone formation with either progesterone or progestins.[13]

For many years, the prime mover behind many of the most important findings regarding progesterone in women has been the Canadian investigator, Jerilynn C. Prior, MD, who is Professor of Endocrinology and Metabolism at the University of British Columbia, Vancouver, BC, and Scientific Director of the Centre for Menstrual Cycle and Ovulation

---

* During pregnancy, the placenta also churns out huge volumes of progesterone, which helps maintain the pregnancy and may also contribute to women's feelings of happiness and serenity during this time.

Research (www.cemcor.ubc.ca). In 1990, Dr. Prior published the first major review of progesterone research in the bones of animals and humans.[13]

Overall, her findings lead us to a startling conclusion: that bone loss actually begins *long before menopause* – sometimes as early your 30s – while your estrogen levels are still essentially normal. Between the ages of 35 and 50, you might lose as much as 75% of your progesterone. So that when you enter the perimenopausal period, with estrogen loss just beginning in earnest, your progesterone has been declining for 15 years.[17, 18, 19, 20]

Thus, it is not uncommon for women to *start* menopause with as little as 25% of their youthful progesterone on board. The decline in progesterone during the *premenopausal* years is associated with a fall in bone mass of about 1% per year. By the time of menopause, that rate accelerates to about 3 to 5% per year. During the postmenopausal years, the rate of bone loss slows to about 1 to 1.5% per year.

Dr. Prior's basic hypothesis is simple: if *bone mineral density* (BMD) – a key index of bone strength – is directly related to progesterone levels, then BMD should rise a little bit during each luteal phase, when progesterone production is at its peak. However, during the early days of the menstrual cycle, before ovulation occurs, when progesterone levels are at their lowest, BMD should decline a little, even though estrogen levels are high. The longer your luteal phase is, the more progesterone you produce each month, and the denser your bones should be. However, if you have a cycle during which no ovulation occurs – ie, no progesterone peak for that cycle – your BMD should decline slightly.

Not only do Dr. Prior's studies demonstrate that progesterone is vital for keeping bones strong, but also that BMD is extraordinarily sensitive to even small, normal, periodic shifts in progesterone level. Recall that the women in her studies were all *pre*menopausal and most were still menstruating on a regular basis. Yet, even small variations in their progesterone levels could significantly impair the growth of new bone tissue.

Now, it's one thing to argue that declining progesterone levels contribute to postmenopausal bone loss, because it places a damper on new bone building. But, it's something altogether different to claim that *progesterone replacement* can prevent – or even reverse – osteoporosis. While the available evidence for the former is strong, the evidence for the latter is unfortunately only suggestive and generally lacking in the factors that make medical studies convincing to the mainstream medical community. Nevertheless, to those physicians who prescribe BHRT on a daily basis, the benefits of progesterone replacement to skeletal health are quite evident.

Does HRT Really Protect Against Osteoporosis?

There's plenty of published evidence related to patented "estrogen" and osteoporosis. Because Big Pharma has always been interested in patented "estrogen" for squelching hot flushes, it never made much sense for them to study its effects on bones. They haven't been all that interested in Provera® (or other progestins) for anything other than blocking Premarin's cancer-causing effects in the uterus. Nearly all clinical trials that have looked at sex steroids' role in postmenopausal bone density have employed Premarin® with "progestins" essentially going along for the ride.

Dr. Prior is one of the few researchers who has given serious attention to the potential role of "progestins" – if not always progesterone – in women with osteoporosis. When she gave Provera® for 10 days a month (simulating an average luteal phase) to healthy, premenopausal women, who were experiencing occasional missed periods, anovulatory cycles, shortened luteal phases and other signs typical of impending menopause, she found that BMD increased by a small amount, just 1.7%.[21]

A Swedish questionnaire-based survey found that, for every year women were on hormone replacement therapy (the types of "hormones" were not specified, although Premarin® + Provera® are rarely used in Sweden), their risk of hip fracture decreased by 6%. The key determining factor was the presence of a progestin. For women who took only "estrogen," the risk declined by 4%, but for women who took "estrogen" + a progestin, the risk declined by 11%, nearly three times more.[13]

Although these large studies suggest that Premarin® + Provera® or Premarin® alone may enhance BMD to a small degree,[25, 26] these patented drugs have so many serious risks and side effects that their use has now been severely limited to the lowest possible dose for the shortest possible time. Thus, they are clearly inappropriate for preventing or treating osteoporosis (or anything else).

The PEPI Study

Of course, large-scale studies of sex steroids and bone health have almost always excluded bio-identical hormones. The only major exception was the NIH-sponsored Postmenopausal Estrogen-Progestin Intervention (PEPI) Study, which employed bio-identical (oral micronized) progesterone as just one of its treatment options.[22, 23]

In the PEPI study, 875 healthy postmenopausal women, took either 1) daily Premarin® alone; 2) Premarin® + Provera®, both daily; 3) Premarin® daily + Provera® 12 days per month; 4) Premarin® daily + *oral micronized progesterone* 12 days per month; or 5) placebo. BMD was measured at the start of treatment (baseline) and again after 12 and 36 months of therapy.

After 36 months, the women in the placebo group had lost 1.8% of the BMD in their spines and 1.7% of the BMD in their hips. By contrast, those treated with Premarin® alone, Premarin® + Provera®, or Premarin® + micronized progesterone *gained* between 3.5 and 5% of spine and hip BMD, respectively. Thus, oral bio-identical progesterone (combined with Premarin®) was at least as effective as Provera® for helping to restore lost BMD.

Given that bio-identical progesterone (taken orally, which is not the ideal way to take it) is virtually guaranteed to be safer than Provera®, one has to marvel at the fact that it has not replaced progestins across the board. In fact, even after this positive finding, real, bio-identical progesterone has been completely ignored. The big news coming out of the PEPI study at the time was, "Estrogen protects against osteoporosis." *Go figure!*

Progesterone and Dr. Lee

In preventing osteoporosis, Big Pharma has never taken Mother Nature seriously, generally feeling they could do a better job – or at least make a much bigger profit – using some patented ersatz "hormones." While the PEPI study provided a strong hint that bio-identical progesterone could offer safe and potentially long-term protection against osteoporotic bone loss – in contrast to Provera® or other patented progestins – mainstream medicine largely ignored this result.

It took a Northern California family physician, 20 years into his conventional medical practice, to wonder why Big Pharma seemed to be interested only in "estrogen" replacement as a means of preventing or treating osteoporosis. This was the late 1970s, and conventional medicine practitioners were finally coming to grips with the fact that the unopposed Premarin® they had been prescribing for the last couple of decades had been responsible for a frightening increase in uterine cancer.

John R. Lee, MD, had been one of those doctors, but instead of going along with patent medicine's approved "solution" to this problem – combining Premarin® with Provera® – he decided to open his mind to other ways his patients might enjoy the benefits of hormone replacement without having to put their health or life on the line.[24]

Although Premarin® was the only "approved" treatment for postmenopausal osteoporosis in those days, it was apparent that women who wanted to use it for that purpose were taking an unacceptable risk. After hearing a lecture about bio-identical progesterone at a medical meeting, Dr. Lee soon came to realize that patent medicines like Provera® could never be an acceptable solution, but that progesterone might have real potential. Despite the fact that progesterone had been available since the 1940s and could be purchased without a prescription, there was virtually no research on its effects in postmenopausal women, especially those with osteoporosis. Nevertheless, there was good reason to believe that it could be beneficial.

So, in 1980, around the same time that we had begun researching triple-estrogen at the Tahoma Clinic, Dr. Lee started prescribing a progesterone skin cream to his own patients with osteoporosis, but who could not take

Premarin® alone. He prescribed about 20 to 30 mg of progesterone per day for about 12 days each month, thus simulating the output of the normal, premenopausal ovarian follicle.

To his amazement, Dr. Lee found that the women using the progesterone cream actually *increased their BMD by about 15%.* By contrast, in women taking Premarin® only, BMD remained stable or declined a bit. As a result, he began prescribing progesterone to all his menopausal patients, whether or not they were taking Premarin®.

Dr. Lee's early findings suggested that progesterone might be even more important than estrogen. While Premarin® might slow or even halt the progress of osteoporosis, progesterone seemed to actually reverse it.

Over a period of about 10 years, Dr. Lee treated 100 women with bio-identical progesterone (usually in combination with Premarin®), regularly measuring BMD in 63 of them. Their average age was about 65 years at the start of Dr. Lee's small study, so most were well past menopause, and many had already experienced considerable bone loss. About 40% used Premarin® + bio-identical progesterone, and the remaining 60% used progesterone only. In addition, he urged his patients to avoid smoking and carbonated beverages; to eat a healthful diet with lots of green leafy vegetables (which contain lots of calcium); to take supplements of vitamins C and D, beta-carotene, and calcium; and to exercise regularly; all of which are known to improve bone density and strength. All but one of the women stayed with the program for at least 3 years, a remarkable feat in its own right, given how many women typically quit conventional HRT regimens due to their unpleasant or dangerous side effects.

When he retired and finally had the time to evaluate and compare the records of his patients, Dr. Lee confirmed the results from his first few patients and then some: regular application of a bio-identical progesterone cream was associated with a remarkable increase in BMD. In some women, the density of their lumbar vertebrae *increased by 20 to 25% in the first year.* Over 3 years, the mean increase in bone density leveled out at 15.4% (Fig. 6-4). This compared quite favorably with the *4% to 5% loss* in BMD that would have been expected in women not using hormone replacement of any kind. Most importantly, not one of Dr. Lee's patients, despite their advanced age, experienced any new fractures during this period.

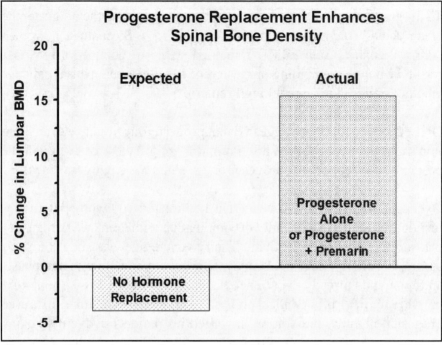

Figure 6-4. This graph shows that there was 15.4% increase in lumbar spine BMD in 63 postmenopausal women with osteoporosis who were treated for up to 3 years with either progesterone cream alone or combined with oral Premarin®. This compares with about a 4.5% decline in vertebral BMD that would be expected in comparable women who did not use any kind of hormone replacement.

Adapted from Lee JR., 1996

Nor was age an obstacle to bone restoration. Women over age 70 made exactly the same gains in bone density as those under 70. Adding "estrogens" to the progesterone made no difference, somewhat supporting Dr. Lee's contention that estrogen was less important for bone health than previously thought. (Unfortunately, we don't know what would have happened had he used bio-identical human estrogens instead of horse estrogens, but the former were not readily available at that time.)

We should point out here that, attractive and exciting as Dr. Lee's results were, they did not *prove* – at least to mainstream medicine's usual standards – that progesterone reverses osteoporosis. Such proof would require a large, double-blind, placebo-controlled study in which one group of women received progesterone and another did not. Moreover, in addition to using progesterone, Dr. Lee's patients altered elements of their lifestyle, diet, and nutritional supplement intake in a rather uncontrolled fashion. Might any of these actions have affected the progress of osteoporosis? Certainly, but we can't tell for sure from these results.

Still, as a practicing physician, Dr. Lee was really in no position to do anything different from what he did. At the time he was treating his patients, he was doing just that – *treating* them – not conducting a controlled clinical trial. He gave them everything he felt they needed to improve their bone strength. He did not try to give some patients some things and others something else as a control to see how they might differ. Controls or no controls, though, the bottom line is that his treatment worked.

Moreover, results like Dr. Lee's haven't been occurring just in the women he treated. In the last 25 years or so, thousands of women working with doctors knowledgeable in natural medicine have achieved comparable results. A 15% increase in BMD may be unheard of in the world of patent medicine research, but every doctor who treats women using bio-identical estrogens and progesterone (along with calcium, magnesium, strontium, vitamins C and D, etc) can document numerous instances of women who have done as well or better.

Is Progesterone Safe?

No doubt about it.

Too much estrogen – especially estradiol or estrone (not to mention equilin and other horse estrogens) – can overstimulate cell growth in the uterine lining and breast and, as a result, have been linked to cancer in both these locations. However, progesterone is not a growth stimulator; quite the opposite. Too much progesterone might make you sleepy, but it does not cause any serious, unpleasant, or dangerous side effects.

Since conventional medicine advocates typically make no distinction between progesterone and Provera®, they "officially" warn us – with absolutely no evidence to support their assertion – that progesterone might have the same adverse side effects as Provera®. Provera® is without question a very dangerous drug, as foreign to the human body as any molecule that might be supplied by a "space alien." As discussed in earlier chapters, women who take Provera® frequently complain of annoying side effects, like breast tenderness, skin irritations, depression, breakthrough bleeding, swelling, and other unpleasantries. Provera® interferes with many of the beneficial effects of estrogen replacement, even those provided by Premarin®. Provera-related side effects may be the main reason so many women quit conventional HRT early.

In addition to being annoying, Provera® can be dangerous. Recent research has confirmed that it increases the risk of heart disease[25] and breast cancer.[26] No such problems have ever been reported, even anecdotally, for the hundreds of thousands of women who have used bio-identical progesterone at physiologic doses. In the PEPI study, the only major NIH-sponsored trial that ever tested bio-identical progesterone (the oral micronized version, which is less than ideal, but still safe), no serious adverse effects associated with its use were reported. This was in sharp contrast to the use of Provera® in the same – and other – large trials.

In premenopausal women, rising levels of progesterone following ovulation prepare the lining of the uterus for pregnancy. (Provera®, of course, would have no such effect on the uterine lining if it could ever to be given to premenopausal women, which it can't because the FDA forbids it, and for once with good reason.) Progesterone has sometimes been given to pregnant women to prevent miscarriages. While there's some question whether this even helps, regardless, Provera® could never be used in this way, because it is known to cause birth defects.

So when the FDA, Wyeth, and their apologists – paid and otherwise – claim there's no difference in safety between Provera® (and other progestins) and bio-identical progesterone, notice that they *never* cite any scientific evidence to support this claim, just vague conjecture based on the supposed lack of any large, prospective, double-blind, controlled trials. Conveniently, they invariably fail to mention the PEPI study. Many critics also raise the specter that bio-identical progesterone *might* not protect against estrogen-caused endometrial overgrowth, while ignoring more than a dozen well-controlled studies clearly demonstrating that it performs that function as well as any patented progestin.[23, 27-39]

Certainly, we would welcome a large, well-controlled, clinical trial of progesterone's safety as well as its effects on bone metabolism. But, given the way Big Pharma dominates medical research and medical education today, no one is holding their breath waiting for a research grant. To those of us who've been recommending progesterone to women, and to the hundreds of thousands of women who've been taking our advice, progesterone's safety could not be more self-evident. In our experience, *it virtually never causes any adverse side effects.*

So, until Big Pharma gets "on the stick" – or until Hell freezes over, whichever comes first – those doctors and patients, who've learned to trust Mother Nature and have gained first-hand experience with progesterone, are likely to remain the only ones who have no doubts about its safety and effectiveness.

Testosterone & DHEA, the Bone-Building Androgens

Testosterone and *DHEA* (*dehydroepiandrosterone*) are generally thought of as "male hormones" or *androgens*, but as explained in previous chapters, women's bodies produce them as well, although in much smaller quantities than do men's bodies. Both hormones are important "bone-builders," since, like progesterone, they stimulate the formation of new bone in both men and women.

The bone building effects of bio-identical testosterone in men are well documented. As with progesterone, though, few studies have been published that document the effects of testosterone on bone in women, and only recently has conventional medicine begun to take these effects seriously.

For example, in one double-blind study,[40] postmenopausal women received sublingual (under the tongue) doses of either micronized estrogen (estradiol) + progesterone, or estrogen + progesterone + testosterone. When BMD in the women's spinal (lumbar) and hip bones were measured after 12 months of treatment, both hormone combinations significantly increased BMD in the spinal vertebrae. Oddly though, hip BMD increased significantly only in those women who were taking the combination that included testosterone.

DHEA is the most abundant steroid hormone in the human body (male or female). Among its other functions, the body uses DHEA to make other androgens and estrogens (See Fig. 4-2, pg. 74). Studies show that DHEA helps keep bones strong by helping to *build new bone tissue* (as progesterone and testosterone do), as well as by inhibiting estrogen-like osteoclastic activity.[41, 42]

Unlike estrogen, progesterone, and testosterone, most of which are produced in the ovaries, the body makes DHEA in the adrenal glands, which sit atop each of the kidneys. Although the adrenals continue secreting DHEA (and its complement, DHEA-S) even after menopause, that secretion begins declining by 1 to 2% per year as early as the 3rd decade of life and is thought to be an important contributor to osteoporosis in both men and women.[43]

Levels of endogenous DHEA and DHEA-S are positively correlated with BMD in both premenopausal and postmenopausal women.[44-47] Low DHEA levels are associated with a higher risk of osteoporotic fractures. In one study, women with the lowest levels of DHEA-S had double the fracture risk of women with the highest levels.[47]

DHEA replacement appears to increase bone strength, as measured by BMD. In a small, but randomized, double-blind, placebo-controlled trial, 58 women and 61 men (aged 60-88 years), who had low serum levels of DHEA-S at the start of the study, took DHEA orally (50 milligrams per day) or placebo. After 12 months of treatment, DHEA replacement significantly increased BMD in the patients' hip and lumbar spine (lower back) bones, compared to placebo. The researchers attributed the bulk of DHEA's bone-building effect to its indirect elevation of serum levels of estradiol.[42]

So strong is the bone-building evidence for DHEA that the FDA has even taken an interest, granting one patent medicine company (Genelabs Technologies, Inc.) the right to develop DHEA as an "orphan drug" (called Prasterone®) for treating women with the disease systemic lupus

erythematosus (SLE), called "lupus" for short. (Of, course, Prasterone®
is exactly the same chemically as bio-identical DHEA, except for the
brand name and the FDA "approval.") Women with lupus are most often
treated with a powerful patent medicine, prednisone, which helps suppress
some of their symptoms for a time. However, a major side effect of
prednisone is severe loss of BMD, leading to osteoporosis. On the other
hand, when women take high doses (100-200 mg/day) of proprietary
DHEA ("Prasterone®") in addition to prednisone, their BMD actually
increases.[48, 49]

Confusing? To be sure, but these studies demonstrate that, should
bone scans, family history, and a genetic predisposition, and other
factors suggest that you may be at risk for osteoporosis, then *complete*
hormone replacement may require androgens in addition to estrogens
and progesterone.

Again, we should emphasize that, because testosterone and DHEA are
androgens, you should be careful to use them at much lower doses than
those that are used by men. Although their presence is very important,
excessive androgens can cause the appearance of secondary male sexual
characteristics, such as acne, growth of body and facial hair, loss of scalp
hair, and deepening of your voice. Excessive testosterone might also
adversely affect your cardiovascular health (in contrast to men, whose
cardiovascular health is often improved by androgens)..

Maintaining and Restoring Bone Strength: Beyond Hormones

While the focus of this book is on hormones, we can't talk about bones
without at least a brief mention of several other very important factors
that interact with steroid hormones to influence your bone health and
strength. These include certain vitamins and minerals, consumed as food
and nutritional supplements, as well as diet, exercise, and lifestyle.

Calcium

Since we were kids, we've heard about the importance of calcium "for
strong teeth and bones." Calcium is the main ingredient in everything
from oyster shells to our bones to our teeth. In bones, calcium is deposited

in a matrix composed of a flexible substance called collagen. As calcium leaches out of that matrix – as it does in osteoporosis – your bones can gradually become softer and weaker.

We normally replenish skeletal calcium by consuming it in foods and nutritional supplements. Calcium-rich foods include green leafy vegetables, beans, nuts, dairy products, sardines, and salmon. Some processed foods are now fortified with extra calcium. Still, the average American diet supplies only between 400 and 800 mg of calcium per day, which is only about one-third to one-half the amount generally recommended for normal, healthy people (1200 - 1500 mg/day). People at risk for osteopenia or osteoporosis probably need even more. In the absence of sufficient dietary calcium, the body slips into "negative calcium balance," which means it is forced to raid its skeletal stores to supply the calcium for its many other needs. This, of course, will weaken your bones if it goes on long enough.

The best way to make up the difference – short of gnawing on bones or oyster shells – is to take calcium supplements, which are inexpensive and widely available. The only catch is that not all calcium supplements are created equal. The most common form is *calcium carbonate*, better known as *chalk*. Calcium carbonate for human consumption comes in the form of capsules and tablets, as well in over-the-counter antacid products like Tums®, Rolaids®, and Maalox®.

While calcium carbonate is generally considered a good source of calcium, it can be problematic for many people, especially those who have low levels of stomach acid (hydrochloric acid, HCl). The potent hydrochloric acid (HCl) produced by special cells in the stomach is a vital early step in the digestion, absorption, and utilization of all kinds of nutrients, including calcium. When we take calcium carbonate supplements, HCl splits the calcium and carbonate molecules apart so that the calcium goes into solution, making it easier for the body to absorb and metabolize it. However, if you have too little HCl in your stomach, it's basically chalk in – chalk out. Very little calcium actually gets absorbed, which obviously does your bones no good at all.

But wait, hold on a second. Too *little* stomach acid? Whoever heard of that? Isn't the bigger problem *too much acid*, causing heartburn and GERD (gastroesophageal reflux disease)? In fact, although mainstream medicine is loathe to admit it, by far the most common problem, especially as people grow older, is *low stomach acid*, which affects at least one-third of the population above the age of 60.[41, 42]

This age-related decline in stomach acid secretion is due to the progressive loss of acid-producing cells in the stomach, a condition known as *atrophic gastritis* or *gastric atrophy*. You'd never know it by watching TV or listening to most conventional doctors, but heartburn and GERD almost always occur in the presence of *too little stomach acid, not too much*. An excess of stomach acid is actually a very rare and dangerous condition.

To make matters worse, how does conventional medicine deal with the symptoms of low stomach acid (eg, heartburn, GERD, and other forms of dyspepsia)? Simple, by making us take powerful drugs, such as Nexium®, Prilosec®, Prevacid®, Protonix®, Aciphex®, Xantac®, Pepcid®, Tagamet®, and Axid®, which do what? They drive our acid levels down even lower, virtually shutting down gastric acid secretion for months or years at a time if used regularly, which is typically what happens. So, who has to worry about low stomach acid? We all do.*

Getting back to calcium supplements, then, to get the most out of a calcium supplement, regardless of how much acid our stomachs may be capable of churning out, it's usually best to avoid calcium carbonate altogether and instead take supplements that supply *calcium citrate* or *calcium malate*. Unlike calcium carbonate, these have no trouble dissolving and dissociating, no matter how much acid your stomach is producing.

Vitamin D

We need vitamin D to, among other things, facilitate the incorporation of calcium into our bones. In the absence of sufficient vitamin D, calcium will not get integrated into bones. As a result, bones become soft, a

---

* The way conventional medicine disregards the role of stomach acid in maintaining normal nutrition and health is a scandal that is only compounded by the widespread promotion and prescription of these very powerful – and extremely profitable – acid suppressing drugs, even for the mildest cases of heartburn. For an eye-opening discussion of this extremely important but poorly appreciated health issue, and also to learn how you can treat heartburn and GERD naturally, without resorting to dangerous drugs, we urge you to read our book, *Why Stomach Acid Is Good for You*, by Jonathan V. Wright, MD, and Lane Lenard, PhD (New York; M. Evans).

condition known in children as *rickets* and in adults as *osteomalacia*. Taking calcium supplements without sufficient vitamin D just wastes the calcium and might actually weaken bones over the long term. In nursing home residents, those taking calcium + vitamin D supplements had a 43% lower risk of a hip fracture and a 32% lower risk of nonvertebral fractures.[50]

Vitamin D is available in many different foods, including fish, dairy, eggs, and liver, as well as supplements. However, vitamin D is unique in that the human body is capable of manufacturing most of what it needs simply through exposure to the sun. We don't absorb any solar "vitamin D rays," but instead, ultraviolet (UV) solar radiation reacts with cholesterol (Yes, *that* cholesterol, again!) in the skin to produce the precursor of vitamin D. Reasonable periods of sun exposure usually supply enough vitamin D to fill most bodily needs.

What is reasonable sun exposure? A lot depends on where you live. Long hours on the beach are not necessary − perhaps 5 to 30 minutes of sun exposure to the face, arms, legs, or back *without sunscreen* between 10 AM and 3 PM at least twice a week − is usually enough to provide sufficient vitamin D synthesis for most people. However, for people living in northern latitudes (or southern latitudes for those of you south of the equator) or regions with excessive smog or cloud cover, who may get little direct sunlight for months at a time, dietary vitamin D becomes very important. Extra dietary vitamin D becomes especially significant as we grow older, because, for a lot of reasons, including increasingly limited sun exposure, elderly people are particularly susceptible to a vitamin D deficiency.

Most nutritionally-oriented physicians now recommend taking 3,000 to 4,000 IU supplemental vitamin D daily, depending on the amount of sunlight exposure. For many individuals, blood tests show that even higher amounts are necessary to achieve optimal levels. However, since taking too much vitamin D for too long can be dangerous, it's always best, when embarking on a serious nutritional supplement program with vitamin D (or any other nutrient) to consult with a physician who is skilled and knowledgeable in natural medicine. (*See Chapter 11 to learn how to locate such a doctor.*)

Strontium: The Miracle Mineral that Prevents and *Reverses* Osteoporosis

Strontium is a mineral that may be just as important for building strong bones and preventing and reversing osteoporosis as BHRT and calcium. Like calcium, strontium is one of the most common elements on earth (chemical symbol, **Sr**). It is found in fresh water and rock formations all over the earth, usually in the form of salts like *strontium sulfate, strontium chloride,* and *strontium carbonate,*[*]and is often found in the same places (and foods) as calcium. Because strontium and calcium are chemically very similar, the body doesn't discriminate and absorbs them both about equally.

Here's the remarkable thing about strontium: once it gets into bone tissue (in *physiologic* amounts), **it slows osteoclastic resorption** while at the same time **enhancing osteoblastic bone building.** In other words, it mimics the effects of estrogen, progesterone, testosterone, and DHEA, but without any other hormonal effects.[51] This means that, all by itself, strontium can help **prevent and even reverse osteoporosis.**

Lots of studies in lab animals have confirmed the bone-building effects of various naturally occurring strontium salts.[3, 45-47] Although strontium salts (unpatentable, of course) have been used safely for a variety of medical purposes since the 1880s, it wasn't until the 1940s and '50s that anyone started to take it seriously as a possible treatment for osteoporosis. During the '50s, strontium salts were commonly used for treating people with osteoporosis.[4, 48]

In 1959, researchers at the Mayo Clinic gave strontium lactate to 22 men and women suffering with severe, painful osteoporosis. Another 10 postmenopausal women took strontium lactate along with "estrogen" (CEEs) and testosterone.[52] In the strontium + "hormones" group, symptoms improved markedly in 9 out of 10 women; the tenth had moderate improvement. In the strontium-only group, 18 of the 22 men and women had marked improvement, while the other 4 had moderate improvement. In other words, *every single person taking strontium lactate in this study had at least moderate improvement*; improvement was rated as *marked* in 84% of the people. Through 3 years of treatment, not one

---

[*]   Since pure strontium is chemically unstable, strontium cannot exist or be ingested except when combined with another atom or molecule to form a salt.

person experienced any side effects. Although today's sophisticated means of measuring bone density were not available in those days, X-ray examinations suggested that bone mass increased in 78% of the people taking strontium (lactate).

It took a quarter century more before another small, but noteworthy study of strontium and bone was conducted. In 1985, McGill University researchers gave daily strontium carbonate supplements to 3 men and 3 women with osteoporosis. After 6 months, bone biopsy samples revealed an *increase in bone formation of 172%*. Moreover, all 6 people reported less bone pain and improved mobility.[53]

Now, this all sounds pretty exciting, and one has to wonder, given the prevalence of osteoporosis and strontium's apparent efficacy, safety, and unique mechanism of action, why conventional medicine has paid so little attention to it in recent years. There are several reasons, none of which have anything to do with strontium's efficacy or safety.

The first has to do with nuclear weapons testing ... really! For readers who grew up in the 1950s and early '60s, the word strontium may have some unpleasant connotations. During those days of above-ground nuclear testing, a radioactive form of the mineral – **strontium-90** – was formed by atomic explosions and carried by air and water all over the globe. Strontium-90 soon came to be recognized as a potentially carcinogenic component of radioactive fallout. When it was taken up by the same plants that also took up ordinary strontium and calcium, it wound up in milk and other foods, and eventually found its way into human bones, making them radioactive and sometimes causing bone cancer. Ordinary strontium is, and always has been, perfectly safe, but the strontium-90 scare irrationally discouraged further use of the mineral for treating osteoporosis.

Strontium also fell out of favor, because it seemed to be associated with certain bone defects in rare cases. However, these were soon found to be related, not to the presence of strontium *per se*, but most likely to a lack of adequate calcium in the diet. Bones need both calcium and strontium to stay strong, with a preference for more calcium than strontium.[4, 54, 55]

Finally, the most enduring reason for the paucity of interest in strontium was that, in all its natural combinations (eg, carbonate, chloride, citrate, gluconate, and lactate), *strontium is not patentable.*

Unpatentability is normally the kiss of death for any potential pharmaceutical product, and for many years, it discouraged widespread testing of strontium compounds by those with the resources to conduct such tests. Nevertheless, positive lab and clinical studies of strontium going back 50 years or more finally piqued Big Pharma's interest. There was only one question they had to answer: How can we make a strontium product that we can patent? As we've mentioned earlier, Big Pharma spends a good deal of its R & D time and dollars trying to outdo Mother Nature, not because they think they can create a superior substitute – they know they can't – but because they know that with the help of the FDA they can make lots of money trying.

In its natural state, strontium always occurs in combination with another common molecule (listed above). All these *naturally occurring* strontium compounds have been shown to build new, healthy bone tissue with no side effects. While there have been no one-on-one comparative studies, so far no one compound seems to have any particular advantage in terms of safety or effectiveness, although some are better absorbed than others. Regardless of which one is used, though, it's invariably the strontium that's doing the heavy lifting, not the other molecule in the compound. To get around this obstacle, patent medicine company researchers decided to create a brand new strontium combination never before seen on this planet.

Strontium Ranelate: The New – *Patented* – Kid on the Block

Into this world was born a new, computer-designed, laboratory-created, and best of all, *patentable* strontium compound named **strontium ranelate,** the product of a chemical marriage between good, old-fashioned natural strontium and a synthetic, patented compound called *ranelic acid.* Strontium ranelate represents one of Big Pharma's latest attempts to go Mother Nature one better, and as these attempts go, it doesn't seem nearly as dangerous as the majority of patent medicines. Based on a couple of clinical trials in a few thousand people for up to 5 years, strontium ranelate appears to be effective and reasonably safe.

Still, aside from the fact that it simply isn't necessary to develop a patented strontium compound, except to earn enormous profits, there may be a few other reasons to take pause. For example, natural strontium compounds typically consist of *a single strontium atom* + 1 or 2 chloride, carbonate, gluconate, citrate, or lactate molecules. (The number of molecules depend on which compound is involved.) By contrast, the strontium ranelate molecule comes out of the test tube looking something like a two-headed monster. Each molecule of strontium ranelate contains *2 atoms of strontium* + 1 molecule of *ranelic acid*, to form a combination that could never occur in Nature, because ranelic acid is an alien molecule that never existed outside of the laboratory.

As the official Prescribing Information for strontium ranelate states, the ranelate portion of the molecule represents "**...the best *compromise* in terms of molecular weight, pharmacokinetics, and acceptability of the medicinal product.**"[56] That's exactly what strontium ranelate is – *a compromise*, something less than optimal for the body in the interests of a higher goal, ie, bigger profits.

Servier, the French company that developed strontium ranelate, has conducted several large, double-blind, placebo-controlled clinical trials that clearly confirm the earlier studies of nonpatented strontium salts in terms of the efficacy of strontium (ranelate, in this case) in stopping and reversing osteoporosis.[57, 58-60]

In the largest and longest of these studies,[59] more than 5,000 elderly postmenopausal women (aged 74 or older, or aged 70-73 and an especially high risk of osteoporotic fracture) took strontium ranelate (2 grams per day) for up to 5 years. (However, almost half of these women dropped out of the study before 5 years.) Of those who remained in the study for the full 5 years, their rate of new vertebral fractures had declined by 24%, compared to the placebo group; the risk of a hip fracture dropped by 43%; and nonvertebral fractures overall – hip, wrist, sacrum, ribs, clavicle (collar bone), and humerus (upper arm bone) – were lower by

15% in the strontium-treated women. The strontium-treated women also had BMD increases of 11% in the femoral neck of the hip; 14% in the hip overall; and 20% in the lumbar spine, compared to placebo.

In a trial in younger women (aged 50-65 years), strontium ranelate was associated with a reduced risk of vertebral fracture of 35% and increases of BMD of 16% in the lumbar spine and 7% in the femoral neck, compared to placebo.[60] In all trials of strontium ranelate, side effects have occurred no more frequently in the strontium group than in the placebo group.

Let us emphasize an important point about these studies: Postmenopausal women without osteoporosis who took no replacement hormones still had increases in BMD when they used strontium. So not only did strontium repair existing damage, it actually helped prevent the women from suffering with osteoporosis in the first place. But, remember this, *it doesn't matter whether it's strontium gluconate, strontium lactate, strontium carbonate, or even strontium ranelate; as long as it's strontium (along with a greater quantity of calcium), it's good for you! Remember, never take strontium without taking more calcium than strontium.*

All of the attention focused on strontium ranelate has sparked interest (and funding) for more strontium-osteoporosis research. True, most current studies are being done on the patented combination, and most will continue to be. Nevertheless, one study we can guarantee Servier (or any other patent medicine company) will never do is to compare its patented strontium-based drug with any other natural strontium compounds in a head-to-head trial, because the results would be embarrassing.

To emphasize, there's no question that it's strontium itself and not the carbonate, not the citrate, not the chloride, not the gluconate, and certainly not the ranelate, that is doing all the bone building. The only thing ranelate offers that the other salts do not is a patent. Therefore, any good news that comes out of strontium ranelate trials can be read as good news for all strontium compounds.

A Note of Caution

Despite its apparent efficacy and safety, experience reminds us that strontium ranelate remains an alien-to-the-human-body molecule. Given its relatively limited exposure to human beings in a few clinical trials, and especially given the ready availability of natural alternatives that are just as good, we should maintain a healthy degree of suspicion about strontium ranelate. A couple of side effects – though uncommon – still deserve an especially careful look:

- One is an elevation of the muscle enzyme *creatine phosphokinase (CPK)*, which strontium ranelate researchers have termed mild, transient, and of "no clinical significance." Now, that may well be true, but if this patent medicine ever becomes available in the United States and you decide to take it, especially over many years, it might be safest to have your CPK levels checked regularly.

A Word about Strontium Dosing

People have taken doses of up to 1,700 mg per day of strontium ranelate in clinical studies with few reports of significant adverse side effects; still, a safe, effective dose was about 680 mg. However, even that dose may be too high for long-term use, because under certain conditions, it might lead over time to osteomalacia, due to the skeleton's failure to incorporate sufficient calcium. From a purely scientific standpoint, this is a predictable result: normal bones contain much more calcium than strontium or any other mineral, so depriving them of what they need – calcium – and then trying to "make up" for it with only one part of the equation – strontium – is bound to present problems.

Dr. Alan Gaby has recently proposed that lower doses of strontium might actually be superior than higher doses for countering osteoporosis.[2] At the very least, the results of animal and clinical studies suggest that we should balance our intake of strontium and calcium.[3, 4]

Fortunately, the typical human diet normally contains much more calcium than strontium, so it's doubtful such an imbalance would occur except when taking supplements (or strontium-containing drugs). To be absolutely safe, then, follow this simple rule: *Always take more calcium than strontium.*

- Another potential problem is a small but *statistically significant* increase (0.7%) in the annual incidence of venous thromboembolism (VTE), a very serious, and potentially fatal condition in which blood clots form in the veins and may travel to the lungs (pulmonary embolism). A 0.7% increase in VTE may not sound like much, but if 10 million women were to take this drug – not an unreasonable number; given the prevalence of osteoporosis, that means that 70,000 of these women might develop VTE. Doctors who prescribe strontium ranelate should always evaluate patients' risk factors for VTE, and those who are vulnerable should probably avoid taking the drug.[56]

So far, strontium ranelate has been marketed only in Europe under the trademark Protelos®, but it's probably only a matter of time before it reaches US shores. Since this new combination has a good deal of profit potential, as opposed to all-natural forms of strontium, we'd be willing to bet that before too long, we'll be hearing that this exciting new osteoporosis drug is the *"only form of strontium that is FDA-approved"* to help rebuild bone tissue. This may be true as far as it goes, but please keep in mind that all FDA-approval really means is that forms have been filled out and money has changed hands. It doesn't guarantee that a substance is safe or that it's the only, or even the best, form of treatment. Based on all the available research, we can see no reason to prefer strontium ranelate over any other strontium compound (*unless, of course, you own stock in Servier*).

Other Nutrients Important to Bone Health

In a book focusing on bio-identical hormones, there just isn't space for a complete discussion of all of the nutrients known to be important to bone health. However, if you're searching for a "comprehensive" anti-osteoporosis formulation, make sure it includes not just calcium, vitamin D, and strontium, but also magnesium, vitamin K2 (as menaquinone), zinc, copper, selenium, manganese, molybdenum, boron, and silicon.

What about Those Other Anti-Osteoporosis Drugs?

At the present time, two major types of patented anti-osteoporosis drugs are currently "approved" and in widespread use: **bisphosphonates** and **SERMs**. Both types mimic, to varying degrees, the effects of estrogen on bone in that they work by inhibiting bone *resorption*. However, like estrogen, neither of these drugs has any ability to build new bone.

A relatively recent addition to the patent medicine anti-osteoporosis armamentarium is Forteo®, a manmade version of natural human parathyroid hormone produced via recombinant technology (genetic modification). Natural human parathyroid hormone is important for helping build new bone tissue, and studies of Forteo® show that it is unique among "FDA-approved" patented drugs; it increases osteoblast activity, rather than suppressing osteoclast activity, and it can indeed increase new bone growth and reduce the risk of fractures in some women and men with osteoporosis. However, Forteo® also has many drawbacks, making it questionable whether its benefits outweigh its risks, especially given the safe and effective natural alternatives. For example, it requires daily self-injection and carries a long list of potential side effects, including light-headedness, fainting, dizziness, orthostatic hypotension,* nausea, vomiting, constipation, leg cramps, joint pain, and muscle weakness. Perhaps most importantly, though, studies in lab animals have demonstrated a propensity for high doses to cause osteosarcoma, a form of bone cancer, which has earned it one of the FDA's dreaded "black box" warnings.[61] Although bone cancer has not been reported in human users of the drug, the safety of Forteo® has not been evaluated beyond 2 years. Consequently, its use for longer than 2 years is not recommended, which would seem to place a serious limitation on its use for treating a chronic progressive disease like osteoporosis.

Bisphosphonates: Bone Strengtheners or Bone Hardeners?

Currently FDA-approved bisphosphonates, including Fosamax® (alendronate), Actonel® (risedronate), Didronel® (etidronate), Boniva® (ibandronate), and Reclast® (Zometa®) (zoledronate), are designed to strengthen bone by inhibiting normal osteoclastic bone resorbing activity, which slows down the loss of BMD, allowing trabecular architecture to stabilize.[62, 63] Notice that this has nothing to do with stabilizing the balance between estrogen and progesterone, restoring calcium levels, or any other natural process.

---

* A transient drop in blood pressure that can cause you to feel lightheaded and dizzy. It can occur immediately after injection or as long as 4 hours later.

Like many other patented drugs, bisphosphonates are synthetic analogs*
of an important natural bone-building chemical, *pyrophosphate*, which
normally helps bind calcium to bone tissue via a process known as
mineralization. Unlike pyrophosphate, however, bisphosphonates actually
block mineralization as well as osteoclastic bone resorption.

Large, placebo-controlled trials generally show that these drugs can indeed
increase BMD and reduce the risk of vertebral, hip, and other nonvertebral
fractures in women with osteoporosis – at least in the short run. That's the
good news. Merck, the company that markets the leading bisphosphonate,
Fosamax® (now also sold generically as alendronate) seized upon results
like these to turn their drug into a blockbuster worth as much as $3.6
billion per year.[64] Use of Fosamax® and other bisphosphonates has been
growing at an especially rapid rate since 2002 when the publication of the
WHI results scared women away from "estrogen" replacement, up until
then the leading conventional method for preventing osteoporosis.

Unfortunately, all may not be so rosy after all. Trials lasting up to 10 years
are beginning to raise doubts about the long-term safety and efficacy of
bisphosphonates.[57, 58] The main problem is that bisphosphonates not only
directly – and unnaturally – inhibit *osteoclastic* bone resorption, they also
indirectly inhibit the other side of the bone-building coin, *osteoblastic*
bone formation. Here's how they work:

As described earlier, in normal bone remodeling, osteoclasts first resorb
bone tissue, forming little pits in the bone structure. In short order,
osteoblasts come along to fill in those pits with healthy new bone. Under
normal circumstances, osteoblasts remain inactive until the osteoclasts
first do their thing. If osteoclastic activity is suppressed enough, though,
as it is by bisphosphonates, osteoblasts have no cavities to fill, and so,
formation of new bone ceases. Although estrogens also inhibit osteoclastic
activity, they do so in a natural way that does not suppress osteoblastic
bone building, which can still be stimulated by agents like progesterone,
testosterone, or strontium.

Thus, the physical cost of bisphosphonate-induced bone stabilization is
to freeze normal bone remodeling – a highly unnatural state of affairs.

---

* Chemical analogs are molecular look-alikes, but with subtle differences, like the substitution of a carbon
atom for an oxygen atom. Bisphosphonates are analogs of the natural substance *pyrophosphate* in the same
way that Provera® is an analog of *progesterone*.

What does this mean for bone health in the long term? This is a crucial question, because there's no such thing as short-term treatment with these drugs. A woman who starts taking bisphosphonates at age 55 could easily still be taking them 25 or 30 years later, if she stays healthy and can tolerate them.

The longest trial so far reported – 10 years with Fosamax® – apparently evidenced no increase in fracture rate in the later years.[65] However, the design of this Merck-sponsored study has been criticized.[58, 60, 61]

Another much smaller, trial – conducted independently of direct drug company influence* – presented a very different story. The researchers selected 9 women with osteopenia or osteoporosis, who had been taking Fosamax® for 3 to 8 years (some had also been taking Premarin®) because, despite the drug treatment, they had still sustained bizarre nonspinal fractures (to the lower back, ribs, hip bones, and femur) while performing normal daily activities, such as walking, standing, or turning around. The locations and circumstances of these fractures were unusual for women with osteopenia or osteoporosis, and none of the fractures was related to a fall or other trauma. The fractures occurred earlier in the women taking both Fosamax® and Premarin®, suggesting an additive effect on bone resorption.[66]

Since the women continued taking Fosamax® while their fractures were healing, the researchers took the opportunity to study the drug's effects on the healing process. What they found was not encouraging. In most of the women, fracture healing slowed down considerably, taking months or even years longer than it should have. One woman's femoral shaft fracture took more than 2 years to heal, despite the fact that her doctors had treated the fracture aggressively, employing metal screws and rods as well as a bone graft. In most of the patients, once the drug treatment was discontinued, the fractures healed satisfactorily.

The researchers also performed bone biopsies at a site away from the fractures, which was intended to give them an idea of the health of the women's bones in general. They found a strikingly severe depression of bone formation – *nearly 100-fold lower* in some of the patients than

---

* The researchers had grants from the US Public Health Service and the University of Texas Southwestern Medical Center, Dallas.

has been found in healthy postmenopausal women. They concluded that the deterioration in bone health was almost certainly due to Fosamax® treatment, and that it was probably exacerbated by the coadministration of Fosamax® with estrogen, since both suppress bone turnover.

One Woman's Experience with Fosamax®

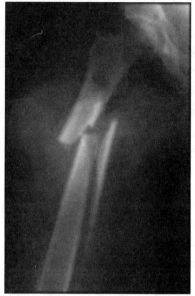

In one case reported in the medical literature, Jennifer P. Schneider, MD, PhD, a physician from Tucson, Arizona, described her personal experience with Fosamax®. At age 59, Dr. Schneider, who had gone into menopause prematurely in her early 40s, was riding in a New York City subway when the car jolted. Although the femur (thigh bone) is normally one of the strongest bones in the body, she reported in the journal *Geriatrics,* that when the car lurched, she "shifted all her weight to one leg, felt the bone snap, and fell to the floor

Figure 6-5.

of the train."[67] Figure 6-5 shows an x-ray of Dr. Schneider's shattered femur.

At the time of her fateful subway ride, Dr. Schneider had been experiencing pain in her right thigh for about 3 months, and a bone scan the week before had shown a stress fracture of her right femur. She had also been taking Fosamax® for about 7 years, in addition to calcium and HRT.

After the fracture, her doctors convinced her to continue taking the drug, dismissing her concerns about its potential for suppressing bone turnover – ie, healing – as only "a theoretical possibility." Yet despite aggressive treatment over more than 9 months, including electrical bone stimulation, surgery to implant a metal rod, and a second surgery to implant a larger rod, her fracture refused to heal. Finally, she halted the drug on her own, and within 6 months, the pieces of her broken thighbone finally began to unite.

Dr. Schneider remained off Fosamax® for 2 years, during which time she was able to regain her normal level of activity. However, since her bone scans were showing that her BMD was beginning to decline somewhat, her doctors advised her to start taking Fosamax® again. Reluctantly she agreed.

About a year later, though, upon getting out of bed one morning, she felt a pain in her right foot with each step. Fearing the possibility of another nontraumatic stress fracture, she again stopped taking the Fosamax®, but a bone scan 2 months later revealed that she had indeed suffered a stress fracture in her foot (the second metatarsal bone).

For the second time in 4 years, Dr. Schneider had fractured a bone due to no particular trauma. This time, instead of Fosamax®, she continued taking calcium supplements and oral estradiol + oral micronized progesterone.* Wearing sturdy shoes to support her foot, she also continued her daily mile-long walks, and after several months, her fractured foot finally healed. Remaining on this regimen ever since, she has not suffered any new fractures.

Dr. Schneider is not alone in her fracture experience. After she published her own "case" history in 2006, she was sent numerous unpublished reports of others who had had similar fractures. Continuing to research the issue, she recently reviewed the current knowledge about this phenomenon.[68] Meanwhile, two other papers – one from doctors in Singapore and the other from the Hospital for Special Surgery in New York – have independently documented a total of 87 men and women, who had had "low-energy," "low-impact," "fragility," or "atypical" fractures associated with use of Fosamax® or other bisphosphonates.[66, 69]

Perhaps the oddest aspect of these Fosamax®-related fractures is that they tend to occur in the upper femur. Remember, this bone is composed primarily of hard, thick *cortical* bone and it is usually the strongest bone in the body. In most healthy people, femoral fractures like these occur only after major, high-energy trauma, like a fall from a high place or an automobile accident. This is in sharp contrast to typical osteoporosis-related fractures, which occur in relatively soft, weakened cancellous

---

* She later switched to a patented combination of oral estradiol + a progestin (norethindrone acetate), brand name Activella®.

bone (eg, trochanter of the hip, wrist, ribs) following (or sometimes preceding) relatively mild trauma, like tripping and falling. As Dr. Schneider points out in her recent review, the femur is "… unlikely to fracture in low-energy trauma unless extreme osteoporosis is present.[69] The reports of multiple cases of low-impact femoral fractures in patients taking alendronate [Fosamax®] for several years, a previously rare event, have therefore called for further study of the possible connection between alendronate and such fractures."[68]

How Bisphosphonates Might Promote New Fractures

Given the way bone remodeling normally takes place, it's easy to see why bisphosphonates might inhibit fracture healing (even though many doctors have been reluctant to admit it), but how they could actually *promote new fractures* while they're supposed to be preventing them seems less obvious. Current thinking on this paradox goes as follows:

The typical stresses of every day life tend to cause bones to develop microcracks. Under normal conditions in otherwise healthy people, these microcracks trigger osteoclasts and osteoblasts to spring into action to repair the damage, unnoticeably and with no ill effects. However, if bone remodeling (turnover) is strongly inhibited, as it unquestionably is by bisphosphonates, the osteoclasts and osteoblasts cannot do their jobs, and so, the microcrack damage – like a well-traveled, but poorly maintained road beaten up by heavy traffic over many years – develops ever-widening cracks and potholes. This hypothesis has recently been supported by Czech researchers, who found that, in women with low BMD, Fosamax® treatment – which keeps the body's "road repair crews" off the job – led to an increase in the accumulation of microcracks.[70]

Let's be clear about something: despite the fact that Fosamax® increases BMD, *it may still make bones more likely to fracture in the long term.* In lab animals, Fosamax-induced oversuppression of bone remodeling increased the appearance of microcracks by a factor of 2- to 7-fold. Accumulation of these microcracks, without subsequent repair – due to the actions of bisphosphonates – appears to increase the risk of fractures while delaying or inhibiting healing.

In summary, even though bone strength *appears* to increase due to Fosamax® treatment, in fact, use of this patent medicine has been associated with a 20% reduction in *bone toughness* (ie, its ability to endure bending pressure without breaking).[71] Dr. Susan M. Ott, of the University of Washington, Seattle, compares bisphosphonate-treated bone to an old tree. Under the stress of a strong wind, younger trees are flexible enough to bend easily without breaking. However, older, denser trees, faced with a serious windstorm, are less able to bend and might just snap in two.[72] "Many people believe that these drugs are '*bone builders*,'" she wrote in a letter to a medical journal, "but the evidence shows they are actually *bone hardeners*."[73]

In an editorial in the *Journal of Endocrinology and Metabolism*, Dr. Ott noted that, once ensconced in bone tissue, bisphosphonates virtually never leave, and in fact, they accumulate with use.[65] "These drugs are not metabolized, but are either excreted renally [in urine] or deposited within bones.... There is no known method of removing the medication from the bones," she wrote.[71]

Dr. Ott urges caution in the long-term use of bisphosphonates, pointing out that research supports their beneficial effects *but only for the first 5 years*. "I believe the current evidence suggests that bisphosphonates should be stopped after 5 years." She adds, "The bisphosphonates in doses used today suppress bone formation to a greater extent than the other anti-resorbing medications, so it is possible that microdamage accumulation would develop after 15 or 20 years – just about the time between menopause and the usual onset of osteoporotic fractures."

More Fosamax® Bad News: It's Not Just in Your Bones

As if these problems weren't bad enough, bisphosphonates have been associated with at least three other serious health problems:

Gastrointestinal Toxicity

Bisphosphonates are potentially destructive to the upper gastrointestinal (GI) tract, including the mouth, esophagus, and stomach. As noted in the official FDA-approved Fosamax® label, "*Fosamax, like other bisphosphonates, may cause local irritation of the upper gastrointestinal mucosa. Esophageal adverse experiences, such as esophagitis, esophageal ulcers, and esophageal erosions, occasionally with bleeding and rarely followed by esophageal stricture or perforation, have been reported in patients receiving treatment with Fosamax. In some cases, these have been severe and required hospitalization."*[74] Recent reports have even linked its use to cancer of the esophagus.[75]

Serious as the bisphosphonate-related GI side effects are, it's pretty simple to prevent them by closely following the recommended procedures for taking the drug, all of which are basically designed to get the pill out of your mouth, through your esophagus, and into and out of your stomach as quickly as possible, with as little contact as possible with the delicate linings of these organs. To accomplish this and also to maximize absorption, Merck recommends the following:

- Take Fosamax® first thing in the morning, right after getting out of bed and at least 30 minutes before any other food, beverage, or medication.

- Take Fosamax® with a full glass (6-8 oz) of ordinary water, *but not mineral water.*

- After swallowing the Fosamax® pill, drink another 2 oz (¼ cup) of water.

- Do not lie down for at least 30 minutes and not until after eating your first food of the day – at least 30 minutes later.

Taking Fosamax® with too little water can expose the esophageal or gastric (stomach) lining to the dangerously irritating drug, which can cause anything from heartburn to perforated ulcers to cancer. Lying down with the drug still in your stomach risks reflux of the acidic, drug-loaded gastric contents back into the esophagus, where they can do serious harm. Moreover, taking Fosamax® while food or other meds are still in your stomach significantly reduces the drug's absorption, thus inhibiting its effectiveness. Even the minerals in mineral water can impede Fosamax® absorption.

Despite these precautions – or maybe because they are so difficult to adhere to – bisphosphonate-related GI pathology turns out to be a common and potentially very serious problem. In fact, the FDA has recently reported receiving more than 40 case reports of cancer of the esophagus related to Fosamax® use, of which 14 resulted in a patient's death.[75] Another 31 cases of esophageal cancer (and 6 deaths) linked to use of Fosamax® and other bisphosphonates have been reported in Europe and Japan. The median time from initial drug exposure to cancer diagnosis was just 2.1 years in the US and 1.3 years in Europe and Japan.[76]

Beware "Jaw Death"

Recently, a new, very disturbing, rare bisphosphonate side effect – osteonecrosis of the jaw (ONJ), also known as "*jaw death*" – has emerged.[77] In ONJ, the bone tissue in the jaw fails to heal after minor trauma, such as a tooth extraction, which leaves the bone exposed and vulnerable to a particularly difficult-to-treat bacterial infection and fracture. Long-term antibiotic therapy and surgery to remove dying bone tissue may be required. Occasionally, a large portion of the jaw may have to be removed.

Ordinarily, ONJ is uncommon and is primarily associated with cancer chemotherapy, radiation of the head or neck, steroid therapy (eg, cortisone), poor dental health, gum disease, dental surgery, alcohol abuse, and other conditions. Accustomed to 1 or 2 cases a year, doctors at one hospital were alarmed to notice that, over a 3-year period, ONJ had been diagnosed in 63 of their patients. The one thing all these patients had in common was bisphosphonate treatment. While 56 of them (89%) had been receiving IV bisphosphonates (pamidronate or zoledronate) as cancer chemotherapy for at least a year, 7 of the patients (11%) had been taking only oral bisphosphonates (alendronate or zoledronic acid) at standard doses for osteoporosis.[78]

There have been numerous subsequent anecdotal reports of bisphosphonate-related ONJ, but Merck, along with the American Dental Association, continue to insist that *oral* Fosamax® (as well as other bisphosphonates) poses minimal risk of ONJ.[79] However, a recent systematic study from researchers at the University of Southern California School of Dentistry suggests otherwise.[80] They evaluated the electronic medical records of patients attending the USC dental school clinic to find out which ones had ever used Fosamax® and which of those later developed ONJ. Of the 208 patients (all women, aged 63-80) with a history of once-a-week Fosamax® use, 9 were being treated for ONJ – about 4%. (Four cases were associated with tooth extractions, and five with ulceration related to poorly fitting dentures.) This was a far higher incidence than had been suggested by most "authorities." By contrast, of the 4,384 USC patients who had undergone dental extraction but had never used Fosamax®, not a single one developed ONJ.

"We've been told that the risk with oral bisphosphonates is negligible, but 4% is not negligible," insisted Dr. Parish Sedghizadeh, who led the USC research team.[81] He points out that most doctors who prescribe bisphosphonates do not tell their patients about the drugs' potential risks, even with short-term use.

The problem is that, as Dr. Ott suggested above, the drug remains locked into bone tissue for a long time (it may take 10 years for levels to drop by half even once you stop taking it). Thus, continuous use allows the drug to build up to levels previously thought to be achievable only by high-dose intravenous administration to cancer patients. The USC results showed that ONJ could develop after taking oral Fosamax® for as little as 1 year.

Several lawsuits have been filed against Merck alleging that Fosamax® causes ONJ and that Merck has known about the risk but has been keeping it under wraps. "We're not quite sure what we're dealing with over the long haul," Dr. Susan Ott told the *Los Angeles Times*. "Side effects like this should make ordinary, healthy women think twice."[82]

Increased Heart Risks, Too

The latest bad news about bisphosphonates concerns their adverse effects on heart function. New research shows that women who have ever used Fosamax® or Reclast® (also called Zometa®) double their risk of developing serious atrial fibrillation (AF), a form of irregular heartbeats. Common symptoms of AF include light-headedness, palpitations, chest pain, and shortness of breath, or no symptoms at all. Left untreated, AF can lead to fluid collecting in the lungs (pulmonary edema), congestive heart failure, and formation of blood clots that may travel to the brain and cause a stroke. An analysis of three studies covering more than 16,000 women, most of whom were taking the drugs for osteoporosis, found that 2.5 to 3% experienced atrial fibrillation; 1 to 2% experienced serious AF, leading to hospitalization or death.[83, 84]

SERMs: The Estrogen Mimics

The other important class of patent medications used to treat osteoporosis is the SERMs, or *selective estrogen-receptor modulators*. These patent medications, of which only one – Evista® (raloxifene) – has so far been FDA-"approved" for preventing or treating osteoporosis in the US, have been shown to significantly increase BMD in the lumbar spine and femoral neck and to reduce the incidence of vertebral fractures by 30% in women with a history of prior fractures, and by 50% in women with no such history.* However, Evista® does not reduce the risk of fractures in the hip and other nonvertebral bones.[85] The reason(s) for this discrepancy are unknown.

Evista® works because, at the molecular level it somewhat resembles estradiol and other bio-identical estrogens – not exactly the same, but close enough to allow it to mimic some typical estrogenic effects. Structurally speaking, Evista® is to estrogen what Provera® is to progesterone, although, based on admittedly limited evidence, Evista® appears to be safer than Provera®.

Evista® acts like estrogens in some ways and unlike them in others. One of the ways Evista® works like estrogens is to inhibit bone resorption; unlike estrogens, Evista® apparently does not stimulate cell growth in breast or endometrial tissue, thus reducing the risk of cancer in these estrogen-sensitive tissues, compared to estradiol or other estrogen-mimicking drugs. Recent research has even led to the FDA-approval of Evista® as a treatment for breast cancer.

---

* The other well-known SERM is a patent medicine called tamoxifen (Nolvadex®), which has been used for treating certain types of breast cancer for more than 25 years. Tamoxifen works by occupying and neutralizing estrogen receptors on breast cells, thus preventing estradiol and estrone from stimulating those cells and possibly fueling the growth of malignant breast cells. Like Evista®, tamoxifen also reduces bone resorption, but it is not approved for that purpose in the US, because, unlike Evista®, tamoxifen stimulates the growth of cells in the uterine lining and thus, can fuel uterine cancer growth. This side effect has understandably limited its utility in treating breast cancer as well. (*More about these drugs in Chapter 7.*)

While Evista® appears to be safer than Fosamax® and the other bisphosphonates, we can see no reason to prefer it over bio-identical estrogens and progesterone and/or strontium. In addition to its apparent inability to prevent fractures of the hip and other nonvertebral bones, it can also cause unpleasant side effects, such as hot flashes and leg cramps. Most importantly, Evista® has been associated with an increased risk of potentially dangerous venous thromboembolism – blood clots that form in the veins of the legs and lungs, a rare but potentially devastating event.85 Moreover, since Evista® is an estrogen-like drug, taking it precludes taking bio-identical estrogens at the same time. Thus, whatever benefits might be gained in terms of preventing osteoporosis (and possibly breast cancer) would be lost in terms of the estrogen's many other skin, genitourinary, and cardiovascular benefits. (For more about SERMs and cancer, see Chapter 7.)

Strengthening Bones the Natural Way

Bio-identical hormones and strontium (along with calcium, vitamin D, magnesium, vitamin K2 – as menaquinone – zinc, copper, selenium, manganese, molybdenum, boron, and silicon) are effective in preventing and treating osteoporosis. Since 2002, when a natural strontium compound (strontium citrate) first became available over-the-counter in the US and Canada, every woman with osteoporosis (and its milder version, osteopenia) has had a significant increase in bone density within a year or less – and even more over the next few years – when using this combination of nutrients, and a bit more when using bio-identical hormones.* And – most importantly – not one woman using BHRT with calcium, strontium, and the other nutrients listed has suffered a new fracture!

Bio-identical hormones and strontium (along with calcium and the other nutrients listed) carry far lower risks than SERMs (although head-to-head studies have never been carried out, nor are they likely ever to be). Given these facts, the choice would seem to be obvious.

---

*   Researchers have pointed out that since strontium is a "denser" mineral than calcium, a proportion of the measured bone density increase should be "discounted" due to this difference in molecular density. While this may be true, even when partially "discounted," the bone density increases I've observed are significant. Other research studies have shown that strontium-containing bone has the same crystalline structure and flexibility as bone without strontium content.

References

1. Tenenhouse A, Joseph L, Kreiger N, et al. Estimation of the prevalence of low bone density in Canadian women and men using a population-specific DXA reference standard: the Canadian Multicentre Osteoporosis Study (CaMos). *Osteoporos Int.* 2000;11:897-904.

2. Gaby A. Strontium for osteoporosis: To dose or to megadose? *Townsend Letter for Doctors & Patients.* May 2006:106-107.

3. Grynpas MD, Marie PJ. Effects of low doses of strontium on bone quality and quantity in rats. *Bone.* 1990;11:313-319.

4. Shorr E, Carter A. The usefulness of strontium as an adjuvant to calcium in the remineralization of the skeleton in man. *Bull Hosp Joint Dis.* 1952;13:59-66.

5. Felson DT, Zhang Y, Hannan MT, Kiel DP, Wilson PW, Anderson JJ. The effect of postmenopausal estrogen therapy on bone density in elderly women. *N Engl J Med.* 1993;329:1141-1146.

6. NHLBI Women's Health Initiative. http://www.nhlbi.nih.gov/whi/whywhi.htm. Accessed March 5, 2006.

7. National Osteoporosis Foundation. Fast Facts. 2006; http://www.nof. org/osteoporosis/ diseasefacts.htm. Accessed March 7, 2006.

8. Compston JE. Sex steroids and bone. *Physiol Rev.* 2001;81:419-447.

9. Cummings SR, Browner WS, Bauer D, et al. Endogenous hormones and the risk of hip and vertebral fractures among older women. Study of Osteoporotic Fractures Research Group. *N Engl J Med.* 1998;339:733-738.

10. Anderson GL, Limacher M, Assaf AR, et al. Effects of conjugated equine estrogen in postmenopausal women with hysterectomy: the Women's Health Initiative randomized controlled trial. *JAMA.* 2004;291:1701-1712.

11. Cauley JA, Robbins J, Chen Z, et al. Effects of estrogen plus progestin on risk of fracture and bone mineral density: the Women's Health Initiative randomized trial. *JAMA.* 2003;290:1729-1738.

12. Orwoll ES, Nelson HD. Does estrogen adequately protect postmenopausal women against osteoporosis: an iconoclastic perspective. *J Clin Endocrinol Metab.* 1999;84:1872-1874.

13. Prior JC. Progesterone as a bone-trophic hormone. *Endocr Rev.* 1990;11:386-398.

14. Michaëlsson K, Baron JA, Farahmand BY, et al. Hormone replacement therapy and risk of hip fracture: population based case-control study. The Swedish Hip Fracture Study Group. *BMJ.* 1998;316:1858-1863.

15. National Institutes of Health. Women's Health Initiative: New Information. http://www.nhlbi.nih.gov/whi/. Accessed March 8, 2006.

16. Barbagallo M, Carbognani A, Palummeri E, et al. The comparative effect of ovarian hormone administration on bone mineral status in oophorectomized rats. *Bone.* 1989;10:113-116.

17. Wepfer S. A review of bioidentical hormone replacement therapy: Part 2. Progesterone. *Int J Pharmaceutical Compounding.* 2002;6:50-54.

18. Prior J. Trabecular bone loss is associated with abnormal luteal phase length: endogenous progesterone deficiency may be a risk factor for osteoporosis. *Int Proc J.* 1989;1:70-73.

19. Prior JC, Vigna YM, Schechter MT, Burgess AE. Spinal bone loss and ovulatory disturbances. *N Engl J Med.* 1990;323:1221-1227.

20. Prior JC, Vigna YM, Barr SI, Kennedy S, Schulzer M, Li DK. Ovulatory premenopausal women lose cancellous spinal bone: a five year prospective study. *Bone.* 1996;18:261-267.

21. Prior JC, Vigna YM, Barr SI, Rexworthy C, Lentle BC. Cyclic medroxyprogesterone treatment increases bone density: a controlled trial in active women with menstrual cycle disturbances. *Am J Med.* 1994;96:521-530.

22. Effects of hormone therapy on bone mineral density: results from the postmenopausal estrogen/progestin interventions (PEPI) trial. The Writing Group for the PEPI. *JAMA.* 1996;276:1389-1396.

23. Effects of hormone replacement therapy on endometrial histology in postmenopausal women. The Postmenopausal Estrogen/Progestin Interventions (PEPI) Trial. The Writing Group for the PEPI Trial. *JAMA.* 1996;275:370-375.

24. Lee J. *What Your Doctor May Not Tell You About Menopause.* New York: Warner Books; 1996.

25. The Writing Group for the PEPI Trial. Effects of estrogen or estrogen/progestin regimens on heart disease risk factors in postmenopausal women. The Postmenopausal Estrogen/Progestin Interventions (PEPI) Trial. *JAMA.* 1995;273:199-208.

26. Schairer C, Lubin J, Troisi R, Sturgeon S, Brinton L, Hoover R. Estrogen-progestin replacement and risk of breast cancer. *JAMA.* 2000;284:691-694.

27. Casanas-Roux F, Nisolle M, Marbaix E, Smets M, Bassil S, Donnez J. Morphometric, immunohistological and three-dimensional evaluation of the endometrium of menopausal women treated by oestrogen and Crinone, a new slow-release vaginal progesterone. *Hum Reprod.* 1996;11:357-363.

28. Dai D, Wolf DM, Litman ES, White MJ, Leslie KK. Progesterone inhibits human endometrial cancer cell growth and invasiveness: down-regulation of cellular adhesion molecules through progesterone B receptors. *Cancer Res.* 2002;62:881-886.

29. Leonetti HB, Anasti JN, Litman ES. Topical progesterone cream: an alternative progestin in hormone replacement therapy. *Obstet & Gynecol.* 2003;101 (4 Suppl):85.

30. Leonetti HB, Landes J, Steinberg D, Anasti JN. Transdermal progesterone cream as an alternative progestin in hormone therapy. *Altern Ther Health Med.* 2005;11:36-38.

31. Leonetti HB, Wilson KJ, Anasti JN. Topical progesterone cream has an antiproliferative effect on estrogen-stimulated endometrium. *Fertil Steril.* 2003;79:221-222.

32. Montz FJ, Bristow RE, Bovicelli A, Tomacruz R, Kurman RJ. Intrauterine progesterone treatment of early endometrial cancer. *Am J Obstet Gynecol.* 2002;186:651-657.

33. Moyer DL, de Lignieres B, Driguez P, Pez JP. Prevention of endometrial hyperplasia by progesterone during long-term estradiol replacement: influence of bleeding pattern and secretory changes. *Fertil Steril.* 1993;59:992-997.

34. Moyer DL, Felix JC. The effects of progesterone and progestins on endometrial proliferation. *Contraception.* 1998;57:399-403.

35. Moyer DL, Felix JC, Kurman RJ, Cuffie CA. Micronized progesterone regulation of the endometrial glandular cycling pool. *Int J Gynecol Pathol.* 2001;20:374-379.

36. Nisolle M, Donnez J. Progesterone receptors (PR) in ectopic endometrium? *Fertil Steril.* 1997;68:943-944.

37. Nisolle M, Gillerot S, Casanas-Roux F, Squifflet J, Berliere M, Donnez J. Immunohistochemical study of the proliferation index, oestrogen receptors and progesterone receptors A and B in leiomyomata and normal myometrium during the menstrual cycle and under gonadotrophin-releasing hormone agonist therapy. *Hum Reprod.* 1999;14:2844-2850.

38. Sager G, Orbo A, Jaeger R, Engstrom C. Non-genomic effects of progestins-- inhibition of cell growth and increased intracellular levels of cyclic nucleotides. *J Steroid Biochem Mol Biol.* 2003;84:1-8.

39. Whitehead MI, Fraser D, Schenkel L, Crook D, Stevenson JC. Transdermal administration of oestrogen/progestagen hormone replacement therapy. *Lancet.* 1990;335:310-312.

40. Miller BE, De Souza MJ, Slade K, Luciano AA. Sublingual administration of micronized estradiol and progesterone, with and without micronized testosterone: effect on biochemical markers of bone metabolism and bone mineral density. *Menopause.* 2000;7:318-326.

41. Villareal DT. Effects of dehydroepiandrosterone on bone mineral density: what implications for therapy? *Treat Endocrinol.* 2002;1:349-357.

42. Jankowski CM, Gozansky WS, Kittelson JM, Van Pelt RE, Schwartz RS, Kohrt WM. Increases in bone mineral density in response to oral dehydroepiandrosterone replacement in older adults appear to be mediated by serum estrogens. *J Clin Endocrinol Metab.* 2008;93:4767-4773.

43. Raven PW, Hinson JP. Dehydroepiandrosterone (DHEA) and the menopause: an update. *Menopause Int.* 2007;13:75-78.

44. Baulieu EE, Thomas G, Legrain S, et al. Dehydroepiandrosterone (DHEA), DHEA sulfate, and aging: contribution of the DHEAge Study to a sociobiomedical issue. *Proc Natl Acad Sci U S A.* 2000;97:4279-4284.

45. Osmanagaoglu MA, Okumus B, Osmanagaoglu T, Bozkaya H. The relationship between serum dehydroepiandrosterone sulfate concentration and bone mineral density, lipids, and hormone replacement therapy in premenopausal and postmenopausal women. *J Womens Health (Larchmt).* 2004;13:993-999.

46. Tok EC, Ertunc D, Oz U, Camdeviren H, Ozdemir G, Dilek S. The effect of circulating androgens on bone mineral density in postmenopausal women. *Maturitas.* 2004;48:235-242.

47. Garnero P, Sornay-Rendu E, Claustrat B, Delmas PD. Biochemical markers of bone turnover, endogenous hormones and the risk of fractures in postmenopausal women: the OFELY study. *J Bone Miner Res.* 2000;15:1526-1536.

48. Kocis P. Prasterone. *Am J Health Syst Pharm.* 2006;63:2201-2210.

49. Petri MA, Mease PJ, Merrill JT, et al. Effects of prasterone on disease activity and symptoms in women with active systemic lupus erythematosus. *Arthritis Rheum.* 2004;50:2858-2868.

50. Chapuy MC, Arlot ME, Duboeuf F, et al. Vitamin D3 and calcium to prevent hip fractures in the elderly women. *N Engl J Med.* 1992;327:1637-1642.

51. Marie PJ, Ammann P, Boivin G, Rey C. Mechanisms of action and therapeutic potential of strontium in bone. *Calcif Tissue Int.* 2001;69:121-129.

52. McCaslin F, James J. The effect of strontium lactate in the treatment of osteoporosis. *Proc Staf Meetings Mayo Clin.* 1959;34:329-334.

53. Marie P, Skoryna S, Pivon R, Chabot G, Glorieux F, Stara J. Histomorphometry of bone changes in stable strontium therapy. In: Hemphill D, ed. *Trace Substances in Environmental Health, XIX.* Columbia, MO: University of Missouri; 1985:193-208.

54. El-Hajj Fuleihan G. Strontium ranelate--a novel therapy for osteoporosis or a permutation of the same? *N Engl J Med.* 2004;350:504-506.

55. Ozgur S, Sumer H, Kocoglu G. Rickets and soil strontium. *Arch Dis Child.* 1996;75:524-526.

56. Protelos: Prescribing Information. http://www.servier.com/pro/osteoporose/ protelos/protelos.asp. Servier: Accessed April 12, 2006.

57. Reginster JY, Deroisy R, Dougados M, Jupsin I, Colette J, Roux C. Prevention of early postmenopausal bone loss by strontium ranelate: the randomized, two-year, double-masked, dose-ranging, placebo-controlled PREVOS trial. *Osteoporos Int.* 2002;13:925-931.

58. Meunier PJ, Roux C, Seeman E, et al. The effects of strontium ranelate on the risk of vertebral fracture in women with postmenopausal osteoporosis. *N Engl J Med.* 2004;350:459-468.

59. Reginster JY, Felsenberg D, Boonen S, et al. Effects of long-term strontium ranelate treatment on the risk of nonvertebral and vertebral fractures in postmenopausal osteoporosis: Results of a five-year, randomized, placebo-controlled trial. *Arthritis Rheum.* 2008;58:1687-1695.

60. Roux C, Fechtenbaum J, Kolta S, Isaia G, Andia JB, Devogelaer JP. Strontium ranelate reduces the risk of vertebral fracture in young postmenopausal women with severe osteoporosis. *Ann Rheum Dis.* 2008;67:1736-1738.

61. US Food and Drug Administration. FORTEO™: teriparatide (rDNA origin) injection. 2004; http://www.fda.gov/MEDwatch/SAFETY/2004/sep_PI/Forteo_ PI.pdf.

62. Hosking D, Chilvers CE, Christiansen C, et al. Prevention of bone loss with alendronate in postmenopausal women under 60 years of age. Early Postmenopausal Intervention Cohort Study Group. *N Engl J Med.* 1998;338:485-492.

63. Rosen CJ. Clinical practice. Postmenopausal osteoporosis. *N Engl J Med.* 2005;353:595-603.

64. Smith A. Merck sales dip; Vioxx blamed. *http://money.cnn.com/2005/04/21/ news/fortune500/merck/index.htm.* CNNMoney.com. Accessed April 24, 2006.

65. Bone HG, Hosking D, Devogelaer JP, et al. Ten years' experience with alendronate for osteoporosis in postmenopausal women. *N Engl J Med.* 2004;350:1189-1199.

66. Odvina CV, Zerwekh JE, Rao DS, Maalouf N, Gottschalk FA, Pak CY. Severely suppressed bone turnover: a potential complication of alendronate therapy. *J Clin Endocrinol Metab.* 2005;90:1294-1301.

67. Schneider J. Should bisphosphonates be continued indefinitely? An unusual fracture in a healthy woman on long-term alendronate. *Geriatrics.* 2006;61:31-33.

68. Schneider J. Bisphosphonates and low-impact femoral fractures: Current evidence on alendronate-fracture risk. *Geriatrics.* 2009;64:18-23.

69. Goh SK, Yang KY, Koh JS, et al. Subtrochanteric insufficiency fractures in patients on alendronate therapy: a caution. *J Bone Joint Surg Br.* 2007;89:349-353.

70. Stepan JJ, Burr DB, Pavo I, et al. Low bone mineral density is associated with bone microdamage accumulation in postmenopausal women with osteoporosis. *Bone.* 2007;41:378-385.

71. Ott SM. Long-term safety of bisphosphonates. *J Clin Endocrinol Metab.* 2005;90:1897-1899.

72. Brody J. Plotting to Save the Structure of Those Aging Bones. *The New York Times.* Vol New YorkJuly 5, 2005.

73. Ott S. New treatments for brittle bones. *Ann Intern Med.* 2004;141:406-407.

74. Fosamax® (alendronate sodium) Prescribing Information. http://www.fosamax. com/alendronate _sodium/fosamax/consumer/product_information/pi/index. jsp?WT.svl=1. *Merck & Co., Inc.*; Accessed April 26, 2006.

75. Wysowski DK. Reports of Esophageal Cancer with Oral Bisphosphonate Use. *N Engl J Med.* 2009;360:89-90.

76. Chustecka Z. Esophageal cancer in patients taking oral bisphosphonates. *Medscape Medical News.* 2008;http://www.medscape.com/viewarticle/586127.

77. Basu N, Reid DM. Bisphosphonate-associated osteonecrosis of the jaw. *Menopause Int.* 2007;13:56-59.

78. Ruggiero SL, Mehrotra B, Rosenberg TJ, Engroff SL. Osteonecrosis of the jaws associated with the use of bisphosphonates: a review of 63 cases. *J Oral Maxillofac Surg.* 2004;62:527-534.

79. Edwards BJ, Hellstein JW, Jacobsen PL, Kaltman S, Mariotti A, Migliorati CA. Updated recommendations for managing the care of patients receiving oral bisphosphonate therapy: an advisory statement from the American Dental Association Council on Scientific Affairs. *J Am Dent Assoc.* 2008;139:1674-1677.

80. Sedghizadeh PP, Stanley K, Caligiuri M, Hofkes S, Lowry B, Shuler CF. Oral bisphosphonate use and the prevalence of osteonecrosis of the jaw: an institutional inquiry. *J Am Dent Assoc.* 2009;140:61-66.

81. Paddock C. Osteoporosis drug linked to bone death in jaw. *Medical News Today.* January 5, 2009; http://www.medicalnewstoday.com/articles/134381.php.

82. Marsa L. Bone drugs' reverse danger. *Los Angeles Times.* April 3, 2006; http:// www.latimes.com/ features/health/la-he-fosamax3apr03,0,3944007,full. story?coll=la-headlines-business:Accessed April 27, 2006.

83. Heckbert SR, Li G, Cummings SR, Smith NL, Psaty BM. Use of alendronate and risk of incident atrial fibrillation in women. *Arch Intern Med.* 2008;168:826-831.

84. Miranda J. Osteoporosis drugs increase risk of heart problems. *CHEST 2008.* Vol Philadelphia, PA: American College of Chest Physicians; 2008.

85. Evista® (raloxifene hydrochloride) Prescribing Information. *http://pi.lilly.com/us/evista-pi.pdf.*Eli Lilly and Co., Indianapolis, IN Accessed April 22, 2006.

CHAPTER 7

DOES HORMONE REPLACEMENT CAUSE CANCER?

This "simple" question turns out to be much more complex than it seems. For example:

- *What types of estrogen?* Some human estrogens, like *estradiol* and *estrone*, as well as nonhuman "estrogens," like horse estrogens (*conjugated equine estrogens, CEEs*) and the highly potent, patented "estrogen" *ethinyl estradiol*, are significantly more carcinogenic in the breast and uterus than others. Horse estrogens, especially, have been solidly linked with the development of breast tumors. However, estriol is different. The more *estriol* a woman has in her body, relative to both *estrone* and *estradiol*, the *smaller her risk of developing breast cancer* seems to be. In the presence of estradiol or estrone, estriol has anticarcinogenic activity – inhibiting carcinogenic actions of the other more carcinogenic estrogens.

- *Progesterone or progestin?* Progesterone-like patent medicines called progestins – usually Provera® (medroxyprogesterone) – have been substituted (by patent medicine companies, of course) for progesterone to "oppose" cancer-causing estrogens (especially Premarin®) as a way of preventing endometrial cancer. However, helpful as they may be in this regard in the uterus, progestins have their own carcinogenic potential in the breast, where they might even contribute to "estrogen"-induced cell proliferation. By contrast, bio-identical progesterone has little or no built-in carcinogenic potential, either in the uterus or breast (or anywhere else), and it also helps modulate the cancer-causing effects of potent estrogens.[1]

- *Which metabolites (changed forms) of estrogen?* "Good" (anticarcinogenic) estrogen metabolites or "bad" (carcinogenic) estrogen metabolites"? Consumption of certain common vegetables and/or nutrient supplements derived from those veggies can improve the ratio of "good" to "bad" estrogen metabolites and so, help reduce the risk of developing breast cancer. On the other hand, use of patented progestin drugs may promote the formation of one of the worst of these "bad" estrogen metabolites.[2] Some anticarcinogenic human estrogen metabolites are currently being tested in clinical trials by patent medicine companies and government agencies to see if they might be useful as safe anticancer "drugs." (Yes, as part of their marketing strategies, it is common practice for patent medicine companies – not to mention most doctors who don't seem to know the difference – to call 100% bio-identical estrogen metabolites "drugs.")

A decade ago, in our previous book on the subject – *Natural Hormone Replacement for Women Over 45*[3] – we argued that there was enough solid scientific evidence to conclude that conventional "hormone" replacement therapy (Premarin® + Provera®) significantly increased the risk of breast cancer. However, the mainstream medicine, for the most part, still felt the jury was out.

Ordinarily, evidence that a patent medicine (or any other substance) might increase the risk of cancer – even if the evidence is not definitive – means banishment from the marketplace. However, conventional HRT has managed to survive the FDA's axe due to the presumption – based on rather weak evidence – that HRT could balance any increased risks of breast and other cancers by providing protection against more common, but also serious risks, such as heart attacks, strokes, osteoporotic bone fractures, and dementia.

Since July 2002, the results of the Women's Health Initiative (WHI) finally put the lie to that presumption, and suddenly, the Empress HRT was revealed in all her not-so-beautiful nakedness. The large, double-blind, placebo-controlled WHI study (as well as other less well-known trials) confirmed that, not only did HRT increase the risk of breast cancer (which was no big surprise), but that it also increased the risks of heart attack, stroke, urinary incontinence, and senility, exactly the opposite of what had been expected and widely promoted for years.[4] Three years later, the International Agency for Research on Cancer, a division of the World Health Organization (WHO), issued a statement declaring that, "*...combined "estrogen"-progestogen contraceptives and menopausal therapy are carcinogenic to humans.*"[5] As described in Chapter 1, the final shoe dropped when researchers from the MD Anderson Cancer

Center in Houston, Texas, produced the "smoking gun," a rock-sold link between the use of conventional HRT and an increased risk of breast cancer.[6-8]

In the 7 years since the WHI revelations, millions of women have turned away from HRT, and many of these have turned to BHRT. Understandably, though, they wonder whether BHRT really has a lower cancer risk than conventional HRT. The loud, powerful, well-coordinated voices of mainstream medicine argue that BHRT is no different from conventional HRT with regard to its risks of cancer promotion and should never be trusted until it is tested "properly." Most "regular" doctors just parrot the FDA's "party line" – heavily influenced by the FDA's Big Pharma patrons – that, in the absence of large "definitive," long-term, double-blind, placebo-controlled studies, BHRT must be considered just as dangerous as HRT.*

We disagree emphatically! There is plenty of evidence, much of it from independent, nonpatent-medicine-related research – some from studies in humans and some in lab studies of human cancer models – all pointing in the same direction, that BHRT has a far lower risk of causing cancer than conventional, patented HRT, and in many instances can contribute to preventing cancer.

"MISSION" Accomplished

We could cite countless reasons why the conventional "party line" is pure nonsense, but perhaps the clearest way to make the point is to refer to the results of a recent large French study (more than 6,700 postmenopausal women) known by its acronym MISSION.[9] The MISSION study compared the incidence of breast cancer in women who had been "exposed" to some form of hormone replacement therapy within the prior 5 years with the breast cancer incidence in women who had never used hormone replacement therapy or had stopped using it more than 5 years before the study. The average exposure to hormones in the MISSION study was 8.3 years, 5 years longer than exposure to conventional HRT in the WHI study. Yet, unlike the WHI, the MISSION study found *no increased risk of breast cancer in women exposed to* hormone replacement therapy.

---

* That Premarin® + Provera® (Prempro®) is still "approved" for treating menopausal symptoms (albeit under much more limited circumstances) is a testament to Big Pharma's political clout, not to mention its incestuous relationship with the Federal agency that's supposed to be regulating it.

Why the difference? The primary reason, according to the MISSION researchers, was likely that women in France for the most part do not use American-style conventional HRT. Instead, at least three-fourths of the participants used *topical estradiol* combined with either *bio-identical progesterone* (44%) or a progestin other than Provera® (56%). Although there were no significant differences in the incidence of breast cancer among the various hormone replacement regimens used in the MISSION study, ***the safest one included topical estradiol + bio-identical progesterone (an oral micronized formulation)***.

While no treatment can ever be considered 100% safe, we believe that a fair reading of the medical literature − the MISSION study is just one of many leading to similar conclusions − leaves little doubt that bio-identical hormones carry far lower cancer (and other) risks than do horse estrogens and other patented, FDA-approved "hormonal" products.

In the 25 years since I (JVW) wrote the first of more than 5,000 prescription for bio-identical estrogens and progesterone for menopausal women (and men with low androgens taking bio-identical testosterone), to the best of my knowledge, only one person subsequently developed a *possibly* hormone-related cancer. Admittedly, this is not "controlled research," but still, based on published statistics, this incidence of cancer is far lower than would have been expected with conventional HRT. Moreover, we can safely multiply my experience by that of thousands of physicians who've decided to re-orient at least part of their practices towards natural therapies, and have had comparable success in prescribing BHRT to hundreds of thousands of satisfied women. Even in the absence of "definitive" FDA-style trials, it's hard to deny the reality of first-hand experiences like these.

But don't take our word for it. Let's examine the role that *published* scientific research has shown that natural and bio-identical estrogens, progesterone, and patented "estrogen" and progestin products might play in the development of cancer.

How *Some* Estrogens Might Cause Cancer

Estrogens are thought to increase the risk of cancer primarily due to their *anabolic* nature. The normal, everyday job of anabolic hormones is to stimulate the growth of new tissue, such as the lining of the uterus each month in preparation for embryo implantation and in the lining of milk ducts and other tissue in the breast in anticipation of lactation.

The dark side of normal anabolic activity is cancer. While stimulating the growth of healthy tissue, there's a possibility that estrogens (or other anabolic hormones, like androgens and human growth hormone) might also stimulate and/or accelerate the growth and progression of tumor cells.

Estrogens have been linked to breast cancer for over a century, since a Scottish surgeon named George Beatson reported on the cases of three premenopausal women whose breast cancer went into remission after he removed their ovaries.[10] Dr. Beatson surmised that something in the ovaries might be fueling cancer growth. However, it was another 10 years (1906) before other British researchers discovered that the ovaries secreted estrogen.[11] Thus, Dr. Beatson's patients probably survived as long as they did, because he had removed the primary source of anabolic estrogens in their bodies.

We have detailed the role estrogens play in promoting normal and abnormal tissue growth in the uterine lining (endometrium) elsewhere in this book (*See Chapter 2.*). Suffice it to say, in the absence of progesterone (or a progestin drug), "unopposed" potent estrogens can promote cellular overgrowth (*hyperplasia*) in the uterine lining, which in some cases may turn cancerous. This is especially true of the more potent "estrogens" like Premarin®, but it can also be true of the "weaker" human estrogens, estradiol, and estrone.

It was this finding back in the 1970s, that led conventional medicine to halt prescribing Premarin® by itself to postmenopausal women and to begin combining it with the patented progestin drug Provera®. Combining Premarin® and Provera® does indeed cut the risk of uterine cancer, but at the same time, it also increases the risk of breast cancer, among other serious problems – a fact it took conventional medicine nearly 30 more years to figure out.

By contrast, the "weak" estrogen estriol has a very low propensity for causing hyperplasia and cancer in the uterus, breast, or anywhere else, even when used "unopposed." This effect is well documented in the medical literature, and some evidence suggests that estriol may even protect against the growth of cancers fueled by more potent estrogens. It is thought that estrogens may induce carcinogenic activity by at least two separate mechanisms:[12]

- Estrogens can trigger cancer cell transformation (*conversion of healthy cells into malignant cells*) either by damaging cellular DNA or by activating cancer-promoting genes (*oncogenes*).

- While stimulating normal tissue growth (*proliferation*) in the uterus or breast, estrogens might also accelerate the growth of a very early, pre-existing malignancy (no matter what started it),

Estrogens influence the growth (or not) of breast cell proliferation and possibly cancer by binding to (and stimulating) two different estrogen receptors, identified as α and β *receptors* – or *ER-α* and *ER-β*.[1] Estrogens that stimulate ER-α tend to promote breast cell proliferation. By contrast, estrogens that stimulate ER-β inhibit breast cell proliferation, and consequently, protect against breast cancer development.

Research has shown that estradiol stimulates ER-α and ER-β receptors about equally, but estrone is about five times more potent in stimulating ER-α vs. ER-β receptors. This helps explain why elevated estrone levels are considered such a high risk for breast cancer. On the other hand, estriol stimulates ER-β receptors about three times more than ER-α receptors, making it less likely to promote breast cancer.

What about horse estrogens? They're worst of all. Not only do CEEs favorably stimulate ER-α receptors, they also *block* (or *downregulate*) ER-β receptors. To make matters worse, one horse estrogen – 4-hydroxequilenin, never found in humans (*See Chapter 1.*) – induces DNA damage, making it a particularly potent carcinogen.

How Risky Is Cumulative Exposure to Estrogens?

Given these dangers, the conventional wisdom has been that the more estrogens a woman is exposed to during her lifetime, the greater the chances she will eventually develop breast cancer. In support of this hypothesis, it is commonly noted that women whose menarche (*first menstrual period*) occurred at a relatively young age and/or whose menopause was later than average might be at increased risk for developing breast cancer, because these women would have had more total months of ovarian estrogen secretion and exposure.[13]

Other research has shown that women with the highest concentrations of estrone and estradiol, as well as of testosterone (and other androgens) had approximately twice the risk of later developing breast cancer compared to those who had the lowest levels.[14] While these conclusions may be valid for estradiol and estrone, they tell us nothing about estriol. For some unexplained reason, these researchers failed to report the concentrations of estriol in these women, which is perhaps a reflection of the disdain conventional medicine has typically shown for this important hormone. Nevertheless, we are quite confident, based on large numbers of other studies, that had they looked at estriol concentrations, they would not have found a comparable relationship between estriol and breast cancer. Moreover, it is quite possible, as we explain later in this chapter, that they might well have found the opposite relationship, because relatively high levels of estriol might have protected them against breast cancer, no matter what their estradiol and estrone levels were.)

In addition to endogenous (ovarian) estrogen secretion, breast cancer risk rises with the extended use of patented "estrogen"-progestin oral contraceptive pills (usually ethinyl estradiol + a progestin) and/or postmenopausal "estrogen"-progestin replacement regimens (usually Premarin® + Provera®). Data from several large studies show that 5 or more years of conventional HRT use increase a woman's risk of breast cancer by 30 to 40%, compared to nonusers. However, as detailed in Chapter 1, once they stop taking their "hormones," removing the "fuel" that breast tumors grow on, their risk declines quite rapidly, and after 1 to 5 years off "hormones," all excess risk has generally evaporated.[8, 12, 15, 16]

While cumulative exposure to some estrogens may be a factor in breast cancer development in some women, it is clearly far from the whole story. For example, the long-term exposure hypothesis is not supported by the following highly valid observation: even as ovarian estrogen secretion falls sharply during and after menopause, women's risk of breast cancer during these years continues to rise. Dr. Richard A. Wiseman of the London School of Hygiene and Tropical Medicine observes that a 75-year-old woman (not on HRT), who has spent her last 25 years without significant ovarian estrogenic stimulation, nevertheless, has a considerably higher risk of breast cancer than a 50-year-old woman, who is just coming to the end of her maximum estrogen-secreting years.[17]

If cumulative estrogen stimulation were important, Dr. Wiseman argues, menopause should signal a decrease in breast cancer risk, not an increase. The postmenopausal decline in carcinogenic estrogens should be analogous to the decline in carcinogen exposure that occurs when people stop smoking. Just as the risk of lung cancer declines with each year off cigarettes, so should the risk of breast cancer decline each year away from estrogen. Plainly, though, that's not what happens when estrogen exposure decreases. "Breast cancer rates in Western societies never fall back to even the highest premenopausal rates, even though estradiol levels [after menopause] fall to less than one-tenth of premenopausal concentration," writes Dr. Wiseman.

Dr. Wiseman further notes that estrogen levels surge during pregnancy, increasing a woman's exposure to the hormone during the last half of the third trimester by 10- to 12-fold. If cumulative estrogen exposure were really an important factor, then pregnancies should increase breast cancer risk.[13] In reality, breast cancer during pregnancy is rare, and repeated pregnancies, with their extremely high cumulative estrogen exposure, actually *reduce* the risk of breast cancer in the long run.

So does long-term estrogen exposure increase the risk of breast cancer? It appears that this is not question we should be asking. Rather, we should be asking, does long-term exposure to *certain estrogens* increase the risk? It seems likely that long-term exposure to potent estrogens – eg, estradiol, estrone, and CEEs – might indeed be dangerous. On the other hand, long-term exposure to estriol actually appears to be protective.

How Pregnancy Might Protect Against Breast Cancer

Women who give birth when they are younger than age 24 have a reduced lifetime risk of breast cancer, and each additional pregnancy thereafter decreases that risk even further.[18] What is it about pregnancy that seems to offer a degree of long-term protection against breast cancer, even though estrogen levels during pregnancy are extraordinarily high?

Both pregnancy and breast cancer are such complex events that nobody knows for sure, although certain suggestive facts stand out as possible explanations. For one, estrogens are not the only hormones that rise dramatically during pregnancy; toward the end of pregnancy, progesterone levels also shoot up by a factor of 7- or 8-fold. Progesterone, of course, has a long and well-documented history of "opposing" the carcinogenic proclivities of potent estrogens. It makes sense that if Mother Nature felt the need to raise estrogen levels during pregnancy, She would also throw in a good complement of progesterone, as well, to mute the estrogens' natural carcinogenicity (much as She does in the uterus for 10 to 14 days each month during menstruation).

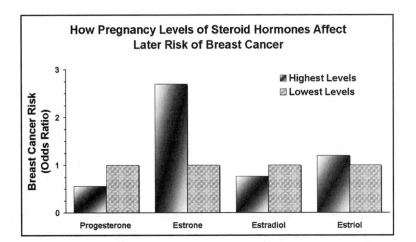

Figure 7-1. Relationship between pregnancy levels of progesterone, estrone, estradiol, and estriol and the later risk (odds ratio) of breast cancer up to 30 years later. The highest levels of progesterone during pregnancy reduced later breast cancer risk by 40-50%, compared to the lowest levels. By contrast, the highest levels of estrone increased that risk by more than 200%.   *Source: Peck et al, 2002*

Only a couple of studies have attempted to correlate sex steroid hormones during pregnancy and the subsequent development of breast cancer. One compared a group of women who had been pregnant between 1959 and 1966 and later developed breast cancer with a matched control group, none of whom had ever developed breast cancer. The results showed that the women's progesterone levels – measured during pregnancy – were strongly and inversely correlated with breast cancer diagnosed at or before (but not after) age 50. Women who had the highest progesterone levels during pregnancy had a risk of later breast cancer that was 40 to 50% lower than in women who had the lowest levels during pregnancy (Fig. 7-1). In other words, the higher a woman's progesterone levels during pregnancy, the lower her risk of developing breast cancer later in life.[19] (Remember we're talking progesterone here, not pseudo-progesterone drugs like Provera®; taking Provera® with Premarin® actually increases the risk of breast cancer.[20])

Another important factor in breast cancer risk may be the nature of the estrogens produced during pregnancy. Estriol is one of the major estrogens women produce during their reproductive years. During pregnancy, estriol, produced primarily by the fetus and placenta, literally floods the body, increasing in volume each month until birth. By the end of the third trimester, estriol levels may rise by as much as 1000%, 10 times higher than estrone and estradiol levels.[21]

If that alone were not confirmation enough of estriol's safety, much other evidence indicates that, compared to other natural or bio-identical estrogens (and patented "estrogens"). As mentioned above, estriol has a very low propensity for stimulating cell growth in places like the uterus and breast, and it may even ameliorate the carcinogenic proliferating tendencies of the other more potent estrogens and "estrogens." It is thought that the extremely high estriol levels that occur during pregnancy may help protect developing fetal tissues from cancer triggered by estrone and/or estradiol, the levels of which are also high at that time.

In the study described above on pregnancy progesterone levels and subsequent breast cancer risk, the researchers also measured estrone, estradiol, and estriol levels during pregnancy. Estrone is often cited as the most carcinogenic of the human estrogens for the breast, and these results support that conclusion. The researchers found a close association between estrone levels (but not with estradiol or estriol levels) and later development of breast cancer; women who had the highest estrone levels during pregnancy had more than double the breast cancer risk of women with the lowest estrone levels (Fig. 7-1).[19]

The benefit of all that estriol floating around during pregnancy was brought home in a study reported by Pentii K. Siiteri, PhD, and colleagues of the US Public Health Service.[22] Women, who had been pregnant at least once between 1959 and 1967, had blood samples taken during their pregnancy, frozen, and stored away. These samples were later thawed and tested for levels of sex steroid hormones.

As shown in Figure 7-2, the USPHS investigators found a strong and statistically significant *inverse association* between estriol levels during pregnancy and the later occurrence of breast cancer. That is, women who had the highest levels of estriol during their pregnancies, had a 77% lower breast cancer risk later in life, while those with the lowest levels of estriol had just a 58% reduction.[*]

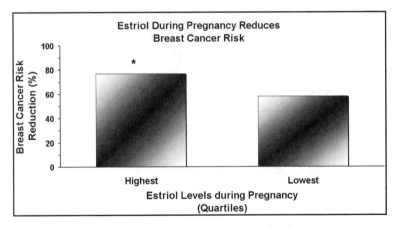

Figure 7-2. Women who had the highest levels of estriol during pregnancy had a significantly lower risk of developing breast cancer over the next 30 years compared with women who had the lowest levels of estriol. * *P* <0.01.
Source: *Siiteri et al. 2002*

---

* Oddly, this research was sponsored by the US Army Medical Research and Materiel Command. The study participants included a sample of 438 women taken from the very large (15,000 women), long-running (40 years) Child Health and Development Studies.

Built-In Cancer Protection

Unlike other "estrogenic" treatments, such as horse estrogens or 100%-estradiol pills, patches, and creams, there is no evidence that estriol, taken at reasonable doses and on a physiologic (close-to-natural) schedule, stimulates abnormally high rates of cell proliferation – a known precursor to cancer – in the uterine lining, breast, or other estrogen-sensitive locations.

Estriol actually antagonizes the proliferative activities of the other more potent estrogens, probably because it competes for and benignly occupies estrogen receptor sites that are targeted by other estrogens. With a "weak" estriol occupying estrogen receptor sites, the more potent, more carcinogenic estrogens are literally crowded out, affording them less opportunity to fuel uterine or breast cell proliferation. Thus, it appears that Mother Nature may use estriol to modulate the actions of these powerful hormones before they can do any serious harm – a kind of built-in cancer protection.

We can illustrate the benign nature of estriol by comparing the dose of each of the estrogens needed to induce the highest rate of cell proliferation in the uterine lining, as if in preparation for embryo implantation. This dose is termed the "proliferative dose." The higher the proliferative dose for a given estrogen, the more benign (some would say "the weaker") the estrogen; the lower the proliferative dose, the more potent (some would say more potentially harmful) the estrogen.

Laboratory studies have shown that the proliferative dose of estriol is at least twice as high as that for horse estrogens (eg, equilin) and estradiol, and 60 to 75 times as high as that of the powerful patented "estrogen," ethinyl estradiol.[23] This means that it takes far more estriol than the other "estrogens" to trigger significant cell proliferation.

For many years, this fact led researchers to dismiss estriol as a "weak estrogen," or just an "inert metabolite" of estrone and estradiol. (One might ask if estriol's weakness might also be its strength. Why else would Mother Nature have designed human estrogens to include a large proportion of estriol during menstruation and an overwhelming majority of estriol during pregnancy, just to take up space?) In fact, compared with its more potent cousins, estriol's relatively benign nature translates into a reduced, or even negligible, risk of cancer.

Even the characterization of estriol as a "weak" estrogen may be misleading. While estriol is certainly less potent for causing proliferation, it has more than enough potency to perform other important estrogenic functions.[24] However, many women have told me [JVW] that it takes them more milligrams of estriol (by itself) than of Tri-Est to "handle" their menopausal symptoms. A very few women say that estriol by itself in any dose "just isn't enough" and that estradiol and estrone must be added – in bio-identical proportions, of course – to "get the job done." For this reason, although estriol has sometimes been used as the sole estrogen in bio-identical hormone replacement regimens, Tri-Est (or Bi-Est) may often be the better choice.

What's Your EQ?

Although ovarian estrogen as a whole has been implicated as a possible cause of breast cancer since the late 19th century, it wasn't until Henry Lemon, MD, came along that anyone had taken the trouble to look at the relative concentrations of the three primary human estrogens to see how each might be related to the development of cancer. During the 1960s and '70s, Dr. Lemon, then the head of the Division of Gynecologic Oncology at the University of Nebraska College of Medicine, began following up on considerable lab research, to investigate the possibility that estriol might provide women with a kind of built-in protection against breast cancer.

Dr. Lemon first got interested in estriol, because of its ability to compete with – or "impede" – estrone and estradiol in their quest to attach to receptor sites, especially in critical areas like the uterine lining and breast, and to do so without stimulating those receptors nearly as much as the other more potent estrogens.[25] Previously published studies had demonstrated that estrone and estradiol were each capable of promoting abnormal cell proliferation, leading to uterine cancer (primarily estradiol) and breast cancer (both estrone and estradiol). However, when natural concentrations of estriol were added to the mix, the ability of estrone and estradiol to stimulate the estrogen-sensitive tissues was significantly inhibited.[26]

The body "expects" estrone and estradiol to have carcinogenic potential, and so, it treats these hormones with extreme care. Estradiol and estrone that are not needed for immediate use may be neutralized by binding them to certain proteins [eg, sex hormone binding globulin (SHBG) or albumin] or by converting them rapidly and irreversibly to estriol, which is virtually noncarcinogenic. Once estrone and estradiol get converted to estriol, they stay estriol.

Dr. Lemon reasoned that, if estriol levels were low relative to estrone and estradiol, these two hormones, now "unimpeded" by not having to compete as much with estriol, might be able to release more of their carcinogenic potential; the less estriol, the greater the risk. Was it possible, he asked, that some women might be developing breast cancer, because their ratio of estriol to estradiol + estrone was too low?

To answer his question, Dr. Lemon ran a preliminary study in which he collected urine from women over a 24-hour period to measure the levels of each of the women's estrogens. From these measurements, he calculated a urinary estrogen quotient (EQ), which was simply the ratio of excreted estriol to the total of excreted estrone + estradiol. If a 24-hour urine collection showed 150 μg of estriol and 50 μg each of estrone and estradiol, the EQ would be 150/100 or 1.5 [arbitrary numbers for illustration only]; the more estriol present relative to estrone + estradiol, the higher the quotient, and perhaps, the lower the risk of breast cancer.[27]

$$\frac{\text{Estriol}}{\text{Estrone} + \text{Estradiol}} = \text{EQ}$$

As part of his review of background research on estriol and breast cancer, Dr. Lemon found that about two-thirds of Caucasian women diagnosed with breast cancer had subnormal urinary EQs (less than 1.0).[25] In his small study, in 34 women with no signs of breast cancer, Dr. Lemon found the median EQ to be 1.3 before menopause and 1.2 postmenopause. The EQ was below 1.0 – a possible danger sign – in only 21% of these healthy women (Fig. 7-3). In 26 other women who had breast cancer, the picture was quite different; their median EQ was low – 0.5 before menopause and 0.8 postmenopause. Nearly two-thirds (62%) of the women with breast cancer had an EQ below 1.0. Thus, relative to the estrone and estradiol, the women without breast cancer seemed to be excreting substantially more estriol than the women with breast cancer.[28]

Considerable published laboratory and clinical evidence from other researchers, as well as from Dr. Lemon himself, has lent credence to the basic concept that estriol has value for preventing breast cancer:

- Laboratory animal studies totaling more than 500 rat-years show estriol to be the most active protective estrogen ever tested against breast cancers induced by several potent carcinogenic agents,[29] including radiation.[30]

- In contrast to estrone, estradiol, equilin, ethinyl estradiol, DES, and other patentable "estrogens," which are routinely found to be carcinogenic and have been "officially" declared as such by the WHO,[5] no appropriate studies have ever shown bio-identical estriol to have any significant carcinogenic activity. It's true that when estriol is taken in excessively high doses (especially orally); is taken continuously (ie, every day without pause); or is implanted as pellets

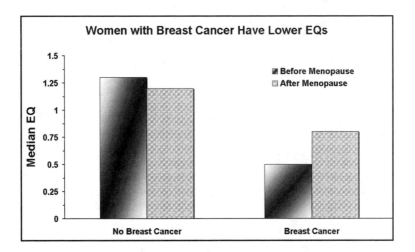

Figure 7- 3. The estrogen quotient (EQ) (the ratio of urinary estriol concentrations to the combined total urinary concentrations of estrone + estradiol) measured in women with no breast cancer was significantly higher than that in women diagnosed with breast cancer, both before and after menopause. $P < 0.01$ *Source: Lemon et al, 1966*

under animals' skin, some carcinogenic activity has been reported.[31, 32] However, these are all highly unphysiologic and unnatural ways of using estriol. When women take estriol in physiologic doses, by a route that mimics Nature, and on a schedule that approximates the body's natural pattern of estrogen secretion and distribution – as they do in BHRT – cancer has never proved to be a serious concern.

- When estriol is given to rats and mice in combination with estrone and estradiol, it inhibits the ability of these more potent estrogens to stimulate uterine cell growth, thus inhibiting a necessary factor in the development of cancer of the uterus.[33]

- Estriol boosts immune function by enhancing the activity of virus- and bacteria-eating cells called phagocytes and other important immune system agents.[34-36]

- In a group of premenopausal women who had noncancerous breast diseases, such as fibroadenoma, sclerosing adenosis, and intraductal hyperplasia, 60% of the women had a rate of estriol excretion that was below normal.[37]

- Dr. Lemon reported a finding of low estriol secretion in three women who had precancerous changes of the breast but who had not yet developed cancer.[27]

- In a small, informal, unpublished study, Dr. Lemon found that when women whose breast cancer had metastasized to their bones, approximately 40% of the women taking high doses of estriol experienced a remission.[38]

Other studies, which have examined the EQ-breast cancer issue from slightly different perspectives, have yielded ambiguous results.[39-42] However, studies in populations of Asian women have been particularly interesting, because they tend to have a relatively low incidence of breast cancer as well as high estriol levels. By contrast, American women have a much higher rate of breast cancer combined with lower levels of estriol.[43, 44] Overall, American women living in the US get breast cancer at rates 4 to 7 times higher than Asian women living in Asia.

However, the more time Asian women spend in the West, the higher their breast cancer risk rises. Appropriately, Asian women living in Hawaii get breast cancer at a rate midway between that of Asian women living in Asia and American women living on the US mainland. These Hawaiian women also had estriol levels midway between those of mainland American women and Asian women living in Asia.[45]

When women migrated to the US from China, Japan, or the Philippines, their incidence of breast cancer rose by 600%. Moreover, Asian American women living in the US have been shown to have a 60% higher risk of developing breast cancer than Asian American women who were born in the East. Finally, immigrant Asian women, who have lived in the US for 10 years or longer, have a risk of breast cancer 80% higher than that of more recent immigrants.[46]

Although estriol levels seem to be at least a partial factor in these cross-cultural differences, many other hormonal, dietary, lifestyle, and genetic factors may help account for the differences in breast cancer risk. As we describe below, part of the cross-cultural difference may be due, not only to differing levels of "good" and "bad" estrogens, but also to "good" and "bad" estrogen *metabolites*.

More Questions than Answers

It's been over 40 years since Dr. Lemon first published his findings and conclusions about estriol and breast cancer, but in the intervening years, they have raised more questions than they answered:

- Does an apparent hormone imbalance indicated by a low EQ open the door to breast cancer (*my conclusion based on evidence so far, but not "absolutely proven"*), or is EQ simply a biologic marker – a chemical sign – of an already existing cancer?

- Could EQ be used to help identify women who might be vulnerable to the disease but have not yet developed it? (*The preponderance of present evidence points that way.*)

- Could restoring an anomalous EQ to normal levels prevent breast cancer from developing (*Yes, in my opinion.*) and perhaps even effectively treat ongoing disease?

- Is an EQ measured at the time of breast cancer less relevant than a deviation from the norm when a woman was young and/or pregnant?

These are all intriguing questions that still lack for good solid scientific answers. It is unfortunate that, although Dr. Lemon's findings clearly demonstrated the potential value of appropriate bio-identical levels of the three estrogens, no other researchers with access to patent medicine or government research grants have ever followed up on them in a systematic way.

The reasons for this are quite evident. Dr. Lemon's research, like that of Dr. John R. Lee on progesterone and osteoporosis and other independent researchers, are typical of the types of studies that are conducted when the future of some new, patented drug is *not* at stake. Because of their relatively small size and limited controls, it is easy for the "opinion leaders," who tend to "speak for" mainstream medicine (and are usually are found by investigators to be on the payroll of one or more patent medicine companies), to dismiss their findings. Quite simply, no patent medicine backing = no research money; no research money = no long-term, double-blind, placebo-controlled trials; no trials = no publications in prestigious journals; no publications = no interest from mainstream medicine and media and, of course, no FDA "approval."

Is the EQ a useful test for assessing a woman's breast cancer risk? It may be, but only large-scale, long-term testing will confirm this to the satisfaction of mainstream medicine. In the mean time, it only makes sense for a woman to have her 24-hour urinary estrogens (the only reliable way of checking estriol and the EQ) checked periodically. It's an easy, inexpensive, noninvasive test that provides her doctor with useful information about the state of her sex hormones, and might help her head off an impending breast cancer years before it shows up on a mammogram or other "approved," expensive, and potentially dangerous test.

Does "re-balancing" estriol, estrone, and estradiol concentrations help prevent or treat ongoing breast disease, as Dr. Lemon's preliminary studies suggested it might? Again, the relevant "approved" studies are lacking, but it's just common sense, that if a woman is at risk for breast cancer, a healthy balance of noncarcinogenic to carcinogenic hormones can only help. When a postmenopausal woman uses BHRT, of course, the balance of hormones she uses is inherently safe, as estriol is always the "majority" replacement estrogen, and other more carcinogenic estrogens are in the minority – just as Mother Nature intended.

While no one has ever "proven" – according to the FDA's double-blind, placebo-controlled standards – that a "re-balancing" of estrogens in favor of a higher EQ could be beneficial for preventing and/or treating breast cancer, neither has anyone ever disproved it. Overall, the level of interest in Dr. Lemon's promising lead by mainstream medical researchers – whose research and reputations live and die with Big Pharma-produced patented drugs and/or Federal government research grants – approaches zero today. *Sure gives us confidence in the future of medicine, doesn't it!*

Progesterone, Progestins, and Breast Cancer

Despite considerable evidence to the contrary, conventional medicine stubbornly refuses to recognize the difference between bio-identical progesterone and patented progestin drugs[*]. This difference is particularly important in the development of breast cancer. Not surprisingly, the evidence – from laboratory animal, "test-tube," and human clinical trials – consistently demonstrates that progesterone decreases the risk of breast cancer, while progestins – especially Provera® – significantly increase that risk. This research has recently been reviewed in detail by Dr. Kent Holtorf.[1]

The most extensive studies (more than 80,000 women) have been done in France based on the E3N cohort.[47, 48] As noted earlier, France is unique in that most postmenopausal women replace estrogen using topical estradiol but use various progestins, as well as bio-identical progesterone. Based on the results of self-administered questionnaires completed between 1990

---

[*] Even the university professor "expert" (later found to be a recipient of patent medicine company funds) on the second Oprah "bio-identical hormone show" of 2009 stated (in front of a national audience) that there is no molecular difference between bio-identical hormones and conventional "hormone" replacement.

and 2002, 2,354 women had developed invasive breast cancer during 8.1 years of postmenopausal follow-up. The E3N study compared the occurrence of breast cancer in women using either estrogen alone or in combination with either progesterone or a patented progestin.

Compared to women who had never used any type of hormone replacement, those who used estrogen + progesterone had a significantly lower risk of invasive breast cancer compared to those who took estrogen alone or estrogen + most progestins. Only one progestin (dyhydrogesterone) came close to bio-identical progesterone in lowering the risk of breast cancer. It is important to note that, except for dyhydrogesterone, every progestin *increased* the risk of breast cancer compared to estrogen alone. By contrast, progesterone *lowered the risk* compared to estrogen alone.

Provera® (medroxyprogesterone acetate), the most commonly used progestin in the US (but rarely in France) may be an important cause of breast cancer. In a study in monkeys (cynomolgus macaques) that had had their ovaries removed, researchers measured the proliferation of breast cells (a marker for potential breast cancer) following treatment with either estradiol, estradiol + bio-identical progesterone, or estradiol + Provera®. The results showed that estradiol + Provera® produced significantly greater breast epithelial cell proliferation, while estradiol + progesterone did not increase breast cell proliferation at all.[49]

In a double-blind, placebo-controlled study in women about to undergo surgery for breast cancer, the women were given topical estradiol, progesterone, estradiol + progesterone, or placebo for 10 to 13 days prior to surgery. The researchers found that estradiol alone more than doubled the rate of breast cell proliferation (230% increase). However, when estradiol was combined with progesterone, proliferation rates *decreased* by 400%.[50]

So the next time you hear some hormone replacement "expert" claim that there's no data to prove that bio-identical progesterone is safer than patented progestin drugs, think about these studies, as well as numerous others reviewed by Dr. Holtorf.[1]

SERMs: Patented Answers to Estriol?

Our friends at the FDA have "approved" two different patent medications – Nolvadex® (tamoxifen) and Evista® (raloxifene) – for preventing and/or treating breast cancer. These drugs, marketed as *selective estrogen receptor modulators* (SERMs), are designed to help prevent or inhibit cancer growth in estrogen-sensitive tumors in the breast.

How do they work? Basically, by competing with estradiol and estrone for estrogen receptor sites and "impeding" the actions of these more active, more carcinogenic estrogens. If this mechanism of action rings a bell, it's because it's essentially the same action by which estriol is thought to work.[51, 52] Both SERM drugs and estriol compete with estradiol and/or estrone for estrogen receptor sites in the breast, but at the same time, they stimulate these receptors with far less intensity than the more potent estrogens. To the extent that a SERM or estriol occupies estrogen receptor sites in breast tissue that would otherwise be occupied by estradiol or estrone, they appear to be able to inhibit the cancer-inducing actions of these estrogens.

The problem with SERMs is that, while they may be relatively benign in the breast, they act very differently in other tissues, such as bone or uterus (*See Chapter 6.*), where they are potent estrogen *agonists* (stimulators). This is fine if your goal is to prevent osteoporosis. However, Nolvadex® and Evista®, even when taken at recommended doses, can and do cause some serious adverse side effects in other estrogen-sensitive tissues, ranging from worsened hot flushes, leg cramps, urinary incontinence, and other menopausal discomforts, to uterine cancer, strokes, and blood clots in the legs and lungs.[51-54] Although Evista® was originally hailed as being safer than Nolvadex® as a potential cause of uterine cancer, a closer look at the results have not supported this conclusion. In fact, Evista® may actually increase the risk of ductal carcinoma *in situ* (DCIS), which is thought to be either a precancerous condition, a risk factor for cancer, or an actual form of breast cancer.[54] Needless to say, no such risks has ever been associated with estriol.

By contrast, estriol's mild stimulatory action is sufficient for a wide range of positive estrogenic effects, like reducing hot flushes and improving genitourinary and cardiovascular function (*See Chapters 5 and 8.*).

At the same time, when taken at doses and according to a schedule that approximates the body's natural estrogen levels, *estriol* has no documented serious side effects or cancer risks (even the FDA admits this). Moreover, when combined with estradiol and estrone, it inhibits the proliferative effects of these more potent estrogens[55]just as Evista® and Nolvadex® are said to do.

Yet, as of this writing, the FDA is still trying to put an end to over 25 years of safe estriol use while "approving" Evista and Nolvadex. There's no logic or science to that, just patent medicine profits!

Remember this important principle: When modern science isn't crystal clear, it's always safest to mimic Mother Nature as exactly as possible. This is why BHRT employs three major human estrogens in proportions similar to those found in women's bodies over tens of thousands of generations. This is undoubtedly safer than using horse hormones, other patentable "estrogens," SERMs, or wrongly dosed, poorly timed, or even incomplete estrogens, such as estradiol.

How Eating Broccoli Might Help Prevent Breast (and Other Types of) Cancer

Although the potential value of estriol and the EQ for breast cancer management have been largely discounted by all but enlightened, natural medicine-oriented doctors, another exciting new area of research has emerged in recent years that looks so promising, even mainstream medicine is having trouble ignoring it.

We're talking about the relative levels of several estrogen metabolites:
* 2-hydroxyestrone
* 16α-hydroxyestrone
* 2-hydroxyestradiol
* 16α-hydroxyestradiol
* 2-methoxyestrone
* 2-methoxyestradiol

Some of these metabolites are known to be highly carcinogenic, whereas others are clearly *anti*carcinogenic. Recent clinical evidence confirms that, by altering the balance between carcinogenic and anticarcinogenic estrogen metabolites, it may be possible to head off or even cure some cancers. While this is most important for premenopausal women, it can be a factor in postmenopausal hormone replacement as well.

A Sermon on the SERMs

The fact is, there is really no such thing as a SERM (selective estrogen receptor modulator), or perhaps more accurately, we should say that *all estrogens are SERMs to some degree.*

"SERM" is essentially a marketing term made up by patent medicine companies to help identify and distinguish their compounds. In reality, since each variety of estrogen, whether natural, bio-identical, or patented, has its own *selective* pattern of estrogen receptor stimulation, all estrogens are *selective* estrogen receptor modulators to varying degrees.

Estrone is more potent in the breast than is estradiol, while estradiol is more potent in the uterus than is estrone. Both of these estrogens are more potent than estriol everywhere.

Like estriol, the SERM Nolvadex® is only mildly active in breast tissue, where it also competes with estrone and estradiol for receptor sites. Unlike estriol, Nolvadex® in the uterus becomes a different "animal" altogether, stimulating hyperplasia and endometrial cancer. Women who take Nolvadex® to protect their breasts necessarily increase their risk of uterine cancer. It's the kind of bargain conventional medicine has regrettably been asking women to make for half a century or more.

The SERM Evista® is like estriol and Nolvadex® in that it has relatively little activity in the breast, where it also competes successfully for receptor sites. However, Evista® and Nolvadex® may actually trigger hot flushes, and other side effects, not suppress them, as estriol does.

Nolvadex® and Evista® are really quite different from estriol, because they are patented and not bio-identical, and because their estrogenic actions can sometimes be dangerous. Do we need any more reasons why bio-identical estriol is a superior SERM?

What kind of sophisticated, high-tech, genetically engineered or patented medicine would be required to accomplish such a miracle? At present, no such patent medicine exists, and even if it did, we have little doubt it would not be as safe or as effective as a natural approach to maintaining or restoring hormone balance, which involves simply eating certain vegetables or taking supplements that contain some of the active ingredients in these vegetables to rebalance some of these metabolites.

Now, we're not talking about some rare Amazon rainforest medicinal plants, here, either. Far from it. We're talking good, old-fashioned cruciferous vegetables or *Brassicas* (members of the mustard family), including:

- Cabbage
- Broccoli
- Brussels sprouts
- Cauliflower
- Bok-choi
- Kale
- Kohlrabi
- Rutabaga
- Turnips

Principal Products and Pathways of Estrogen Metabolism

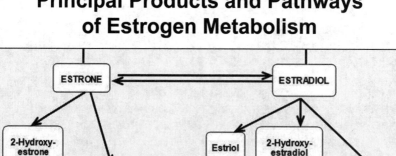

Figure 7-4.

Just a few servings per week of these common veggies may provide significant protection against breast and other hormonally mediated cancers.

But, we're getting ahead of ourselves. To understand how this could possibly be true, let's take a step back and look again at how estrogens get metabolized in the human body. Back in Chapter 4, we described the metabolism of sex steroids, as summarized in Figure 4-2 (page 74). Figure 7-4 focuses on a portion of that chart to highlight the relevant events.

Now, let's focus our attention briefly on the major metabolites and metabolic pathways of the estrogens. First, notice in Figure 7-4 that *estrone* and *estradiol* can each be converted into each other, which helps keep the levels of these hormones in balance. *Estradiol* molecules that do not get changed into *estrone* can have three different possible destinies; they may get turned into either 1) *estriol*, 2) *2-hydroxyestradiol*, or 3) *16α-hydroxyestradiol*. Finally, some of the resulting *2-hydroxyestradiol* can, in turn, be changed into a metabolite called *2-methoxyestradiol*.

Switching over to the *estrone* side of the chart, we see a similar pattern. *Estrone* that doesn't become *estradiol* may be metabolized to either *2-hydroxyestrone* or to *16α-hydroxyestrone*. Importantly, since there is a fixed amount of estrone to work from, if the body makes more *2-hydroxyestrone*, then it winds up making less *16α-hydroxyestrone* and vice versa. Some of the resulting *2-hydroxyestrone* may be converted to *2-methoxyestrone*, while some of the *16α-hydroxyestrone* is metabolized to *estriol*.

Note that *estriol* is a byproduct of both *estrone* and *estradiol* metabolism.

"Good" vs. "Bad" Estrogen Metabolites
It wasn't long ago that conventional medicine dismissed these metabolites – including estriol – as mere "breakdown products" of estrogen, assuming they played little or no useful role in the body. Now it is becoming undeniable that they have vital functions in the body's cancer protection system.

H. Leon Bradlow, MD, and his research group at the Strang-Cornell Cancer Research Laboratory of Rockefeller University in New York, and other researchers, have provided a large body of very convincing evidence indicating that *2-hydroxyestrone* should be considered a *"good"* *estrogen metabolite*, whereas *16α-hydroxyestrone* is a *"bad" estrogen metabolite.* "Evidence from a long series of studies has demonstrated a specific role for *16α-hydroxyestrone* as a *transforming*[*] estrogen, which is [a more potent carcinogen] than estradiol itself," wrote Dr. Bradlow.[56] By contrast, *2-hydroxyestrone* is *noncarcinogenic* and may even be *anticarcinogenic.*

To summarize (as shown in Figure 7-4), estrone can be metabolized to either of two different estrogens that have opposing biologic properties:

- *16α-hydroxyestrone* is a potent "bad" estrogen; in test-tube experiments, it is a more potent carcinogen than estradiol and is about as toxic to DNA as a synthetic chemical often used in animal studies to *induce* breast tumors.[57]

- *2-hydroxyestrone* is estriol-like in that it is a weak, "good" estrogen that may even be *anticarcinogenic. 2-hydroxyestrone* has about 1/10 the estrogenic activity of *16α-hydroxyestrone.*[58]

Anything that alters the *balance* of "good" to "bad" estrogens – the *2-hydroxyestrone/16α-hydroxyestrone ratio* (also called the *2/16 ratio*, for short) – may alter the risk of estrogen-related cancer. The optimal ratio (as measured in samples of urine) appears to be about 2:1 (ie, twice as much "good" estrogen to "bad" estrogen).

In *premenopausal* women, ratios around 1:1 or lower have been consistently linked to an increased breast cancer risk.[59] Increasing the ratio – ie, raising levels of *2-hydroxyestrone* relative to *16α-hydroxyestrone* – has also been shown to reverse the growth of human laryngeal papillomas, abnormal growths on the larynx (voice box) caused by human papilloma

---

[*] "Transforming" refers to the tendency of an agent – 16α-hydroxyestrone in this case – to promote cellular growth, proliferation, and transformation of normal cells to malignant cells in estrogen-responsive tissues.

virus (HPV), the same family of viruses that causes cervical cancers. In addition to the cervix, the *2/16 ratio* may also affect cancer growth in the breast, uterus, prostate, liver, and kidney.[60, 61]

Research on *2-hydroxyestrone* and *16α-hydroxyestrone* is accelerating at an exciting pace. For example, in one study of premenopausal Asian women, urinary levels of *2-hydroxyestrone* and the *2/16 ratio* were both significantly lower, and the level of *16α-hydroxyestrone* was significantly higher in those women who had breast cancer, compared to a control group of women without cancer. The *2/16 ratio* was *the most significant factor predictive of breast cancer.*[62]

Lots of scientific findings from both lab and clinical research support the relationship between breast cancer and these estrogen metabolites.[63] For example:

- In women who had breast cancer, the formation of *16α-hydroxyestrone* ("bad" estrogen) was found to have been elevated by 50%.[64]

- In women who were cancer-free but who had a family history of breast cancer, levels of *16α-hydroxyestrone* were significantly higher.[63]

- Women who had low *2/16 ratios* (below 1.0) had an increased risk of developing breast cancer and a poorer prognosis once it developed. Conversely, women with higher ratios (above 1.0) had a lower risk and an improved prognosis.[65, 66]

- In two US studies, researchers compared urine samples from women with or without breast cancer. In one study, in the women with breast cancer, all urinary estrogens *except for estriol* were elevated. Furthermore, women with the lowest *2/16 ratios* had the highest relative cancer risk.[66, 67]

In summary, accumulating evidence supports the hypothesis that the ratio of *2-hydroxyestrone* ("good" estrogen) to *16α-hydroxyestrone* ("bad" estrogen) is an important marker and/or risk factor, not only for breast cancer, but for any estrogen-related cancer, including cancers of the ovary, uterus in *premenopausal* women, and possibly the prostate in men. Quite simply, the theory states, a *higher ratio is better* for preventing (or even treating) cancer, and a *lower ratio is worse*.

We should emphasize that the evidence to support the 2/16 hypothesis is clear for *premenopausal* women, but this hypothesis does not appear to apply to *postmenopausal* women not taking replacement hormones. Although it seems entirely logical and predictable that the 2/16 hypothesis would also apply to postmenopausal women taking enough BHRT to achieve premenopausal levels of estrogens, there is as yet no research on this point.

It is also worth noting that, unlike most standard risk factors for breast cancer, such as giving birth later in life or not at all and a genetic predisposition, risks related to estrogen metabolism appear to be modifiable via diet and exercise. As we show in the next section, altering the all-important *2/16 ratio* in a favorable direction can be a relatively simple matter of consuming the right nutrients.

Eat Veggies, Reduce Cancer Risk

In premenopausal women, eating cruciferous vegetables – or taking supplements containing the key nutrients in these vegetables – can help maintain or restore a *positive 2/16 ratio*, and in so doing, reduce your risk of breast and other estrogen-related cancers. This is neither health food store hype nor vegetarian rumor; it is well-documented *scientific fact*.

For every 10 grams of cruciferous vegetables you eat each day, your *2/16 ratio* increases by 8%.[68] Swedish researchers compared the consumption of cruciferous and noncruciferous vegetables in women with breast cancer and a group of matched control women without cancer. As you can see in Figure 7-5, women who ate the most *Brassicas* - about 1.5 servings/ day - had a 42% lower cancer risk than women who ate the least veggies - about 0.1 servings/day.[69]

What is the "magic ingredient" that makes these vegetables such potent and promising anticancer weapons? Cruciferous vegetables are rich sources of a variety of phytochemicals, including some with proven

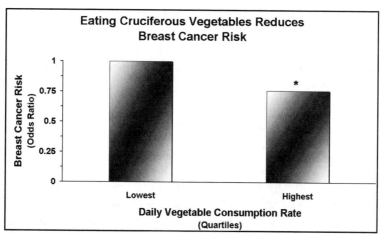

Figure 7-5. Swedish women with the highest daily consumption of *Brassica* vegetables (1.5 servings/day) had a significantly lower risk of developing breast cancer than women with the lowest daily consumption (0.1 servings/day). * *P* = 0.003 *Source: Terry et al, 2001*

anticancer activity. The phytochemical that seems to be most effective against estrogen-based cancers (eg, breast, uterine, ovary) in lab animals is called ***indole-3-carbinol (I3C)***.

When placed in an acidic environment, like a healthy stomach, I3C molecules chemically bond together to form a variety of different biologically active products, the most prominent of which is ***3,3'-diindolylmethane (DIM).*** Each DIM molecule has 10 times the potency of an individual I3C molecule, making it *the most powerful natural inducer of 2-hydroxyestrone production known,* thus a great way to raise the ***2/16 ratio.***[61, 70]

Dietary I3C/DIM has been termed a "negative regulator of estrogen."[71] While estrogens typically promote the growth and survival of tumors, I3C/DIM does the opposite; it halts tumor growth and hastens the death of cancer cells, thus ameliorating the carcinogenic tendencies of potent estrogens.[61]

When researchers looked at I3C in the lab, they found that at the same time that it boosts levels of the anticarcinogenic metabolite *2-hydroxyestrone,* it also squelches the production of the potent carcinogenic metabolite *16α-hydroxyestrone.* As a result, it increases the ***2/16 ratio.***

Daily oral doses of 300 to 400 mg of I3C per week - equivalent to about 300 to 400 grams of raw vegetables (about one-third of a head of cabbage) – significantly improved the *2/16 ratios* in women who were at increased risk for breast cancer.[72-75] If eating I3C/DIM raises our *2/16 ratios*, and if raising the ratio reduces our risk of cancer, is it possible to cut our risk of cancer simply by consuming more I3C/DIM? It would seem so; if A = B and B = C, then shouldn't A = C?

So far only one clinical trial has investigated this crucial question, and its results were extremely encouraging. Maria C. Bell, MD, and colleagues gave I3C supplements to women with biopsy-proven *cervical intraepithelial neoplasia* (*CIN*), an abnormal growth in the cervix that is a precursor to cervical cancer.[76] CIN (and consequently, cervical cancer) is caused primarily by infection with the sexually transmitted human papillomavirus (HPV).

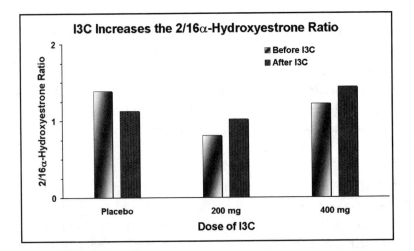

Figure 7-6. Thirty women with CIN, a precancerous condition of the cervix, took 200 mg or 400 mg of I3C or placebo for 12 weeks. In urine samples taken at the 4-week mark, I3C increased the 2/16α-hydroxyestrone ratio at both doses, while the ratio declined slightly in the placebo group.

Source: Bell et al, 2000

Note that this was a "gold standard" trial – double-blinded and placebo-controlled. For 12 weeks, the women took either I3C supplements (200 or 400 mg per day) or a placebo. After 4 weeks of treatment, tests revealed that in the women taking I3C, *2/16 ratios* had generally increased; the higher the dose, the higher the ratio. In the placebo group, the ratio declined somewhat after treatment (Fig. 7-6).

After 12 weeks, Dr. Bell's research team performed cervical biopsies on the study participants to evaluate disease progression. They found that 47% of the women (8/17) who had taken I3C had a *complete CIN regression* (4 at each dose). The precancerous growths in these women had completely disappeared! This contrasted with the placebo group, where not one of the 10 women had any CIN regression (Fig. 7-7). Needless to say, none of Dr. Bell's patients experienced any adverse side effects from their treatment, a finding that is typical in people taking I3C or DIM, or, of course, eating cruciferous vegetables.

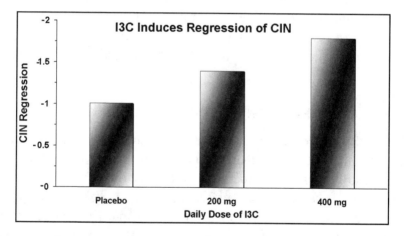

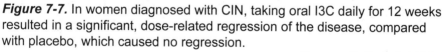

Figure 7-7. In women diagnosed with CIN, taking oral I3C daily for 12 weeks resulted in a significant, dose-related regression of the disease, compared with placebo, which caused no regression.

Source: Bell et al, 2000

This was only one small study, but its implications are enormous. It showed that a simple, harmless intervention using a phytochemical that occurs naturally in common vegetables can induce regression of a dangerous precancerous condition in half the women who use it. It suggests that eating moderate amounts of broccoli, cabbage, etc – just three or four servings per week – might be able to head off at least half of all cases of cervical cancer.

(We suspect you haven't heard or read about this in the "mainstream" media, probably because it doesn't relate to a patented drug!)

Can I3C/DIM really prevent cervical cancer? What about uterine cancer, ovarian cancer, and breast cancer? Logic says it might help, but only more careful clinical studies will prove how well it works. In the meantime, remember that until the significance and utility of the *2/16 ratio* is firmly established, enough research is certainly already available to allow us to modify our risks of estrogen-related cancers using diet and supplements.

We should also point out that some studies in lab animals have shown that long-term use of I3C *supplements* (but not DIM) can actually promote or enhance the growth of some cancers. However, this effect has never been seen in humans or with the consumption of cruciferous vegetables. Nevertheless, it has led some researchers to caution against the use of I3C supplements until their risks and benefits are more clearly spelled out.[77]

Two More Possible Anticancer Metabolites

In addition to *2-hydroxyestrone*, medical researchers have recently shown considerable interest in two other estrogen metabolites, *2-methoxyestrone* and, especially *2-methoxyestradiol*. Note that these metabolites are derived from *2-hydroxyestrone* and *2-hydroxyestradiol*, respectively (Fig. 7-4). Test-tube and lab animal studies have shown that *2-methoxyestradiol* inhibits cancers of the uterus,[78] endothelial cells,[79] pituitary gland,[80] prostate,[81, 82] and thyroid.[83]

How well does it work in people? The National Cancer Institute is currently recruiting patients with advanced solid tumors for a clinical trial of 2-methoxyestradiol.[84] Not surprisingly, two different patent medicine companies, in their never-ending quest to outdo Mother

Nature, have synthesized patented analogs of 2-methoxyestradiol (2-methoxymethylestradiol)[85] and 2-methoxyestrone (2-methoxyestrone-3-O-sulphamate)[86] and are currently testing them.

But patent medicine companies can see enormous financial potential in bio-identical hormones, too, if they can somehow get "exclusive rights" to them. So one patent medicine company is conducting trials of bio-identical 2-methoxyestradiol (name carefully changed to "Panzem®") with an eye on ultimate FDA "approval." Another patent medication company is conducting clinical trials with bio-identical estriol (name changed to "Trimesta®"), also anticipating FDA "approval."

But how can exclusivity be possible if bio-identical hormones are totally unpatentable? By remarkable coincidence (no doubt), the FDA is trying to outlaw the over 25-year use of estriol through hundreds of compounding pharmacies, and to prevent these same compounding pharmacies from using 2-methoxyestradiol or any other bio-identical estrogens (except estradiol) without specific FDA "approval." (*For further details, see Chapter 12.*)

Premarin®, Alcohol, and Breast Cancer

As we have shown, certain estrogens, especially those supplied by conventional patented HRT, can be a significant factor in breast cancer. The risk is even higher, though, if women taking Premarin® also drink alcohol. Evidence shows that oral CEEs can combine with even modest alcohol consumption to increase a woman's risk of breast cancer. The reason seems to be that drinking alcohol raises estrogen levels.

As little as two drinks (about 30 grams of alcohol) per day can increase estrone levels by 7.5%.[87] This may not sound like much, but just 5 grams a day (2/3 oz of whiskey or 3 oz of wine) may be enough to boost estrogen levels well over the threshold for promoting breast cancer.[88] Drinking 30 grams a day has been shown to increase the risk of breast cancer overall by 80% and to increase the risk of the relatively uncommon ductal form of breast cancer by 330%. The authors of this study surmised a 65% increase in lobular breast cancer documented over the past decade may be due to the increased use of conventional HRT, as described in Chapter 1.[89]

Hormones and Ovarian Cancer

Ovarian cancer occurs far less frequently than breast cancer (lifetime risk is about 1.7%[90]), but it is often deadly. Since the ovary is the source of most estrogens and progesterone in the female body, the presumption has long been that ovarian cancer, like breast and endometrial cancer, was related to the activity of sex steroid hormones. However, the precise relationship between sex steroids, especially the exogenous "hormones" used in patented HRT, and ovarian cancer still remains somewhat of a puzzle.

The risk of developing ovarian cancer as a result of "hormone" replacement has not been investigated nearly as intensively as the risk of breast or other gynecologic cancers. Those studies that have been published have yielded conflicting results, although more recent studies seem to be leading toward a consensus that patented HRT increases the risk of developing ovarian cancer by as much as 50%, with the risk increasing with longer duration of use.[91]

A large *prospective* study of hormone replacement and ovarian cancer was conducted by researchers under the auspices of the American Cancer Society (ACS).[92] The study began in 1982 and, by 2001, included data from more than 211,000 postmenopausal women. In 14 years of follow-up, the investigators recorded 944 deaths due to ovarian cancer. They found that, among women using conventional "estrogen" replacement therapy (ERT) at the start of the study, typically Premarin®, the overall death rate was 51% higher than among non-Premarin users. Those who used "estrogen" for 10 or more years had more than double the risk of developing ovarian cancer (a 220% increase). Unlike breast cancer, where halting "estrogen" replacement typically leads to a relatively rapid decline in risk, after 10 or more years of "estrogen" replacement, the risk of ovarian cancer persisted for up to 29 years after cessation of treatment.

Another study, published in the same issue of the *Journal of the American Medical Association* as the original WHI data, followed women using conventional ERT or HRT for 20 years or more. The results showed that the overall use of "estrogen"-only (Premarin® again) was associated with an average increase in ovarian cancer risk of 60%, compared to no "estrogen" use. Like the ACS study (above), the longer women used "estrogen," the higher their risk, which rose at a rate of 7% per year. For those using it for 20 years or more, the risk was 320% higher. Like uterine cancer, concomitant use of a progestin appeared to offer a large degree of protection against ovarian cancer. However, in "women without a uterus," who were thought not to require a progestin, the risk of ovarian cancer after 20 years was the highest of all – 340%![93]

No specific studies have evaluated the effects of BHRT on ovarian cancer, although the results of one study suggested that "non-CEE" estrogen (eg, bio-identical estradiol) had less of a propensity to cause ovarian cancer than did CEEs.[94] No alarms have ever been raised indicating an increase in risk among women who use BHRT. This is to be expected, given the *natural* mode of action of these hormones and their perfect fit into the body's normal physiology – these are, after all, the same hormones the ovary itself secretes.

References

1. Holtorf K. The bioidentical hormone debate: are bioidentical hormones (estradiol, estriol, and progesterone) safer or more efficacious than commonly used synthetic versions in hormone replacement therapy? *Postgrad Med.* 2009;121:73-85.

2. Seeger H, Mueck AO, Lippert TH. Effect of norethisterone acetate on estrogen metabolism in postmenopausal women. *Horm Metab Res.* 2000;32:436-439.

3. Wright J, Morgenthaler J. *Natural Hormone Replacement for Women Over 45.* Petaluma, CA: Smart Publications; 1997.

4. Pradhan AD, Manson JE, Rossouw JE, et al. Inflammatory biomarkers, hormone replacement therapy, and incident coronary heart disease: prospective analysis from the Women's Health Initiative observational study. *JAMA.* 2002;288:980-987.

5. International Agency for Research on Cancer. IARC monographs programme finds combined estrogen-progestogen contraceptives and menopausal therapy are carcinogenic to humans. *http://www.iarc.fr/ENG/Press_Releases/pr167a. html.* July 29, 2005;Press Release No. 167:Accessed June 13, 2006.

6. Glass AG, Lacey JV, Jr., Carreon JD, Hoover RN. Breast cancer incidence, 1980-2006: Combined roles of menopausal hormone therapy, screening mammography, and estrogen receptor status. *J. Natl. Cancer Inst.* 2007;99:1152-1161.

7. Ravdin PM, Cronin KA, Howlader N, et al. The decrease in breast-cancer incidence in 2003 in the United States. *N Engl J Med.* 2007;356:1670-1674.

8. Chlebowski RT, Kuller LH, Prentice RL, et al. Breast cancer after use of estrogen plus progestin in postmenopausal women. *N Engl J Med.* 2009;360:573-587.

9. Espie M, Daures JP, Chevallier T, Mares P, Micheletti MC, de Reilhac P. Breast cancer incidence and hormone replacement therapy: Results from the MISSION study, prospective phase. *Gynecol Endocrinol.* 2007;23:391-397.

10. Beatson G. On the treatment of inoperable cases of carcinoma of the mamma: Suggestions for a new method of treatment, with illustrative cases. *Lancet.* 1896;2:104-107.

11. Marshall F, Jolley W. The ovary as an organ of internal secretion. *Phil Trans R Soc.* 1906;198:99-141.

12. Yager JD, Davidson NE. Estrogen carcinogenesis in breast cancer. *N Engl J Med.* 2006;354:270-282.

13. Henderson BE, Bernstein L. Endogenous and exogenous hormonal factors. In: Harris J, Lippman M, Morrow M, Hellman S, eds. *Diseases of the Breast, 1st Edition.* Philadelphia: Lippincott-Raven; 1996:185-200.

14. Key T, Appleby P, Barnes I, Reeves G. Endogenous sex hormones and breast cancer in postmenopausal women: reanalysis of nine prospective studies. *J Natl Cancer Inst.* 2002;94:606-616.

15. Breast cancer and hormone replacement therapy: collaborative reanalysis of data from 51 epidemiological studies of 52,705 women with breast cancer and 108,411 women without breast cancer. Collaborative Group on Hormonal Factors in Breast Cancer. *Lancet.* 1997;350:1047-1059.

16. Fournier A, Berrino F, Riboli E, Avenel V, Clavel-Chapelon F. Breast cancer risk in relation to different types of hormone replacement therapy in the E3N-EPIC cohort. *Int J Cancer.* 2004.

17. Wiseman RA. Breast cancer: critical data analysis concludes that estrogens are not the cause, however lifestyle changes can alter risk rapidly. *J Clin Epidemiol.* 2004;57:766-772.

18. Lambe M, Hsieh CC, Chan HW, Ekbom A, Trichopoulos D, Adami HO. Parity, age at first and last birth, and risk of breast cancer: a population-based study in Sweden. *Breast Cancer Res Treat.* 1996;38:305-311.

19. Peck JD, Hulka BS, Poole C, Savitz DA, Baird D, Richardson BE. Steroid hormone levels during pregnancy and incidence of maternal breast cancer. *Cancer Epidemiol Biomarkers Prev.* 2002;11:361-368.

20. Clemons M, Goss P. Estrogen and the risk of breast cancer. *N Engl J Med.* 2001;344:276-285.

21. Eik-Nes KB, Hall PF. Secretion of steroid hormones in vivo. *Vitam Horm.* 1965;23:153-208.

22. Siiteri PK, Sholtz RI, Cirillo PM, et al. Prospective study of estrogens during pregnancy and risk of breast cancer. *Department of Defense Breast Cancer Research Meeting.* 2009; http://cdmrp.army.mil/bcrp/era/abstracts2002/p13%5F chemoprevention/9919358%5Fabs.pdf.

23. Utian W. The place of oestriol therapy after menopause. *Acta Endocrinol.* 1980;233 (suppl):51-56.

24. Esposito G. Estriol: a weak estrogen or a different hormone? *Gynecol Endocrinol.* 1991;5:131-153.

25. Lemon HM. Endocrine influences on human mammary cancer formation. A critique. *Cancer.* 1969;23:781-790.

26. Lemon HM. Pathophysiologic considerations in the treatment of menopausal patients with oestrogens; the role of oestriol in the prevention of mammary carcinoma. *Acta Endocrinol Suppl (Copenh).* 1980;233:17-27.

27. Lemon H, Wotiz H, Parsons L, Mozden P. Reduced estriol secretion in patients with breast cancer prior to endocrine therapy. *JAMA.* 1966;196:112-120.

28. Lemon HM, Wotiz HH, Parsons L, Mozden PJ. Reduced estriol excretion in patients with breast cancer prior to endocrine therapy. *JAMA*. 1966;196:1128-1136.

29. Lemon H. Oestriol and prevention of breast cancer. *Lancet*. 1973;1:546-547.

30. Lemon HM, Heidel JW, Rodriguez-Sierra JF. Principles of breast cancer prevention. *Annual Meeting of the AACR*. Vol 1991.

31. Noble RL, Hochachka BC, King D. Spontaneous and estrogen-produced tumors in Nb rats and their behavior after transplantation. *Cancer Res*. 1975;35:766-780.

32. Rudali G, Apiou F, Muel B. Mammary cancer produced in mice with estriol. *Eur J Cancer*. 1975;11:39-41.

33. Hisaw FL, Velardo JT, Goolsby CM. Interaction of estrogens on uterine growth. *J Clin Endocrinol Metab*. 1954;14:1134-1143.

34. Jacobs AA, Selvardj RJ, Strauss RR, Paul BB, Mitchell GW, Jr., Sbarra AJ. The role of the phagocyte in host-parasite interactions. XXXIX. Stimulation of bactericidal activity of myeloperoxidase-containing leukocytic fractions by estrogens. *Am J Obstet Gynecol*. 1973;117:671-678.

35. Zuckerman SH, Ahmari SE, Bryan-Poole N, Evans GF, Short L, Glasebrook AL. Estriol: a potent regulator of TNF and IL-6 expression in a murine model of endotoxemia. *Inflammation*. 1996;20:581-597.

36. Nicol T, Vernon-Roberts B, Quantock DC. Oestrogenic and anti-oestrogenic effects of oestriol, 16-epi-oestriol, 2-methoxyoestrone and 2-hydroxyoestradiol-17β on the reticulo-endothelial system and reproductive tract. *J Endocrinol*. 1966;35:119-120.

37. Bacigalupo G, Schubert K. Untersuchungen uber die oestrogen auscheidung im urin bei mastopathie. *Klin Worsch*. 1960;38:804-805.

38. Follingstad A. Estriol, the forgotten estrogen? *JAMA*. 1978;239:29-30.

39. Trichopoulos D, Brown J, MacMahon B. Urine estrogens and breast cancer risk factors among post-menopausal women. *Int J Cancer*. 1987;40:721-725.

40. Fishman J, Fukushima DK, O'Connor J, Lynch HT. Low urinary estrogen glucuronides in women at risk for familial breast cancer. *Science*. 1979;204:1089-1091.

41. Morgan RW, Vakil DV, Brown JB, Elinson L. Estrogen profiles in young women: effect of maternal history of breast cancer. *J Natl Cancer Inst*. 1978;60:965-967.

42. Pike MC, Casagrande JT, Brown JB, Gerkins V, Henderson BE. Comparison of urinary and plasma hormone levels in daughters of breast cancer patients and controls. *J Natl Cancer Inst*. 1977;59:1351-1355.

43. Lemon HM. Genetic predisposition to carcinoma of the breast: multiple human genotypes for estrogen 16α-hydroxylase activity in Caucasians. *J Surg Oncol.* 1972;4:255-273.

44. MacMahon B, Cole P, Brown JB, et al. Oestrogen profiles of Asian and North American women. *Lancet.* 1971;2:900-902.

45. Dickinson LE, MacMahon B, Cole P, Brown JB. Estrogen profiles of Oriental and Caucasian women in Hawaii. *N Engl J Med.* 1974;291:1211-1213.

46. Ziegler RG, Hoover RN, Pike MC, et al. Migration patterns and breast cancer risk in Asian-American women. *J Natl Cancer Inst.* 1993;85:1819-1827.

47. Fournier A, Berrino F, Clavel-Chapelon F. Unequal risks for breast cancer associated with different hormone replacement therapies: results from the E3N cohort study. *Breast Cancer Res Treat.* 2008;107:103-111.

48. Fournier A, Fabre A, Mesrine S, Boutron-Ruault MC, Berrino F, Clavel-Chapelon F. Use of different postmenopausal hormone therapies and risk of histology- and hormone receptor-defined invasive breast cancer. *J Clin Oncol.* 2008;26:1260-1268.

49. Wood CE, Register TC, Lees CJ, Chen H, Kimrey S, Cline JM. Effects of estradiol with micronized progesterone or medroxyprogesterone acetate on risk markers for breast cancer in postmenopausal monkeys. *Breast Cancer Res Treat.* 2007;101:125-134.

50. Chang KJ, Lee TT, Linares-Cruz G, Fournier S, de Lignieres B. Influences of percutaneous administration of estradiol and progesterone on human breast epithelial cell cycle in vivo. *Fertil Steril.* 1995;63:785-791.

51. Evista® (raloxifene hydrochloride) Prescribing Information. *http://pi.lilly.com/us/evista-pi.pdf.* Eli Lilly and Co., Indianapolis, IN Accessed April 22, 2006.

52. Nolvadex® (tamoxifen citrate). Prescribing Information. *http://www.astrazeneca-us.com/pi/Nolvadex.pdf.*AstraZeneca Pharmaceuticals:Acessed July 7, 2006.

53. Barrett-Connor E, Mosca L, Collins P, et al. Effects of raloxifene on cardiovascular events and breast cancer in postmenopausal women. *N Engl J Med.* 2006;355:125-137.

54. Vogel VG, Costantino JP, Wickerham DL, et al. Effects of Tamoxifen vs Raloxifene on the Risk of Developing Invasive Breast Cancer and Other Disease Outcomes: The NSABP Study of Tamoxifen and Raloxifene (STAR) P-2 Trial. *JAMA.* 2006;295:2727-2741.

55. Melamed M, Castano E, Notides AC, Sasson S. Molecular and kinetic basis for the mixed agonist/antagonist activity of estriol. *Mol Endocrinol.* 1997;11:1868-1878.

56. Bradlow HL, Telang NT, Sepkovic DW, Osborne MP. 2-hydroxyestrone: the 'good' estrogen. *J Endocrinol.* 1996;150 Suppl:S259-265.

57. Telang NT, Suto A, Wong GY, Osborne MP, Bradlow HL. Induction by estrogen metabolite 16 α-hydroxyestrone of genotoxic damage and aberrant proliferation in mouse mammary epithelial cells. *J Natl Cancer Inst.* 1992;84:634-638.

58. Grodon S, Cantrall E, Cekleniak W, et al. Steroid and lipid metabolism. The hypocholesterolemic effect of estrogen metabolism. *Steroids.* 1964;4:267-271.

59. Persson I. The risk of endometrial and breast cancer after estrogen treatment. A review of epidemiological studies. *Acta Obstet Gynecol Scand Suppl.* 1985;130:59-66.

60. Brignall MS. Prevention and treatment of cancer with indole-3-carbinol. *Altern Med Rev.* 2001;6:580-589.

61. Lord RS, Bongiovanni B, Bralley JA. Estrogen metabolism and the diet-cancer connection: rationale for assessing the ratio of urinary hydroxylated estrogen metabolites. *Altern Med Rev.* 2002;7:112-129.

62. Ho GH, Luo XW, Ji CY, Foo SC, Ng EH. Urinary 2/16α-hydroxyestrone ratio: correlation with serum insulin-like growth factor binding protein-3 and a potential biomarker of breast cancer risk. *Ann Acad Med Singapore.* 1998;27:294-299.

63. Zumoff B. Hormonal profiles in women with breast cancer. *Obstet Gynecol Clin North Am.* 1994;21:751-772.

64. Schneider J, Kinne D, Fracchia A, et al. Abnormal oxidative metabolism of estradiol in women with breast cancer. *Proc Natl Acad Sci U S A.* 1982;79:3047-3051.

65. Kabat GC, Chang CJ, Sparano JA, et al. Urinary estrogen metabolites and breast cancer: a case-control study. *Cancer Epidemiol Biomarkers Prev.* 1997;6:505-509.

66. Kabat GC, O'Leary ES, Gammon MD, et al. Estrogen metabolism and breast cancer. *Epidemiology.* 2006;17:80-88.

67. Ursin G, London S, Stanczyk FZ, et al. Urinary 2-hydroxyestrone/16α-hydroxyestrone ratio and risk of breast cancer in postmenopausal women. *J Natl Cancer Inst.* 1999;91:1067-1072.

68. Fowke JH, Longcope C, Hebert JR. Brassica vegetable consumption shifts estrogen metabolism in healthy postmenopausal women. *Cancer Epidemiol Biomarkers Prev.* 2000;9:773-779.

69. Terry P, Wolk A, Persson I, Magnusson C. *Brassica* vegetables and breast cancer risk. *JAMA.* 2001;285:2975-2977.

70. Jellinck PH, Forkert PG, Riddick DS, Okey AB, Michnovicz JJ, Bradlow HL. Ah receptor binding properties of indole carbinols and induction of hepatic estradiol hydroxylation. *Biochem Pharmacol.* 1993;45:1129-1136.

71. Auborn KJ, Fan S, Rosen EM, et al. Indole-3-carbinol is a negative regulator of estrogen. *J Nutr.* 2003;133:2470S-2475S.

72. Wong GY, Bradlow L, Sepkovic D, Mehl S, Mailman J, Osborne MP. Dose-ranging study of indole-3-carbinol for breast cancer prevention. *J Cell Biochem Suppl.* 1997;28-29:111-116.

73. Bradlow HL, Michnovicz JJ, Halper M, Miller DG, Wong GY, Osborne MP. Long-term responses of women to indole-3-carbinol or a high fiber diet. *Cancer Epidemiol Biomarkers Prev.* 1994;3:591-595.

74. Bradlow HL, Sepkovic DW, Telang NT, Osborne MP. Indole-3-carbinol. A novel approach to breast cancer prevention. *Ann N Y Acad Sci.* 1995;768:180-200.

75. Kall MA, Vang O, Clausen J. Effects of dietary broccoli on human drug metabolising activity. *Cancer Lett.* 1997;114:169-170.

76. Bell MC, Crowley-Nowick P, Bradlow HL, et al. Placebo-controlled trial of indole-3-carbinol in the treatment of CIN. *Gynecol Oncol.* 2000;78:123-129.

77. Linus Pauling Institute. Indole-3-Carbinol. *http://lpi.oregonstate.edu/infocenter/ phytochemicals/i3c/.*Oregon State University:Accessed July 22, 2006.

78. Amant F, Lottering ML, Joubert A, Thaver V, Vergote I, Lindeque BG. 2-methoxyestradiol strongly inhibits human uterine sarcomatous cell growth. *Gynecol Oncol.* 2003;91:299-308.

79. Arbiser JL, Panigrathy D, Klauber N, et al. The antiangiogenic agents TNP-470 and 2-methoxyestradiol inhibit the growth of angiosarcoma in mice. *J Am Acad Dermatol.* 1999;40:925-929.

80. Banerjeei SK, Zoubine MN, Sarkar DK, Weston AP, Shah JH, Campbell DR. 2-Methoxyestradiol blocks estrogen-induced rat pituitary tumor growth and tumor angiogenesis: possible role of vascular endothelial growth factor. *Anticancer Res.* 2000;20:2641-2645.

81. Bu S, Blaukat A, Fu X, Heldin NE, Landstrom M. Mechanisms for 2-methoxyestradiol-induced apoptosis of prostate cancer cells. *FEBS Lett.* 2002;531:141-151.

82. Garcia GE, Wisniewski HG, Lucia MS, et al. 2-Methoxyestradiol inhibits prostate tumor development in transgenic adenocarcinoma of mouse prostate: role of tumor necrosis factor-alpha-stimulated gene 6. *Clin Cancer Res.* 2006;12:980-988.

83. Roswall P, Bu S, Rubin K, Landstrom M, Heldin NE. 2-methoxyestradiol induces apoptosis in cultured human anaplastic thyroid carcinoma cells. *Thyroid.* 2006;16:143-150.

84. National Cancer Institute. 2-Methoxyestradiol in Treating Patients with Advanced Solid Tumors. *www.clinicaltrials.gov/ct/show/NCT00024609.* 2006;NCI - Center for Cancer Research, Bethesda, Maryland, 20892:Accessed July 21, 2006.

85. Brueggemeier RW, Bhat AS, Lovely CJ, et al. 2-Methoxymethylestradiol: a new 2-methoxy estrogen analog that exhibits antiproliferative activity and alters tubulin dynamics. *J Steroid Biochem Mol Biol.* 2001;78:145-156.

86. Purohit A, Hejaz HA, Walden L, et al. The effect of 2-methoxyoestrone-3-O-sulphamate on the growth of breast cancer cells and induced mammary tumours. *Int J Cancer.* 2000;85:584-589.

87. Dorgan JF, Baer DJ, Albert PS, et al. Serum hormones and the alcohol-breast cancer association in postmenopausal women. *J Natl Cancer Inst.* 2001;93:710-715.

88. Zumoff B. Does postmenopausal estrogen administration increase the risk of breast cancer? Contributions of animal, biochemical, and clinical investigative studies to a resolution of the controversy. *Proc Soc Exp Biol Med.* 1998;217:30-37.

89. Li CI, Anderson BO, Daling JR, Moe RE. Trends in incidence rates of invasive lobular and ductal breast carcinoma. *JAMA.* 2003;289:1421-1424.

90. Ries L, Kosary C, Hankey B, Miller B, Edwards B. SEER Cancer Statistics Review, 1973-1996Bethesda, MD: National Cancer Institute; 1999.

91. Riman T, Nilsson S, Persson IR. Review of epidemiological evidence for reproductive and hormonal factors in relation to the risk of epithelial ovarian malignancies. *Acta Obstet Gynecol Scand.* 2004;83:783-795.

92. Rodriguez C, Patel AV, Calle EE, Jacob EJ, Thun MJ. Estrogen replacement therapy and ovarian cancer mortality in a large prospective study of US women. *Jama.* 2001;285:1460-1465.

93. Lacey JV, Jr., Mink PJ, Lubin JH, et al. Menopausal hormone replacement therapy and risk of ovarian cancer. *JAMA.* 2002;288:334-341.

94. Sit AS, Modugno F, Weissfeld JL, Berga SL, Ness RB. Hormone replacement therapy formulations and risk of epithelial ovarian carcinoma. *Gynecol Oncol.* 2002;86:118-123.

CHAPTER 8

ESTROGEN IS GOOD FOR A WOMAN'S HEART
...OR IS IT?

Based on large, "gold-standard" studies from the 1980s and '90s, medical "authorities" proclaimed that *"Estrogen is good for a woman's heart."*[1] A couple of years ago, based on more recent studies, like the Women's Health Initiative (WHI) and others, they proclaimed that "estrogen" is *not good* for a woman's heart.[2] Then, after re-examining the WHI data, they thought better of it and decided that estrogen might indeed be *good for a woman's heart*, as long as she wasn't too old when she started taking it and didn't take it for too many years.[3]

If women and their physicians are now thoroughly confused about the safety and efficacy of "hormone replacement" for their hearts, it is with good reason.

As we will show in this chapter, it is quite evident that the confusion of these "authorities" – and of the women who depend on them for advice – derives from the fact that these studies all tested Premarin® + Provera® (or Premarin® alone) almost exclusively, alien "hormones" that have been amply demonstrated to be problematic in the human body. By contrast, when *human bio-identical hormones* are properly used in human bodies, the cardiovascular problems seen in these studies – increased risks of heart attacks, strokes, blood clots, and others – seem to magically disappear, and cardiovascular risk is actually diminished.

It's been over 100 years since medical researchers first noticed that, compared with men of about the same age, women generally had less risk of coronary heart disease, including heart attacks and strokes. The principal exceptions to this rule were women who had had their ovaries surgically removed before menopause (*surgically induced menopause*). Having been thrown into menopause literally overnight, these women soon found themselves at markedly increased risk for premature heart attacks and strokes.

Over the next half-century or so, these and other observations increasingly supported the hypothesis that women's premenopausal protection against heart disease derived from the estrogens secreted by their ovaries.* As long as women's estrogens were flowing normally, they appeared to shield their cardiovascular systems. But once estrogen flow mostly dried up, at around age 50 (or earlier in women following surgically induced menopause), that protection soon dissipated.

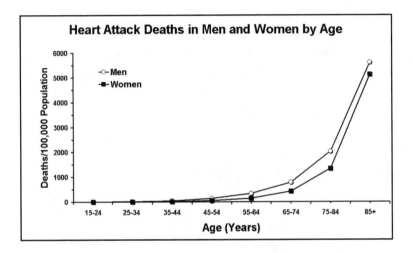

Figure 8-1. **As men and women age, their risk of dying from a heart attack increases with each succeeding decade beginning in their mid-40s. The primary reason for the lower death rate in women is the protection provided by the secretion of estrogen up until menopause.**

Source: US Centers for Disease Control and Prevention

As Figure 8-1 illustrates, young men and women tend to have about the same very low risk of dying from a heart attack. Beginning in their mid-40s, though, men's risk starts to climb, the rate accelerating with each succeeding decade. Women's risk starts to climb also, although the increase begins about a decade later and the rate continues to lag

---

*   Estrogens secreted by the ovaries are of course human estrogens, not horse estrogens. Logic and common sense tells us that hormone replacement, which precisely duplicates estrogens and other hormones secreted by human ovaries – bio-identical hormone replacement (BHRT) – will do the same job.

slightly behind men's for a few decades, until they eventually catch up.[4] The difference in risk between the genders is due largely to estrogen's cardioprotective effects in women.[*]

WHI: "HRT" Increases Cardiovascular Risks

The belief (unsupported by well-controlled research) that conventional patented "hormone" replacement therapy (Premarin® + Provera®) helped women maintain estrogen's natural cardioprotection in the years after menopause was exposed as false in the summer of 2002, when the results of the WHI study first became public.

The finding that cast the deepest shadow over conventional HRT at that time was not the 24% increase in breast cancer risk caused by "hormone" replacement[2] – that was pretty much a "given" based on prior research. Rather, what forced WHI researchers to pull the plug on their study after only 5.2 years (it had been scheduled to run 8.5 years), was a *29% increase in the risk of death from coronary heart disease, including a 78% increase in death during the first year of treatment; a 31% increase in the risk of ischemic[†] stroke;* and a *2- to 3-fold increase in venous thromboembolism* (VTE, dangerous blood clots in the limbs and lungs). All these events occurred in postmenopausal women participating in the WHI, who had been generally healthy – no signs of heart disease or increased risk of stroke – just a few years earlier, before they started HRT.[2, 5, 6]

The WHI also found that the HRT-related risk of stroke was 46% higher in younger women (aged 50-59 years). A more recent British pooled analysis (meta-analysis) of data combined from 28 different clinical trials, encompassing nearly 40,000 postmenopausal women, confirmed the WHI's finding of an increase in stroke risk (29%) linked to HRT.

---

[*]   Although conventional medicine has yet to really come to grips with this fact, the rise in heart disease risk in men beginning in their mid-40s is due in part to a gradual decline in their testosterone levels, which begins around that time. Testosterone seems to provide men with essentially the same type of cardiovascular protection that estrogens provide women. Increasing evidence also shows that replacing testosterone in men (with bio-identical testosterone, of course) may significantly lower their risk of suffering heart attacks or strokes. (See Chapter 10 *"Hormones for Him: Why Men Need BHRT, Too"* and our book on male hormone replacement therapy, *Maximize Your Vitality and Potency,* Smart Publications, 1999, for more about the vastly underappreciated value of testosterone for men's cardiovascular health.)

[†]   There are two major types of stroke: 1) *Ischemic* strokes, sometimes called "brain attacks," are the most common type (83%). They are analogous to heart attacks (myocardial infarctions) in that they occur when a blood clot obstructs the flow of blood to a region of the brain, which then dies from lack of oxygen-carrying blood (ischemia). 2) *Hemorrhagic strokes* (17% of all strokes) occur when a weakened artery in the brain ruptures and bleeds into the surrounding brain, compressing and eventually killing the surrounding brain tissue.

Moreover, among women who suffered a stroke in these studies, those taking HRT had a 56% worse outcome, in terms of death, disability, and dependency combined.[7]

These findings came as a complete surprise to most conventional doctors. Up until that point, the official rationalization for forcing women on HRT to "live with" an increased risk of breast cancer was the substantial protection HRT supposedly offered them against other long-term consequences of a postmenopausal estrogen deficiency, such as osteoporosis, dementia/Alzheimer's disease, incontinence, and most importantly, heart attacks and strokes. After all, heart attacks and strokes kill or disable at least twice as many postmenopausal women as breast, uterine, and ovarian cancers combined.

In a medical world governed by risk/benefit analyses, a "small" increased cancer risk was deemed an acceptable price for women to pay if they wanted to protect their cardiovascular systems after menopause. Because heart disease is so common, even a minimal improvement in risk here was thought to more than compensate – statistically speaking – for a risk of breast cancer that would be unacceptable under other circumstances. As an old philosopher once said, *"You pays yer money, you takes yer choice!"*

But, when the WHI results finally came in, that choice didn't look so good after all. The WHI confirmed that HRT not only didn't improve cardiovascular risk as presumed, but it actually made it worse. The only *positive* effects HRT appeared to offer, besides eliminating hot flushes, etc, was a slight decline in the risk of hip fractures due to osteoporosis and a small decrease in the risk of colon cancer. These benefits were necessarily short-lived and inconsequential, though, since the "official" response to the WHI findings was that extended use of HRT (for more than a few years) was not recommended (*See Chapter 5.*) – that old breast cancer problem again.

These days, the conventional medical wisdom about "hormones" and cardiovascular disease goes something like this: "Although we've been telling you for decades – with complete confidence – that *HRT was good for your heart*, it is now evident we were wrong. In fact, the conclusions drawn from most of our large clinical trials were wrong, the product of design deficiencies infused with heavy doses of wishful thinking. Now that we have new, trustworthy data from large, prospective, long-term, randomized, double-blind, placebo-controlled trials (the WHI and couple of others), we can tell you – with complete confidence – that *HRT is not good for your heart,* unless you start it right after menopause and quit it once your hot flushes have gone away for good."

Are we confused yet? (*Since you've read this far, you probably aren't, but mainstream medicine certainly is!*)

"A Nearly Unshakeable Belief"

In the years preceding the WHI (2002), large, patent medicine industry- or government-sponsored clinical studies were nearly uniformly positive in their apparent validation of "hormone" replacement's cardiovascular benefits, demonstrating that "estrogen" users* had a 30 to 50% lower risk of coronary heart disease compared to nonusers.[8]

Patent medicine companies were only too happy to disseminate this news far and wide, making sure every doctor and every woman in her menopausal years knew all about it. HRT's supposed cardiovascular benefits became part of the conventional wisdom, and some women even took Premarin® + Provera® – with their doctors' blessings – with the sole aim of reducing their chances of suffering a heart attack or stroke.

In a post-WHI editorial in the *New England Journal of Medicine,* David M. Herrington, MD, and Timothy D. Howard, PhD, of the Wake-Forest University School of Medicine, exposed the long-running deception. They wrote that, until about 1998, when mainstream medicine first began to awaken to the truth about HRT and cardiovascular disease, it had adopted *"a nearly unshakeable belief"* in the cardioprotective benefits of "hormone" replacement therapy.[9]

This "nearly unshakeable belief" was bolstered by an impressive body of evidence, albeit almost entirely *indirect,* that was magnified out of all proportion by Big Pharma's extraordinary marketing and public relations apparatus. "As a result," wrote Herrington and Howard, *"...**many**

---

* The early studies typically employed Premarin® only, without progesterone, Provera®, or some other progestin. Provera® was added in later studies (mostly post-1975) in "women with a uterus" to reduce the risk of Premarin-induced uterine cancer.

people suspended ordinary standards of evidence concerning medical interventions and concluded that hormone therapy was the right thing to prevent heart disease in millions of postmenopausal women – despite the absence of any large-scale clinical trials quantifying the overall risk-benefit ratio."

Although the belief that ERT/HRT was safe and beneficial for the heart had pervaded conventional medicine throughout the 1970s, '80s, and '90s, if doctors, journalists, or anyone else really wanted to know, they could have easily seen how misguided this belief was. For example, placebo-controlled studies dating as far back as the late '60s had shown that women taking HRT's chemical cousins, oral contraceptives (usually ethinyl estradiol + a progestin) had a well-documented elevated risk of coronary heart disease.[8] You'd have thought data like these might at least trigger some serious doubts, but for the most part, they were ignored.

In 1997, British researchers pooled data from 22 separate *placebo-controlled* trials conducted between 1989 and 1995. In these studies, postmenopausal women had taken "estrogen" (in any form) for at least 3 months, with or without a progestin. Although most of the trials were small, in total they included more than 1,800 women, who took some form of ERT or HRT, and a comparable number who took a placebo. Putting all the data together, the researchers found that "estrogen"-treated women had a *39% higher cardiovascular risk,* compared with placebo-treated women, a far cry from the *30-to-50% lower risk* reported in most observational studies, that had been driving the conventional medical wisdom.[10] Since placebo-controlled trials usually carry more weight, scientifically speaking, than observational studies, these results were very telling.

A close analysis of the results from these 22 studies is also quite telling. The studies reported overall 16 cardiovascular disease "events" (eg, heart attacks); 6 events occurred in studies using horse-derived CEEs (Premarin®); 2 in studies using high-dose estradiol (2 milligrams/day (taken orally), which is clearly more than occurs in any woman with normal menstrual cycles); 1 in a study using a form of estrone; 4 in placebo or other control groups; and 3 in a study using mestranol, a potent, patented, man-made "estrogen" related to the "estrogen" ethinyl estradiol. On the other hand, no cardiovascular events occurred in 3 small studies (~25 women each) that employed regimens containing *estradiol* + *estriol* (even though the dosages used were not always what would be considered "bio-identical" today).

Yet, these findings were so different from what most doctors were accustomed to hearing, that it was easy to brush them under the rug, if that was one's mindset, and that's essentially what most doctors did with them. As Herrington and Howard observed, "Not surprisingly, when the initial randomized clinical trials failed to show a cardiovascular benefit, *the results were heavily criticized and, in some cases, disregarded in lieu of the less credible evidence that fit the prevailing paradigm.*"[9]

Most importantly, since this was not the "good news" Big Pharma and the rest of conventional medicine wanted us to hear, hardly any doctors – nor anyone else – ever heard it. All they heard – thanks to Big Pharma's well-tuned PR machine – was the "good news" about ERT/HRT, which was based on "less credible evidence."

Studies that raised doubts about ERT/HRT's cardiovascular benefits lay buried amongst the thousands of other medical research articles that get published each year, unpromoted by Big Pharma sales reps, unmentioned in slick drug ads in prestigious journals or know-nothing media outlets that respond on cue to Big Pharma PR, never to be heard from again, except by the relatively few motivated doctors and researchers who actually read the journals.

However, to the relatively small number of physicians, who recognize that "*Copy Nature*" is always the best path to health, these results, like those from the WHI to follow a few years later, were entirely predictable and vitally important.

The HERS Study: A Red Flag Finally Goes Up

In 1998, the publication of the results of the HERS study finally began to set off some alarms. HERS (*Heart and Estrogen/Progestin Replacement Study*) had the right pedigree: it was a *large, prospective, double-blind, placebo-controlled, NIH-sponsored* trial in which 2,763 women who had *proven coronary heart disease* at the start of the trial, randomly received either Premarin® + Provera® or placebo. If HRT were really beneficial for women's hearts, the NIH investigators reasoned, the "hormone"-treated women should fair significantly better – in terms of their cardiovascular health – than the placebo controls.

Needless to say, that's not what HERS found. After a mean of 4.1 years (later extended to 6.8 years), HRT had done nothing either to slow the progression of atherosclerosis or to reduce the rate of heart attacks or deaths due to heart disease. Moreover, HRT actually made things worse for some women by increasing their risk of serious blood clots (VTEs) and gallbladder disease (eg, gallstones). The HERS investigators concluded that "… *postmenopausal ['hormone'] therapy should not be used to reduce the risk of CHD [coronary heart disease] events in women with CHD.*"[11-13]

This was certainly disheartening news to the conventional medical community, and it led some physicians to start being more careful and selective in prescribing HRT. However, because HERS was limited to women who already had heart disease at the start of treatment, it left open the possibility that "hormone" replacement might still benefit postmenopausal women whose cardiovascular health was still good. That's where the WHI came in; the 160,000+ women who participated in this study were all heart disease-free at the start of the trial.

Because most doctors and news media people hadn't been paying much attention to HERS or to any of the other pre-WHI placebo-controlled trials of HRT and heart disease,[13] the soon-to-follow WHI results came as a complete shock, raising many difficult questions: Why did the WHI findings vary so much from nearly all the other large clinical studies that had preceded them? How could all those hundreds of nonclinical lab and animal studies, which had strongly suggested that hormone replacement *should* be beneficial, have been so far off the mark? Would WHI be the last word on this subject?

The "Healthy Woman Effect"

To those who really understood that hormone replacement means replacement of exactly identical hormones that follows Nature's "original blueprints" for types, quantities, timing, and methods of use, the WHI results were no surprise at all. They were well aware that the WHI, like most other controlled clinical trials, used only one "hormone" treatment: Premarin® (with or without Provera®). This factor alone could have explained the apparently anomalous findings. They were also aware that most of these pre-WHI studies were subject to a long list of potential biases, which, in the case of ERT/HRT, left the supposed cardiovascular benefits open to serious question.

Key among these biases is the "healthy woman effect." This well-known bias can affect study results this way: Women who voluntarily choose HRT, compared to women who do not use HRT, also tend to pay closer attention to other aspects of their health. For example, women who choose HRT are usually better educated, better informed about health, take much more responsibility for their own health, are leaner, healthier, eat a more nutritious diet, and are more likely to reliably "follow doctor's orders" and "take their 'meds,' as instructed."

So, can we conclude that HRT-treated women's superior cardiovascular health during clinical studies derives from their HRT use? Not necessarily. Perhaps it's due to a more nutritious diet. Or maybe it's a result of their generally better health or healthier lifestyle. Researchers can apply various statistical "tricks" to minimize the influence of these and other variables, but you can never know for sure.

We can usually draw more clinically valid conclusions from *randomized, double-blind, placebo-controlled trials,* which is why they are considered the "gold standard" among clinical studies.* In these trials, a population of postmenopausal women would be randomly divided into at least two groups; one group gets "hormones," while the other gets an inactive but identical-looking placebo, but neither the participants nor the researchers know who is getting which treatment until the end of the study – a classic "double-blind" design. Since both groups are treated exactly the same except for the primary variable – "hormones" vs. placebo – any subsequent differences in health between the two groups should be attributable to their specific treatment with a known degree of statistical reliability.

---

* There are exceptions to this general rule. For example, a relatively recent article in the *British Medical Journal* has pointed out that randomized, double-blind, placebo-controlled research is unnecessary to determine whether jumping out of an airplane is safer with a parachute than without a parachute. Smith GC, Pell JP. *Parachute use to prevent death and major trauma related to gravitational challenge: systematic review of randomised controlled trials. BMJ.* 2003; 327: 1459-1461.

The WHI, which met the "gold standard" criteria, confirmed what many of the other, less stringently controlled – but largely ignored – trials had been showing for decades: when conventional HRT is evaluated on a level, unbiased "playing field," its risk of causing cardiovascular events rises by at least 25%.

The Plausibility Factor

But does this mean that *all* hormone replacement regimens – not just Premarin® + Provera® – should be considered dangerous for women's cardiovascular health, as the FDA now states? *Hardly!* There's no logic that says that horse estrogens = bio-identical estrogens or that a patented pseudoprogesterone = bio-identical progesterone. Well-designed as the WHI may have been, its results and conclusions apply only to the materials used in that study.

Nevertheless, from the FDA's narrow-minded Big Pharma-driven viewpoint, one implication of studies like HERS and the WHI was that estrogen replacement – any kind of estrogen – may not play a significant role in preventing cardiovascular disease in women after all; or it might even make it worse. As a result, in the immediate aftermath of these studies – which, again, were limited to the use of horse estrogens – doctors were "officially" discouraged from prescribing estrogens *of all kinds* for women for the sole purpose of reducing their cardiovascular risk.

In fact, though, despite this faulty logic, and despite what the WHI results seemed to imply, there is every reason to expect that real, ovarian or bio-identical estrogen replacement should be cardioprotective, a factor that Elizabeth Barrett-Connor, MD, a leading sex hormone researcher from the University of California, San Diego, has referred to as its *plausibility*. "Cardioprotection is plausible," she wrote in 1998. "The fact that estrogen has been found [in decades of laboratory and clinical studies] to be associated with so many potentially favorable biologic and physiologic changes gives biological plausibility to the thesis that estrogen prevents CHD [coronary heart disease]."[8, 14] These potentially favorable biologic and physiologic changes include the following:

Lipidemic effects. Natural human estrogen's best appreciated cardioprotective actions concern blood lipid (*fatty acid*) levels, which account for about 30% of its known clinical benefits:[15]

- Decreases in *low-density lipoprotein (LDL)-cholesterol* (the "bad" cholesterol).

- Decreases in *lipoprotein(a) [Lp(a)]* and *triglycerides* (both also "bad").

- Increases in *high-density lipoprotein (HDL)-cholesterol* (the "good" cholesterol).

Direct vascular effects. Natural human estrogen also contributes to cardioprotection by acting directly on blood vessels to:

- Increase dilation of arteries (lowering blood pressure).

- Inhibit progression of atherosclerosis (slowing the clogging of arteries by cholesterol-laden plaques).

- Favorably affect the multiple factors that control blood coagulation, clotting, and the formation of thrombi (obstructive blood clots), all of which contribute to heart attacks and strokes.[*]

Arterial contraction, dilation, and blood clotting. Natural human estrogen acts on both the outer *smooth muscle* layers of arteries and the slick *endothelial* layers that line their inner surfaces (lumens):

- As noted above, as arterial smooth muscle contracts and dilates, it varies the vessel's inner diameter, and consequently, controls the volume of blood flow while raising and lowering blood pressure.

- Under the influence of natural human estrogen, arterial endothelial cells secrete a variety of bioactive substances, key among which is *nitric oxide (NO)*. When microdrops of NO come in contact with nearby arterial smooth muscle cells, the cells respond by relaxing, which dilates the artery and lowers blood pressure.

---

[*] A partial list of blood factors that are favorably affected by estrogens includes fibrinogen, the anticoagulant proteins antithrombin III and protein S, and the antifibrinolytic protein PAI-1.

- NO in the arterial lumen also inhibits platelet activation, an early step in blood clotting and thrombus formation and a factor in endothelial dysfunction. *Endothelial dysfunction*, which has come to be seen in recent years as a major contributor to atherosclerotic disease, is a direct consequence of estrogen deficiency. Endothelial dysfunction, among its many other actions, impedes arterial NO secretion, leading to high blood pressure (*hypertension*) and coronary artery disease.[15]

Antioxidant effects. Oxidation is an important metabolic process that can be destructive if not adequately controlled by substances with *antioxidant* properties:

- For example, oxidation of LDL-cholesterol is a crucial step in the formation of arterial plaque and the progression of atherosclerosis. Nutrients like vitamins C and E, and hormones, including estradiol, are all powerful antioxidants, which can inhibit LDL-cholesterol oxidation and so slow the progression of atherosclerosis.[15]

- The relative absence of estradiol and/or antioxidant vitamins is an important risk factor in the development of coronary heart disease.

Bio-identical Hormones and HRT Go Head-to-Head

Although the FDA and other powers of conventional medicine constantly repeat the meme that there's no proof that BHRT is better or safer than patented HRT, it started to become apparent as far back as the mid-1980s that a large percentage of the cardiovascular difficulties attributed to HRT could be traced to the unique actions of horse estrogens and Provera®. Moreover, on the few occasions that Premarin® and/or progestins have been compared head-to-head with bio-identical estrogens and/or progesterone in controlled trials, it has been no contest; bio-identical hormones were unquestionably safer and more effective.

Most of these studies did not look directly at clinical cardiovascular events – eg, heart attacks, strokes, and angina pectoris – but rather at various risk factors and physiologic changes, like cholesterol levels, blood clotting, atherosclerosis progression, venous thrombosis, and other signs of vascular disease, all of which are known to predispose to cardiovascular events. Many of these studies have recently been reviewed by Holtorf.[16] He shows, for example, that progesterone by itself, or combined with estrogen inhibited atherosclerotic plaque formation in primates. However, patented progestins had the exact opposite effect, promoting plaque formation and preventing the plaque-inhibiting and lipid-lowering actions of estrogen.

In another example, a 1985 Swedish study measured levels of HDL-cholesterol in 58 postmenopausal women following different "hormone" replacement regimens.[17] The women first received 3 "cycles" (28 days per cycle) of an "unopposed" estrogen: *estradiol valerate*. During the next 3 "cycles," the women received estradiol plus either *Provera®*, *levonorgestrel* (another patented progestin), or bio-identical *progesterone* (oral micronized formulation). In order to simulate the hormonal environment of a natural premenopausal menstrual cycle, the progestins and progesterone were given only during the last 10 days of each cycle. The results showed that, compared with estradiol alone, estradiol + Provera® and estradiol + levonorgestrel caused significant *decreases in HDL levels* – an undesirable result, because high HDL is considered to be cardioprotective. On the other hand, estradiol + progesterone had no adverse effect on HDL levels.

Since higher HDL levels are associated with a lower risk of coronary artery disease, this finding suggested that progestins – *but not progesterone* – can increase the risk of a heart attack or stroke. The Swedish investigators concluded, "Apart from the protection against endometrial hyperproliferation [overgrowth in the uterine lining], most of the effects of [Provera® and levonorgestrel] during ERT are basically *unwanted and of little benefit to the patient*."

Ten years later, the NIH published the results of the watershed Postmenopausal Estrogen/Progestin Interventions (PEPI) trial in the *Journal of the American Medical Association (JAMA)*. PEPI essentially replicated and extended the findings of the Swedish study. It also did something few, if any, major US studies have done so far; it included a treatment group receiving a bio-identical hormone – *oral micronized progesterone*. Specifically, PEPI compared the effects of Premarin® + Provera® with those of Premarin® + progesterone on levels of LDL, HDL, and other factors.[18]

The PEPI trial was a "gold-standard," double-blind, placebo-controlled study in which 875 *healthy* postmenopausal women randomly received one of four treatments: 1) Placebo; 2) Premarin® "unopposed"; 3) Premarin® + Provera®; or 4) Premarin® + oral micronized progesterone.

After 3 years of treatment, the results showed that "unopposed" Premarin® treatment resulted in a large increase in HDL levels, compared to placebo (Fig. 8-2). However, the shock came when Premarin® was combined with Provera®. In the women receiving this treatment, Premarin's lipidemic benefit (increased HDL) was nearly completely erased. By contrast, in those women who received Premarin® + real, bio-identical progesterone, HDL levels remained elevated.

From these data, then, it's obvious that "estrogen" + progesterone is far superior to "estrogen" + Provera® for producing a favorable effect on HDL-cholesterol. (*Isn't it a shame the researchers didn't include a group of women taking bio-identical estrogens + progesterone, especially considering all the taxpayer money used to conduct this study?*)

Although the PEPI researchers could see the significance of their findings as well as we can, they declared the major finding of the study to be *"Estrogen is good for a woman's heart."*[1] They barely mentioned the startling progesterone finding, burying it in the very last sentence of the paper. Wrote the authors: "[For women with a uterus], estrogen [ie, Premarin®] plus [progesterone] appears to spare the endometrium and to preserve the bulk of estrogen's favorable effects on [heart disease] risk factors including HDL-C." Of course, they avoided recommending progesterone for "women without a uterus" (*Osteoporosis, anyone?*).

In an interview posted on the American Medical Association's (AMA) website designed to coincide with the *JAMA* publication of the PEPI results, the study's principal investigator, Dr. Elizabeth Barrett-Connor, did take note of the progesterone result. "If I were treating a woman primarily because she was worried about heart disease or because she had dyslipidemia [abnormal blood levels of cholesterol] and low HDL-cholesterol, *I would probably see if she wanted to take micronized progesterone. I was quite impressed with the better effect,*" she said. (Emphasis added.) She then added, "I would like to see micronized

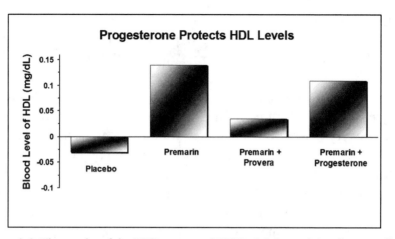

Figure 8-2. The results of the NIH-sponsored PEPI trial showed that "estrogen" (Premarin®) administered to postmenopausal women resulted in a large increase in HDL levels, compared with placebo. However, this benefit was lost when "estrogen" was combined with Provera® but not when combined with bio-identical progesterone.
Adapted from PEPI Trial. *JAMA.1996;273:199-208*

progesterone included as a treatment in the big studies like the Women's Health Initiative" (Not yet completed at that time.) The president of the American Heart Association at the time speculated that women who followed Dr. Barrett-Connor's advice and took progesterone instead of Provera® might reduce their heart disease risk by 12%.[19]

Unfortunately, Dr. Barrett-Connor's wish regarding the use of progesterone in the WHI never came true. As noted above, a few years later, after the WHI results came out, one of the recommendations of the FDA and other authorities was that conventional HRT *not* be prescribed for women specifically because they were worried about heart disease, which made sense, given that it clearly didn't work. What about using progesterone instead of Provera®? It seems to have been forgotten.

Although the "official message" of the PEPI study was that "estrogen is good for a woman's heart," a closer look at the result raised new questions about the safety of Premarin® as well as Provera®. Yes, "unopposed" Premarin® did raise HDL levels, but at the same time, five new cases of heart disease developed during the first 3 years of the study, all in patients taking Premarin®, compared with zero cases in the placebo group. This suggests that Premarin® might actually be *causing* heart disease in some postmenopausal women. Moreover, 10 women who took Premarin®

developed blood clots (VTEs), which in four cases were considered serious; no women in the placebo group developed VTE. These serious risks of Premarin® were later confirmed in the WHI study.

If Tri-Est, Bi-Est, or even estriol alone had been used instead of horse estrogens in the PEPI study, would these same problems have occurred? We have every reason to believe they would not, but actual studies are obviously required. The same question was apparently on the minds of the PEPI researchers, though. During the AMA Internet discussion, Dr. Barrett-Connor was asked, "Do you have a suspicion that we haven't adequately explored what preparations we should be using in the first place? For example, some people complain that *estriol* was not available in our preparations yet. *It's available in Europe. It's a mild estrogen, and it may have anti-breast cancer effects. It may, if anything, inhibit and certainly will not increase the risk of breast cancer.*"

However, Dr. Barrett-Connor, who had earlier voiced her desire to see progesterone explored further in the WHI, seemed less enthusiastic about estriol. "Although I'm not opposed to new studies of new *drugs** ..." she said, and then went on to enumerate all the obstacles in the way of doing them.

Progesterone (*but Not* Provera®) Improves Coronary Blood Flow

As the PEPI study demonstrated, the closer we look at conventional HRT, the more dangerous it seems to be for the heart. Yet, when bio-identical hormones are used in similar studies, the dangers seem to vanish.

Heart muscle requires an uninterrupted supply of blood bearing lots of oxygen and nutrients, especially in times of physical or emotional stress. Disruption of this blood supply, even for a few minutes – a condition known as *myocardial ischemia* (literal English translation: "not enough blood flow to the heart muscle") could leave the heart muscle severely and permanently damaged. This is what happens in a heart attack. The value of bio-identical hormones is again demonstrated in its ability to

---

*   As do most conventional physicians, Dr. Barrett-Connor unfortunately persists in describing natural substances, like bio-identical hormones, as "drugs," again demonstrating how Big Pharma distorts the language of medicine to suit its own goals and motives.

facilitate the dilation and constriction of coronary arteries in response to normal stimuli so that the heart muscle gets the blood it needs when it needs it.

Arteries that get clogged with atherosclerotic plaque or are hyperreactive to normal stimuli may constrict too much or for too long (*vasospasm*), which can deprive the heart muscle of blood just when it needs it most. Ischemia due to coronary vasospasm can cause heart pain (*angina pectoris*), arrhythmia, heart failure, and heart attack.

The reactivity of coronary arteries is partially under the control of estrogen and progesterone, which relax arterial smooth muscle so that blood flow to heart muscle tissue increases.[20, 21] It should come as no surprise by now that bio-identical estrogen and progesterone promote healthy vasodilation and coronary blood flow in postmenopausal women, but what about an alien-to-the-human body pseudohormone like Provera®? Can we expect it to support normal vasodilation as well?

Guess what? It doesn't even come close.[22]

The advantage of progesterone over patented *medroxy*progesterone (Provera®) was confirmed in a study in which surgically menopausal (ovaries removed) rhesus monkeys were put on "hormone replacement" consisting of either 1) estradiol + Provera® or 2) estradiol + progesterone. At one point during their treatment, the monkeys were exposed to a chemical toxin that triggers a rapid constriction, or vasospasm, in their coronary arteries, producing what is essentially a simulated heart attack.

The monkeys receiving progesterone resisted the toxin-induced vasospasm, allowing their coronary blood flow to quickly return to normal. However, Provera® offered no such protection, and actually *increased the risk of vasospasm*. The researchers observed that, had the Provera-treated monkeys not been given a special protective antidote, they would have died within minutes.[23]

Ethically, you couldn't run a comparable study in humans, but one randomized, double-blind study in postmenopausal women, who had confirmed coronary artery disease came to a similar conclusion:

progesterone, but not Provera® significantly enhances the beneficial vasodilatory effects of estradiol on stress-induced myocardial ischemia, just as it had done in the monkeys exposed to a coronary toxin.[24] The primary measure of coronary blood flow in this study was the amount of time the women could exercise on a treadmill before experiencing myocardial ischemia.*

As shown in Figure 8-3, compared to baseline (no treatment), women taking estradiol alone significantly increased their exercise time, However, the addition of Provera® to estradiol provided no further advantage. But when women took both estradiol and progesterone, their exercise time increased significantly. As the authors concluded, "The results of the present study indicate *a synergistic effect of estrogen and progesterone, but not estrogen and MPA [Provera®],* on exercise time to myocardial ischemia. This is a novel finding in the setting of CAD [coronary artery disease].[24]

As one researcher pointed out later, in terms of heart disease protection, *"Provera® is worse than no treatment at all."*

HRT (but *Not* BHRT) Promotes Atherosclerosis, Venous Thrombosis, and Abnormal Blood Clotting

Bio-identical estrogens – especially estradiol (which is the most tested bio-identical estrogen in mainstream research) – have generally been found to be effective at slowing the progression of atherosclerosis.[15] However, when women take Premarin® and/or Provera®, all bets are off. Here are just a few examples of research findings that demonstrate this distinction:

- "Unopposed" estradiol slows the progression of atherosclerosis in the carotid artery (the main artery that carries blood to the brain) in postmenopausal women, reducing the risk of a stroke.[25]

- In a double-blind, placebo-controlled trial of postmenopausal women with coronary artery disease, estradiol lost its ability to inhibit atherosclerosis progression when combined with Provera®.[26]

---

* **Myocardial ischemia was assessed by a characteristic electrocardiogram (ECG) effect** known as ST segment depression, a classic sign that the heart muscle is not getting enough oxygen.

- Estradiol reduces the risk of thrombus (obstructive blood clot) formation by favorably affecting blood clotting and coagulation factors – known as *hemostatic markers.*[27, 28]

- In rhesus monkeys placed on a diet designed to promote atherosclerosis, estradiol plus progesterone nevertheless reduced the formation of atherosclerotic plaque in coronary arteries by 50%.[29]

- Premarin® + Provera® increased the risk of VTEs by more than 400% in women aged 60 to 69 years, and by 750% in women aged 70 or older.[30]

- Unopposed Premarin® use resulted in a 65% increase in the risk of VTE; adding Provera® increased the risk by another 60%. By contrast, use of estradiol did not increase the risk of VTE, and actually decreased it by 8%.[31]

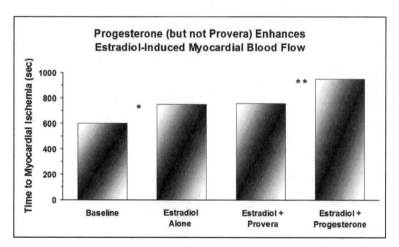

Figure 8-3. In a study comparing the effects of progesterone with Provera®, postmenopausal women with coronary artery disease exercised on a treadmill until ECG signs of myocardial ischemia appeared. Estradiol + progesterone allowed the women to exercise significantly longer than did estradiol + Provera® before ischemia occurred. These results show that progesterone, but not Provera®, improves blood flow to heart muscle during physical stress.

*   *P* <0.001 estradiol alone vs. baseline (no treatment)
** *P* <0.001 estradiol + Provera® vs. estradiol + progesterone

Adapted from Rosano et al, 2000

- Although estradiol has been the bio-identical alternative to Premarin® used in most clinical studies, one Japanese study did investigate the effects of estriol in elderly women (aged 80+). They found that estriol significantly improved the women's vascular endothelial function (an important sign of cardiovascular health) as well as their bone mineral density (signifying stronger bones), with no serious adverse side effects.[32]

In June 2007, nearly 5 years after the original WHI results were first revealed, the WHI research team came out with a re-analysis of some data purporting to show that, perhaps Premarin® wasn't so bad for women's hearts after all. The re-analysis, which was confined to "women without a uterus," who had been taking Premarin® alone or with placebo, employed CT scans of the women's hearts to look for coronary-artery calcification, evidence of atherosclerosis. They found that, among younger women (aged 50-59), those taking Premarin® had less calcification, suggesting a lower risk of heart attacks, compared to those taking placebo.[3]

Of course, the media – with lots of encouragement from the friendly folks at Wyeth Pharmaceuticals – jumped all over this apparent "good news" story. Lost in the details, though, were such "unimportant" facts as the limited study population (women with surgically induced menopause); the fact that the treatment did nothing about reducing the risks of stroke, abnormal blood clotting, breast cancer, senility, and all the other long-term consequences of Premarin® use; or the fact that women in the 50- to 59-year age range have a relatively low risk of coronary heart disease to begin with. Since the FDA presently recommends that women use the lowest dose of HRT for the shortest duration possible, by the time these women reached age 60 and beyond, when their vulnerability to heart disease really begins to accelerate, they would have long stopped taking Premarin®, and there's no reason to expect that any cardiovascular benefits accrued during the few years of early use would carry over once they stopped therapy.

Taking HRT for a few years to suppress hot flushes does nothing for the long-term health of postmenopausal women. In order to improve their health long-term, they need to take their hormones long-term, and the only safe way to accomplish that is with BHRT.

Whither BHRT and the Heart?

If conventional HRT is no good for women's hearts, a conclusion that still stands, what does this mean for BHRT?

Just listen to what hormone "experts" are essentially saying today: "Since horse estrogens and pseudohormone progestin drugs are demonstrably dangerous in women, therefore, we must assume that *bio-identical human estrogens and progesterone* are also potentially dangerous in human females, *despite the lack of any evidence to support this assumption.*"

Conventional medicine "authorities" make the tortured, double-negative argument that there's "no proof" that bio-identical hormones are *not* just as dangerous for women as horse hormones and patented pseudohormone drugs. Aside from the fact that this contention is demonstrably false, as illustrated by a casual browse through the preceding chapters, not to mention the scientific literature of the last 40 or so years on which they're based, this line of reasoning is, as Mr. Spock might have said, "*Illogical!*"

Although the WHI results exposed the cardiovascular risks of Premarin® and Provera®, they told us nothing about the potential benefits or risks of bio-identical human hormones. As we've said before, and will say again, because it's so easy to forget, especially if you depend on conventional medicine or media as sources of information:

- Horse estrogens (ie, Premarin®) are *not natural human ovarian estrogens.*

- Patented progestins (eg, Provera®) are *not natural human ovarian progesterone.*

- So-called "natural," FDA-"approved" estrogen replacement products (eg, 100% estradiol pills, skin patches, gels, or creams) are *a very incomplete attempt at bio-identical hormone replacement for women, even though the hormone estradiol itself is one of many bio-identical hormones.* But the recommended dose of estradiol in these products – 1 to 2 *milli*grams daily – is usually much too high (a physiologic dose of BHRT typically contains no more than 0.25 milligrams of estradiol daily), making the FDA-"approved" products potentially dangerous. Moreover, they lack estriol, which acts as an essential buffer against estradiol's and estrone's procarcinogenic proclivities.

- Physicians who prescribe 100% estradiol products typically combine them with Provera® or some other patented progestin drug, not with progesterone.

- Conventional physicians smart enough to avoid Premarin® + Provera® often opt for *oral* formulations of estradiol (and a progestin). Yet, there's no doubt that taking steroid hormones by mouth can increase the risks of many serious diseases that are easily avoided by topical use. (*See Chapter 9 for more about optimal use of bio-identical hormones.*)

Menopausal symptoms, as well as heart disease, osteoporosis, and other long-term consequences of menopause, are largely a result of deficiencies in the production of ovarian estrogens and progesterone, not of horse hormones or pseudohormone patent medicines. Hard as this concept may be for many doctors to grasp, in all of human history, there has never been a woman whose body suffered due to a deficiency in horse estrogens and/or patented progestins.

Thus, *substituting* alien pseudohormone patent medicines that may be similar to – but not exactly the same as – Mother Nature's built-in hormones for these deficient hormones defies common sense. True, they may help suppress symptoms like hot flushes and vaginal soreness in the short term, in the long run, the only benefits of these products are to patent medicine companies' bottom lines.

On the other hand, doing the *logical* thing – replacing deficient estrogens and progesterone with bio-identical versions of themselves – not only minimizes the short-term symptoms, but also reduces the long-term consequences of hormone deficiencies, all without raising the risks of cancer or heart disease.

Here's another point conventional medicine "experts" find difficult to grasp: the familiar pathologies associated with HRT derive, not from their "estrogenic" or "progestogenic" properties, but rather from the fact that these alien "hormones" are different in molecular structure – and therefore their function and metabolism (molecular processing) – from the bio-identical human ideal. There is no question about this; it has been demonstrated in dozens of scientific studies.

Although the requisite large-scale, double-blind, placebo-controlled trials proving the cardiovascular safety and efficacy of BHRT are yet to be done, decades of other research and clinical experience convincingly argue that bio-identical hormones, when used at physiologic doses and administered via a route and on a schedule that closely mimics Mother Nature's design, carry all the cardiovascular benefits of the naturally-secreted ovarian hormones and none of the risks of their patented alien molecular cousins.

Whenever studies related to cardiovascular diseases employ bio-identical hormones – including most lab studies and many smaller clinical trials – the results almost invariably show them to be safe and effective. We have absolutely no doubt that should a large "gold-standard" trial ever somehow get around to testing BHRT,* the results would confirm what has already been demonstrated in the earlier studies.

As we have asserted in other contexts in this book, with regard to the actual cardiovascular effects of bio-identical hormones, we might as well take all the clinical research using horse estrogens and other pseudohormone patent medicines and throw them in the trash. *That's how much all that "research" is worth!*

---

* Actually, Nature and Creation have "run a study" for at least 200,000 years about precisely which estrogens and other hormones, in what quantities, by what route of administration, and by which timing are all best for human females. But that common-sense point of view – a very logical one – is often called "non-scientific"!

References

1. Healy B. PEPI in perspective. Good answers spawn pressing questions. *JAMA*. 1995;273:240-241.

2. Rossouw JE, Anderson GL, Prentice RL, et al. Risks and benefits of estrogen plus progestin in healthy postmenopausal women: principal results From the Women's Health Initiative randomized controlled trial. *JAMA*. 2002;288:321-333.

3. Manson JE, Allison MA, Rossouw JE, et al. Estrogen therapy and coronary-artery calcification. *N Engl J Med*. 2007;356:2591-2602.

4. National Center for Health Statistics. Health, United States, 2005. *http://www.cdc.gov/nchs/data/hus/hus05.pdf#036*. 2005;Hyattsville, Maryland.

5. Wassertheil-Smoller S, Hendrix SL, Limacher M, et al. Effect of estrogen plus progestin on stroke in postmenopausal women: the Women's Health Initiative: a randomized trial. *JAMA*. 2003;289:2673-2684.

6. Manson JE, Hsia J, Johnson KC, et al. Estrogen plus progestin and the risk of coronary heart disease. *N Engl J Med*. 2003;349:523-534.

7. Bath PM, Gray LJ. Association between hormone replacement therapy and subsequent stroke: a meta-analysis. *BMJ*. 2005;330:342.

8. Barrett-Connor E, Grady D. Hormone replacement therapy, heart disease, and other considerations. *Annu Rev Public Health*. 1998;19:55-72.

9. Herrington DM, Howard TD. From presumed benefit to potential harm--hormone therapy and heart disease. *N Engl J Med*. 2003;349:519-521.

10. Hemminki E, McPherson K. Impact of postmenopausal hormone therapy on cardiovascular events and cancer: pooled data from clinical trials. *BMJ*. 1997;315:149-153.

11. Hulley S, Grady D, Bush T, et al. Randomized trial of estrogen plus progestin for secondary prevention of coronary heart disease in postmenopausal women. Heart and Estrogen/progestin Replacement Study (HERS) Research Group. *JAMA*. 1998;280:605-613.

12. Grady D, Herrington D, Bittner V, et al. Cardiovascular disease outcomes during 6.8 years of hormone therapy: Heart and Estrogen/progestin Replacement Study follow-up (HERS II). *JAMA*. 2002;288:49-57.

13. Herrington DM, Reboussin DM, Brosnihan KB, et al. Effects of estrogen replacement on the progression of coronary-artery atherosclerosis. *N Engl J Med*. 2000;343:522-529.

14. Barrett-Connor E. Hormone replacement therapy. *BMJ*. 1998;317:457-461.

15. Mendelsohn ME, Karas RH. The protective effects of estrogen on the cardiovascular system. *N Engl J Med*. 1999;340:1801-1811.

16. Holtorf K. The bioidentical hormone debate: are bioidentical hormones (estradiol, estriol, and progesterone) safer or more efficacious than commonly used synthetic versions in hormone replacement therapy? *Postgrad Med.* 2009;121:73-85.

17. Ottosson UB, Johansson BG, von Schoultz B. Subfractions of high-density lipoprotein cholesterol during estrogen replacement therapy: a comparison between progestogens and natural progesterone. *Am J Obstet Gynecol.* 1985;151:746-750.

18. The Writing Group for the PEPI Trial. Effects of estrogen or estrogen/progestin regimens on heart disease risk factors in postmenopausal women. The Postmenopausal Estrogen/Progestin Interventions (PEPI) Trial. *JAMA.* 1995;273:199-208.

19. Archives Journal Club/Women's Health Roundtable. Estrogen Replacement Therapy and Heart Disease: A Discussion of the PEPI Trial. *www.ama-assn.org/ sci-pubs/journals/archive /womh/vol_1/no_1/jcr.htm.* Accessed May 19, 1996 (no longer available).

20. Rosano GM, Caixeta AM, Chierchia S, et al. Short-term anti-ischemic effect of 17β-estradiol in postmenopausal women with coronary artery disease. *Circulation.* 1997;96:2837-2841.

21. Rosano GM, Sarrel PM, Poole-Wilson PA, Collins P. Beneficial effect of oestrogen on exercise-induced myocardial ischaemia in women with coronary artery disease. *Lancet.* 1993;342:133-136.

22. Kawano H, Motoyama T, Hirai N, et al. Effect of medroxyprogesterone acetate plus estradiol on endothelium-dependent vasodilation in postmenopausal women. *Am J Cardiol.* 2001;87:238-240, A239.

23. Miyagawa K, Rösch J, Stanczyk F, Hermsmeyer K. Medroxyprogesterone interferes with ovarian steroid protection against coronary vasospasm. *Nature Med.* 1997;3:324-327.

24. Rosano GM, Webb CM, Chierchia S, et al. Natural progesterone, but not medroxyprogesterone acetate, enhances the beneficial effect of estrogen on exercise-induced myocardial ischemia in postmenopausal women. *J Am Coll Cardiol.* 2000;36:2154-2159.

25. Karim R, Mack WJ, Lobo RA, et al. Determinants of the effect of estrogen on the progression of subclinical atherosclerosis: Estrogen in the Prevention of Atherosclerosis Trial. *Menopause.* 2005;12:366-373.

26. Hodis HN, Mack WJ, Azen SP, et al. Hormone therapy and the progression of coronary-artery atherosclerosis in postmenopausal women. *N Engl J Med.* 2003;349:535-545.

27. Basurto L, Saucedo R, Zarate A, et al. Effect of pulsed estrogen therapy on hemostatic markers in comparison with oral estrogen regimen in postmenopausal women. *Gynecol Obstet Invest.* 2006;61:61-64.

28. Sowers MR, Matthews KA, Jannausch M, et al. Hemostatic factors and estrogen during the menopausal transition. *J Clin Endocrinol Metab.* 2005;90:5942-5948.

29. Minshall RD, Stanczyk FZ, Miyagawa K, et al. Ovarian steroid protection against coronary artery hyperreactivity in rhesus monkeys. *J Clin Endocrinol Metab.* 1998;83:649-659.

30. Cushman M, Kuller LH, Prentice R, et al. Estrogen plus progestin and risk of venous thrombosis. *JAMA.* 2004;292:1573-1580.

31. Smith NL, Heckbert SR, Lemaitre RN, et al. Esterified estrogens and conjugated equine estrogens and the risk of venous thrombosis. *JAMA.* 2004;292:1581-1587.

32. Hayashi T, Ito I, Kano H, Endo H, Iguchi A. Estriol (E3) replacement improves endothelial function and bone mineral density in very elderly women. *J Gerontol A Biol Sci Med Sci.* 2000;55:B183-190; discussion B191-183.

CHAPTER 9

GETTING THE MOST OUT OF BHRT:
HOW MUCH TO USE AND HOW BEST TO USE IT

One of the principal benefits of the Women's Health Initiative (WHI) study has been to scare millions of women away from conventional patented hormone replacement therapy – Premarin® + Provera® (HRT). Some quit altogether, choosing to endure the hot flushes, etc, until they went away on their own. Others switched to one of the increasing numbers of "hormone" replacement regimens that combine only the bio-identical hormone estradiol with a variety of other patent medicine pseudohormones. Others have switched to entirely patented pseudohormones which aren't Premarin® and/or Provera® (at least the old fashioned, high-dose versions), the only "hormone treatments" tested in the WHI.

Most of these "alternative" HRT regimens consist of a combination of *estradiol,* the most potent of the bio-identical estrogens, combined with a patented progestin. While some doctors still prescribe Provera® (medroxyprogesterone, MPA), more "enlightened" ones have switched to other progestins, such as norgestimate, norethindrone, or levonorgestrel, all of which have been commonly used in oral contraceptive (OC) drug combinations and are generally considered to be somewhat less dangerous than Provera®. Better yet, some enlightened doctors have chosen to prescribe bio-identical progesterone instead.

Fortunately, an unprecedented number of women have also turned to bio-identical hormone replacement therapy (BHRT). This swing toward BHRT received a huge boost a few years back with the publication of *The Sexy Years,* and subsequent books, *Ageless: The Naked Truth About Bioidentical Hormones*, and *Breakthrough: Eight Steps to Wellness,* in which Hollywood celebrity and natural-health-and-fitness advocate Suzanne Somers writes of her success using variations of BHRT, and interviews physicians expert in their use.

But while a giant step in the right direction, the "BHRT" recommended in *The Sexy Years* was not "complete" BHRT, prescribed, and carefully monitored as we describe it in this book. Although we enthusiastically applaud the increased use and acceptance of BHRT that her books have initiated, it is with a note of caution, since many physicians who *think* they are prescribing BHRT may be doing so in the absence of any real understanding of its scientific foundation. So in the habit are they of simply prescribing prepackaged pills and expecting (hoping for?) the best outcome, they often fail to appreciate that proper use of BHRT requires a very different approach to hormone replacement.

BHRT is not simply a less toxic form of Prempro®, nor is it a "fountain of youth" capable of transforming 60-year-olds into 20-year-olds again. BHRT can certainly have important anti-aging properties, but turning the hormonal clock back 3 or 4 *decades*, as some advocate, may be a little too much to ask. Trying to do so by taking excessive doses of the wrong hormones, or an incomplete pattern of hormones – especially without careful monitoring – may be putting some women at unnecessary risk.

On a larger, political scale, needless and preventable adverse events related to uninformed or incorrect use of BHRT could well encourage overeager government regulators to further ally with patent medicine companies, anxious to protect their deeply flawed but still lucrative pseudohormone franchises. They would just love to pounce on some apparent "hazards" of BHRT related to improper use, and then try to tar all bio-identical hormones with the same brush as their dangerous patented products, without so much as a single clinical trial result to back up their claims. You can read more about these important issues in Chapter 12, *"The Politics of Bio-Identical Hormones: How They're Trying to Take Them Away."*

It's Simple Really: Just Follow Mother Nature's Hormone Recipe

Some doctors and patients think they are using genuine BHRT just by taking pills containing bio-identical estradiol and progesterone. Although estradiol is a primary estrogen produced by the premenopausal ovary, normal metabolic processes eventually result in several primary circulating estrogens, including *estrone, estradiol, estriol, and 2-hydroxyestrone.*

Estradiol is the most potent and most carcinogenic of these; estrone is a carcinogen, too, especially in the breast. Fortunately, most premenopausal women metabolize their internally secreted estrone and estradiol into sufficient estriol (and other anticarcinogenic estrogen metabolites) to buffer the effects of the procarcinogenic estrogens, thus avoiding "estrogen-related" cancer. But when women "replace" deficient ovarian hormones with 100% estradiol but without adding anticarcinogenic estriol, they badly distort the natural balance of circulating estrogens. Since there's no guarantee that their natural metabolic processes will produce sufficient estriol from these replacements to counteract the inherent carcinogenicity of estradiol and the estrone that the body almost always forms from estradiol, it's always safest to include estriol, too, in any replacement regimen.

In *true* BHRT, potentially carcinogenic estrogens, like estrone and estradiol, are more than balanced by relatively high doses of the more benign, *anticarcinogenic* estriol, which inhibits the expression of their carcinogenic properties. In order to best approximate the natural premenopausal hormonal environment, it's best to take (at a minimum) estriol and estradiol; sometimes estrone can be left out, especially by women whose bodies tend to be very efficient at metabolizing estradiol into estrone. These women may be better off taking just estradiol and estriol (Bi-Est).

Conventional HRT: At Odds with Nature

Contrary to most conventional doctors' erroneous belief, safe and effective use of BHRT demands a philosophical approach to medicine that is probably alien to what they have been taught throughout their entire careers. The key misconception was clearly expressed by the author of a recent review of "hormone" replacement regimens: "The aim of any [conventional] hormonal treatment of postmenopausal women is *not to restore the physiological serum levels occurring in ovulatory cycles of fertile women, but **to prevent or improve complaints and symptoms caused by estrogen deficiency**.*"[1]

That pretty much says it all. The conventional medical approach – *see a symptom, suppress a symptom, with a patent medication* – is at odds with Nature and completely inappropriate for BHRT. Whatever might be causing those symptoms is typically of secondary concern; as long as the treatment works and is not too toxic, it is deemed acceptable. This is the kind of thinking that makes it not only acceptable but *preferable* to treat women in menopause with estrogens from a pregnant horse. Moreover, the way the FDA's drug "approval" process is structured, the treatment need not be better or safer than a natural or bio-identical alternative; it only needs to be more efficacious at removing said complaints and symptoms and not significantly more toxic than an inactive dummy pill, or placebo, the proverbial "sugar pill" (although they're usually not made of sugar any more).

Rather than merely suppressing hot flushes using any *patent medicine* or pseudohormone that seems to work,* ***the primary goal of BHRT is to restore a hormonal environment as close to the natural, premenopausal state as possible.***

BHRT requires that we follow the hormonal recipe Mother Nature has worked out over millions of years of evolution in the *human* female. The closer that recipe is followed, the happier and healthier you will be. If symptoms are caused by an imbalance in a complex, integrated physiologic system, like the one that controls sex steroid secretion and activity, rather than ignoring and/or overriding that control – as conventional treatments almost always do – natural medicine aims to restore the natural balance of hormones to which the body is accustomed.

Since menopausal complaints and symptoms are largely a result of a "hormone deficiency," once that deficiency is resolved by replacing the deficient hormones with bio-identical copies, the complaints and symptoms generally go away of their own accord. There is no need to suppress them artificially. This may seem like a subtle distinction, but when it comes to the overall health of women using hormone replacement, it makes all the difference in the world.

Most importantly, BHRT works well and it works safely. I and a few thousand like-minded doctors and hundreds of thousands of healthy, satisfied women will vouch for it. In fact, last year, when Wyeth petitioned the FDA to essentially eliminate BHRT, more than 70,000 such women

---

* In recent years, many doctors have tried giving drugs, such as SSRIs ("selective serotonin re-uptake inhibitors" – Prozac®, Zoloft®, etc), to women with hot flushes under the assumption that these drugs are safer than conventional HRT. SSRIs are FDA-"approved" for treating anxiety and depression, but do they also work against symptoms of menopause? Perhaps in some women, but do they have anything to do with restoring normal hormonal balance? Absolutely not, nor do they provide any of the other long-term benefits of bio-identical hormone replacement. It is pure symptom suppression.

wrote to the FDA in protest (*See Chapter 12*). All the FDA and Wyeth and the rest of conventional patent medicine can argue is, "BHRT *might* be as dangerous as patented horse hormones and pseudoprogesterones, but we don't really know, because we've never tested it."

Maximizing the value of BHRT requires that doctors have a real appreciation of the way these hormones are metabolized and how much the body actually needs and can safely handle at any one time. Using too little may yield unsatisfactory results, while using too much may carry unacceptable risks. In this regard, what often gets lost in the translation from conventional HRT to BHRT is any serious attention to the dose, timing, route of administration, and metabolic processing of the replacement hormones.

If BHRT has any disadvantages, it is that it asks women to do more than just pop a pill every morning. It also requires doctors to monitor their patients' doses and hormone levels, and to make sure those hormones are safely metabolized. (*What good is giving a bio-identical estrogen such as estradiol – a procarcinogenic estrogen itself – if too much of it gets metabolized to other carcinogenic estrogens, such as estrone, 16a-hydroxyestrone or the stongly carcinogenic 4-hydroxyestrone, and/or not enough of it is metabolized into "balancing" anticarcinogenic estrogens, such as estriol, 2-hydroxyestrone, or that most potent anticarcinogenic estrogen, 2-methoxyestradiol?*)

More than 25 years of experience with BHRT have taught us that close attention to these and other factors is essential if women are to achieve the highest degrees of safety and effectiveness from BHRT. As we shall see in this chapter, proper use of BHRT demands:

- The correct mix of human bio-identical hormones.

- The optimal amount of each hormone.

- Taking hormones by the safest, most natural route.

- Approximating the natural timing of hormone secretion.

- Close monitoring of the levels of hormones and their metabolites for safety.

How Much Estrogen Is Too Much?

As we discussed in Chapter 7, more and more doctors and researchers are coming to the realization that a woman's risk of developing an estrogen-related cancer is directly related to the dose and type of replacement estrogen she uses, the way her body handles (metabolizes) those estrogens, and the balance between pro- and anticancer metabolites that ultimately results. These factors may be at least partially inborn, and every woman's body is unique in this way.[2] Nevertheless, any risks are usually manageable.

Unfortunately, women – and their doctors – who *think* they are using BHRT by limiting their estrogen replacement to high doses of bio-identical but procarcinogenic estradiol and ignoring the use of anticarcinogenic estriol or progesterone, are failing to restore a *natural* female hormonal environment and may possibly be increasing their risk of dangerous side effects, including cancer. While Suzanne Somers has brought an enormous amount of public attention to BHRT (*Thank you very much, Suzanne!*) the use of 1 milligram or more of estradiol daily (without estriol, as described in *The Sexy Years* in 2004) may have put her at unnecessary risk. But after we discussed estriol for her 2008 book *Breakthrough,* I suspect she may be balancing her estradiol with estriol now. Most women can achieve the same effects with considerably smaller quantities of estradiol along with estriol, which offsets the carcinogenic tendencies of estradiol (and in some cases estrone, which the body naturally forms from estradiol).

100% Bio-Identical Estradiol Products Are Risky

A 1994 study[3] showed what happens when doctors opt for "estrogen replacement" using estradiol alone, treating it like a patent medicine and paying little or no attention to women's natural hormone levels. In this study, 26 women, who had had "surgically induced menopause" (surgical removal of the ovaries) took a single, standard, FDA-"approved" 2-millgram dose of oral estradiol. Over the next 24 hours, the researchers periodically measured the women's serum levels of estradiol (serum = the liquid portion of blood, minus all the red and white blood cells, etc). They found these levels to be "excessively high" in 57% of the women. Based on their results, they cautioned, "…monitoring estradiol levels and ***individualizing estrogen replacement therapy***, to avoid the long-term exposure of postmenopausal patients to superphysiological estradiol levels."

Yet more than 14 years later, replacing estrogen with pills or topical creams/gels that provide 100% estradiol at doses of 1 or 2 milligrams per day has become increasingly popular, especially in the wake of the WHI study. Proprietary 100% estradiol products are often promoted as an FDA-"approved" bio-identical alternative to HRT, despite the fact that this practice flies in the face of research showing them to be far from bio-identical in their effects. Use of 100% estradiol products at these doses can lead to levels of estradiol and estrone in the body that are *5- to 10-fold above normal*, without adequate levels of estriol to buffer them and thus protect uterus and breast tissue against potentially carcinogenic overstimulation.

Premarin® and the Incredibly Shrinking Dose

Excessively high doses have always been an important part of the Premarin® story. In the early days of estrogen replacement therapy (ERT), before the protective value of progestins was realized, the most commonly recommended dose of Premarin® was 1.25 milligrams per day. Most of that 1.25 milligrams consisted of the potentially carcinogenic human estrogen estrone; the potent horse estrogen, equilin (which the body metabolizes to the highly carcinogenic 4-hydroxyequilin); a small amount of estradiol; and at least 10 other potent horse estrogens that have no natural, built-in metabolic pathways in the human body and consequently, no business being there. The increases in cancer and heart disease risk associated with this dose of Premarin® have been well-documented.

Why was this original dose chosen? Certainly not because it could reproduce a close-to-natural hormonal milieu in women's bodies; the "natural" levels of unique-to-horse estrogens in the human body are, of course, *zero*. Rather, the dose was based – like that of every other patented drug – on an "educated guesstimate" of the balance between benefits (eg, fewer hot flushes) and risks (eg, more physical discomforts, breast and endometrial cancer); not a very good estimate, at that, it turned out, especially in the absence of any "opposing" progesterone (or patented progestin drugs) during the earliest days of ERT.

With the cancer risk looming, the FDA decreed in 1988 that henceforth, the "approved" dose of Premarin® (+ Provera®) would be cut in half; women *really needed* only 0.625 milligrams of horse estrogens per day, anyway they said. Then, in 2003, after the Women's Health Initiative (WHI) showed that, even at this dose, Prempro® was still causing cancer and heart disease at an unacceptable rate, the FDA, in consultation with Wyeth Pharmaceuticals (the manufacturer of Premarin® and Provera®), decided that the dose of Premarin® (+ Provera®) should be halved again, to 0.3 milligrams per day – one quarter of the original dose.

How did they know these new lower doses would be safer? No clinical trials or testing were ever done! Basically because it *seemed like they ought to be safer,* even though they could cite no reliable clinical trial data to support any claim that the new lower Premarin® dose was significantly safer than the 0.625-milligram or 1.25-milligram doses. It wouldn't surprise us in the least if in 5 or so years hence, they would conclude that the dose should be halved again – or better yet, that the dangerous horse estrogens be finally banned.

Determining a Safe Dose of Estrogen

Using bio-identical estrogens makes it a lot easier to determine what the correct dose should be, because it allows us to measure *meaningful* changes in the body's hormonal environment. We know what the natural premenopausal range of estrogen and progesterone levels should be, so we can easily devise dosage regimens that yield hormone levels that fall somewhere within that range.

It's a rather simple question: What dose of estradiol would reproduce a natural level of estradiol (and other estrogens) in the average woman's body?

Researchers at the Tahoma Clinic and Meridian Valley Labs (both in Renton, Washington) decided to find out by testing 35 postmenopausal women (15 of whom had had hysterectomies), who had been taking varying doses of *oral* estradiol for up to a year.[4] (Oral dosing is generally a bad idea that's still favored by some mostly "mainstream" physicians). In this study, the women (aged 43 - 80) took estradiol pills at doses ranging from 0.025 to 2 milligrams per day. Throughout the year, their levels of estrone, estradiol, and estriol were measured periodically via urine samples collected over a 24-hour period. (*See below for more about the importance of 24-hour urine testing.*)

The results showed that the women's estradiol levels rose in direct proportion to the dose of oral estradiol they had been taking. The more hormone they took in, the more they excreted; no big surprise here.

The most important findings are shown in Figures 9-1 and 9-2. The dotted horizontal line in each graph represents the *highest levels* of estradiol or estrone, respectively, that are typically found in 24-hour urine samples

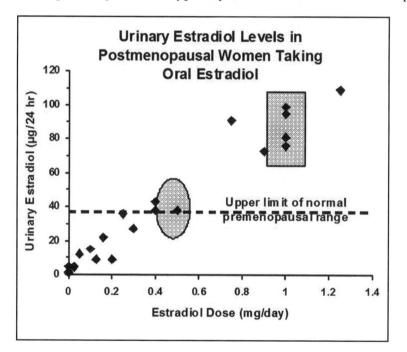

Figure 9-1. 24-hour urinary levels of estradiol rise in direct proportion to the increase in the oral dose of estradiol. Any levels above the dotted line (representing the upper range of "normal" urinary estradiol levels) are deemed above normal and may increase the risk of cancer and other serious adverse effects. These data indicate that the FDA-approved dose of estradiol (1 mg per day) can result in excessively high urinary levels of estradiol (rectangle). The estradiol dosage that reproduces normal urinary estradiol levels is about 0.5 mg per day (oval). (µg = micrograms; mg = milligrams)

Adapted from Freil, Hinchcliffe, & Wright, 2005

taken from normal, nonpregnant, premenopausal women. (This level is known as the "upper limit of normal."). For both hormones, the upper limit of normal was about 40 micrograms. In other words, 24 hours' worth of urine in normal, nonpregnant, premenopausal women should contain no more than 40 micrograms each of estradiol and estrone. Because

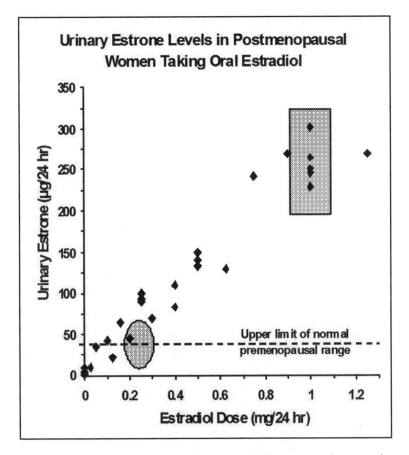

Figure 9-2. 24-hour urinary levels of estrone rise in direct proportion to an increase in the oral dose of estradiol. Any points above the dotted line (representing the upper range of "normal" 24-hour urinary estrone levels) are above normal and may increase the risk of cancer, especially of the breast. These data indicate that the FDA-approved dose of estradiol (1 mg per day) can produce excessively high urinary estrone levels (rectangle), while the estradiol dosage that results in approximately normal levels appears to be about 0.25 mg per day or lower (oval). (μg = micrograms; mg = milligrams)

Adapted from Freil, Hinchcliffe, & Wright, 2005

excessive amounts of estradiol and estrone are potentially carcinogenic, women who have 24-hour urinary levels of these hormones above the 40-microgram line may be at increased risk for breast cancer.

A close look at Figure 9-1 reveals that urinary levels of estradiol close to the upper limit of normal occurred when the women took oral estradiol at doses between 0.2 and 0.5 milligrams. At the FDA-recommended daily dose of 1 milligram, urinary estradiol levels rose to about 70 to 100 micrograms – *2- to 3-fold higher than the normal level.*

With estrone the picture only gets worse. Recall that estradiol and estrone have a harmonic relationship, whereby estradiol readily converts to estrone, which acts as a kind of storage depot for estradiol. As estradiol gets used up and levels drop, some of that stored estrone gets converted back to estradiol to make up the deficit. This action is especially prominent in postmenopausal women. Recall also that, although estrone is less potent than estradiol, high estrone levels are believed to be a particularly important factor in the development of breast cancer.[5]

Figure 9-2 shows what happened to 24-hour urinary estrone levels as the daily dose of oral estradiol increased in the Tahoma Clinic study. Thanks to the interconversion of estradiol and estrone, oral doses of estradiol led to estrone levels that were actually higher than estradiol levels. While estradiol doses as high as 0.5 milligrams per day produced safe levels of estradiol, this same dose produced estrone levels that were about 3 times higher. In other words, the 1-milligram *FDA-"approved"* dose of estradiol resulted in estrone levels *4 to 6 times above safe, normal levels.* Thus, a safe dose of oral estradiol turns out to be about 0.25 milligrams (or 250 micrograms) per day – about 4 times lower than the FDA-"approved" level found in commercial "drugstore" varieties, the kind touted as FDA-"approved" BHRT.

Lest some readers doubt the validity of the findings from our small Tahoma Clinic/Meridian Valley Labs trial, these results have been essentially replicated in a large, controlled study conducted by the patent medicine company Novo Nordisk in support of its product Activella®, a pill that combines 1 milligram of estradiol with the patented progestin norethindrone acetate.[6] As shown in Figure 9-3, a single dose of Activella® resulted in essentially normal *serum* estradiol levels, but it also produced a prolonged elevation of estrone levels over 24 hours.* By comparison, a study using a sensitive assay of hormone levels in *normal, nonpregnant, premenopausal women* found serum estrone levels ranging from 62 to 123 picograms per milliliter, depending on the phase of the menstrual cycle (horizontal broken line in Fig. 9-3). Thus, the recommended oral dose of Activella® produced serum levels of estrone that were about *5 times higher* than safe, normal levels.

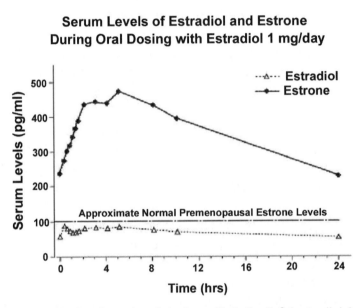

Serum Levels of Estradiol and Estrone During Oral Dosing with Estradiol 1 mg/day

Figure 9-3. Following 2 weeks of dosing with Activella® (estradiol 1 mg + norethindrone), serum levels of *estrone* rose to peak levels 5 times higher than normal premenopausal levels. These results also indicate that most of the ingested estradiol is quickly converted to estrone.

Adapted from Activella ® Prescribing Information, 2006

OK, It's Safe but Does It Work?

Estradiol dose levels of 0.25 milligrams per day may be safe, but are they sufficient to deliver any clinical benefits? (*Given that Mother Nature built in these hormone levels, this may seem like a silly question, but please bear with us, because BHRT critics sometimes question whether bio-identical hormones even work!*) In fact, the basic Tri-Est

---

* The reason these results were measured in picograms per milliliter and those in the Tahoma Clinic study in micrograms per milliliter is that these levels were measured in *serum samples* rather than *24-hour urine samples*. (1 microgram = 1 million picograms) Because urine is collected over 24 hours, it contains far more of the hormone than a single milliliter of blood.

(or Bi-Est) prescriptions that I and thousands of other doctors write each month include 0.25 milligrams of estradiol, and we find that it (along with appropriate quantities of estriol and estrone) is usually sufficient to restore a close-to-natural hormonal environment that eliminates menopausal symptoms without increasing the risks of cancer, heart disease, or any other serious concerns. (*However, please note that, for the reasons explained below, all the prescriptions I write are for the topical – "transdermal" or "transmucosal" – formulations, **not for oral dosing**, as were used in these early studies (see below for explanation). Follow-up observations and hormone-level testing have shown that a topical estrogen combination that includes an estradiol dose of 0.25 milligrams is safe and effective for the large majority of women.*)

Our observations on dose have been confirmed by a recent study at the University of Connecticut Health Center. These investigators compared the effects on bone mineral density (BMD) of 3 years of *oral* estradiol treatment (0.25 milligrams per day) vs. placebo in 167 women, aged 65 or older. The women taking what the investigators considered a "low-dose" of estradiol had significantly higher BMD in their hip, spine, wrist, and total body than did women taking a placebo. The side effects were the same in the estradiol group as they were in the placebo group, ie, none.[7]

To summarize these important findings, oral estradiol at doses greater than 0.25 milligrams per day produces excessively high urinary levels of estrone, which could indicate an increased risk for breast cancer. It seems clear that, in order to minimize the risk of estrogen-related breast cancer, the highest dose of oral estradiol women should normally be taking is 0.25 milligrams per day.

Reminder: The widely recommended, commercially available, FDA-"approved" dose of oral estradiol – considered by some to be an FDA-"approved" version of BHRT – is 1 to 2 milligrams per day – which results in circulating estradiol and estrone levels *4 to 8 times higher* than the upper limit of normal (safe natural level).

Such high levels of estrone and estradiol *might* be more acceptable if they were combined with higher levels of estriol in these women's bodies, because, as confirmed by a host of studies, estriol modulates the carcinogenic impact of the other two estrogens.[8, 9] Thus, raising a woman's levels of estradiol and/or estrone without also raising her estriol levels may set her on the road to breast cancer.

Even though estriol has long been viewed by conventional medicine as a "weak estrogen" or a "waste product" of estrogen metabolism that is important only during pregnancy (much as DHEA – the most common steroid hormone in the body – was also considered, until relatively recently, an "unimportant steroid"), we conclude that Mother Nature must have a "purpose" for the presence of relatively large proportions of estriol, even in healthy, nonpregnant women.

It is for these reasons that Tri-Est and Bi-Est formulations always contain a relatively high dose of estriol (2.0-2.25 milligrams) and very small doses of the carcinogenic estrogens, estradiol (0.25 milligrams) and sometimes estrone (0.25 milligrams). The experience of hundreds of thousands of women using these or similar doses over more than 25 years confirms that they can achieve the same beneficial effects as those taking excessively high doses of FDA-approved estradiol products by closely replicating the natural hormonal environment but with far lower risks of breast cancer or other serious adverse effects.

What's the Best Way to Take Bio-Identical Hormones?

You can take bio-identical hormones via one of several routes:

- *Creams or gels.* You can rub hormone-containing creams or gels into your skin (*transdermal*), or preferably your vaginal mucosa or the inner surfaces of your labia (*transmucosal or transvaginal*). Based on more than 25 years of personal experience at the Tahoma Clinic, we have found these *topical* methods (especially *transmucosal/transvaginal*) to be the preferred ways of using bio-identical hormones, especially if they are personally formulated by a compounding pharmacist.

- *Suppositories.* You insert the hormone, formed into a suppository by a compounding pharmacist, either into the vagina or the rectum for rapid *transmucosal* absorption.

- *Oral capsules.* Nothing unusual here (although I don't recommend it!). Like most patent medicines and nutritional supplements, just swallow the compounded bio-identical hormone put into capsules and the body does the rest, although as we shall see, not always for the best. Oral administration of steroid hormones has distinct disadvantages, because, as discussed below, it brings the gastrointestinal (GI) system and liver into play where they do not belong.

- *Lozenges (troches) and sublingual (under-the-tongue) drops.* You allow the hormone-containing lozenge or drop to dissolve in your mouth, *but try not to swallow,* so that a large portion of the hormones gets absorbed directly into your blood stream through the mucous membranes that line your mouth. Lozenges and sublingual drops are technically considered *transmucosal* methods, because they are designed to avoid having the hormones pass through the GI tract. The problem is that, due to normal saliva formation, it can be hard not to swallow, and usually 50% or more of the hormone winds up getting into your GI tract anyway. (I don't recommend these methods either.)

- *"Pellets" implanted under the skin.* Although this method avoids sending the hormones from the mouth to the stomach and intestines, the timing of hormone release by the pellets is nowhere close to Nature's pattern, which follows a monthly cycle of hormonal secretion, varying from very little for a few days to considerably more the rest of the month. Even when the anticarcinogenic estriol is used alone, animal research shows that "overriding" the normal cycle with daily use for a prolonged time can lead to higher cancer risk.

No matter what "route of administration" is chosen, it is essential that your doctor employ follow-up testing – as described later in this chapter – to confirm that the hormones are being properly absorbed and that your levels are within optimal ranges.

How you take your bio-identical hormones may seem at first to be largely a matter of convenience or personal preference. On the contrary, though, the route of administration can make a huge difference in how well the hormones work, how safe they are, and how good you feel while using them. By virtually every measure, topical application beats out oral administration every time.

Patent medicine companies, usually more interested in marketing and profits than safety and efficacy, almost always try to formulate their drugs as pills or capsules to be swallowed. There are lots of reasons for this practice, hardly any of which have anything to do with how well the drugs work or how safe they may be.

Drugs formulated for oral administration are generally easier to package, easier to market, easier for the pharmacist to deliver to the customer, and easier for the individual to use: We all know how it goes: "Take 1 tablet 3 times a day." *The bottom line:* making hormones *easier* to use ultimately translates into making them *more profitable,* but does not necessarily make them better or safer, quite the opposite.

Oral administration works reasonably well for some patented medicines and nutritional supplements, but with sex steroids, oral administration can seriously detract from their optimal use. In fact, oral administration of steroid hormones is Exhibit A when it comes to demonstrating how profitability trumps safety and efficacy. To prove our point that taking sex steroids by mouth may not be the best idea, all we have to do is look again at the way the human body is designed.

Running the GI-Liver Gauntlet

Now, if Mother Nature had only thought to locate the ovaries in the stomach or somewhere else within the GI tract, it might make sense for women to take their hormone replacements by mouth. With ovaries inside the GI tract, the body would certainly have evolved a way to process them safely and efficiently so that everything worked out the way it was supposed to.

Of course, the ovaries are not inside the GI tract; they're located in the pelvic region of the lower abdomen, *outside the GI tract*, and connected to the uterus and vagina via the fallopian tubes. (*See Fig. 3-1, page 53.*) In this location, the ovaries have direct access to the circulatory system via a *pelvic plexus of veins*, which delivers their hormone secretions directly to the heart, which in turn pumps them – unchanged – to estrogen-, progesterone-, and testosterone-sensitive cells all over the body.

Taking most steroid hormones by mouth badly distorts their natural metabolism. Whenever we ingest something, whether food, medications, or hormones, it must first run a gauntlet of potent stomach acid and destructive digestive enzymes. Should it survive this, those portions absorbed by the small intestine flow directly to the liver, where they undergo a process called "first pass metabolism."

The liver acts like a physiologic "customs service," screening all molecules that enter the bloodstream, passing some onward, modifying or detoxifying others, and rejecting a few. Only after they have been processed by the liver are *oral* replacement hormones released into the general circulation. It turns out that the liver is very efficient at metabolizing – and often neutralizing – steroid hormones, so that very little of a swallowed dose actually makes it into the bloodstream in its original form.

This "routing" of hormones through the liver is in sharp contrast to the way Mother Nature intended them to be "routed": first secreted directly into the bloodstream, next to the heart, and then – *still in their original, unchanged form* – to every steroid-using cell in the body. Only after that do natural or bio-identical steroid hormones pass through the liver – on *"secondary pass" metabolism* – where a large proportion is neutralized and excreted from the body, thus keeping the hormones at normal – and safe – levels.

When "alien" molecules – those not created in Nature but in a horse's ovaries or in some company's research labs – are swallowed and go through first-pass metabolism, the liver – lacking any inborn enzymes to work on the aliens – does the best it can with them. Sometimes, though, things can go dangerously awry, leading to the formation of toxic or otherwise destructive metabolites. For example, when women take oral Premarin®, the liver converts the already quite potent horse estrogens into even more potent metabolites. As noted earlier, one metabolite of equilin formed in the liver is *8 times more potent* than equilin itself, which itself is far more potent, and therefore potentially more carcinogenic, than any combination of ovarian or bio-identical estradiol, estrone, and estriol.[10]

Like their counterparts secreted by the ovaries, bio-identical steroid hormones were never intended to withstand the rigors of first-pass metabolism. Although they can be taken by mouth, very high doses are typically required, and their metabolism differs significantly from topically applied versions. For example, although the liver has no trouble metabolizing bio-identical estradiol, Mother Nature designed the liver to handle only the small amounts of the hormone that normally pass through during secondary-pass metabolism. If you take the high doses of estradiol usually prescribed for *oral* administration, you can push your liver to its metabolic limits during first-pass metabolism.

Even though first-pass metabolism of oral estradiol does not produce any overtly toxic metabolites (as it does with Premarin®), the liver rapidly and extensively transforms most of an oral estradiol dose into estrone, which then circulates in the blood stream, serving as an inert reservoir for continuous re-supply of estradiol. Circulating estrone – which has been linked to increased risk of breast cancer – can remain at excessively high levels for more than 12 hours after dosing, and only slowly decline over time. (See Figs. 9-1, 9-2, and 9-3.)[1, 10]

In addition, FDA-"approved" oral doses of estradiol (1-2 milligrams) can cause the liver to produce dangerously high levels of substances, such as C-reactive protein and blood clotting factors, which increase the risks of heart attacks, strokes, and deep vein thromboses (blood clots). By contrast, topical estrogens have no such effects. (*See below for more about these important differences between oral and topical dosing.*)

If you take progesterone by mouth, liver enzymes break it down into more than 30 different metabolites, but very little of the original progesterone, which is what your body really needs, actually ever makes it into the bloodstream.[1]

Researchers have found that by formulating the progesterone into extremely small particles – a process known as *micronization* – it's possible to increase the quantity of progesterone that makes it through first-pass metabolism unscathed. Nevertheless, in order for you to achieve close-to-normal physiologic effects from orally dosed progesterone, you still need to take *extra-high doses* of micronized progesterone. Such doses are usually considered safe, although they can cause certain side effects, especially sleepiness.

Topical Dosing: Do Not Pass the Liver, Do Not Collect Unwanted Metabolites!

If we want to copy Nature and reproduce a hormonal environment that most closely resembles that of the normal, premenopausal woman, the first step has to be transporting the replacement hormones into the bloodstream. The ovaries easily accomplish this because they have direct access to the circulatory system. In fact, it is a defining characteristic of all endocrine glands (eg, ovaries, testes, adrenals, pituitary, thyroid, pancreas) that *they secrete their hormones directly into the bloodstream.*

Viewed from this perspective, taking hormones by mouth is just about the most *unnatural* way imaginable for sex steroids to gain entry to the body. In fact, copying ovarian hormone secretion by delivering bio-identical hormones in physiologic doses directly into the bloodstream is a lot simpler than we might imagine.

Hormones, carefully measured and formulated in an appropriate cream or gel, need only be rubbed once or twice a day into the skin, or preferably, mucous (epithelial) membranes, especially those that line the labia or vagina. The hormones diffuse through the skin or epithelial tissue and pass easily *and directly* into the bloodstream. With no destructive detours through the GI tract and liver, bio-identical estrogens, progesterone, DHEA, and testosterone applied topically enter the blood stream *metabolically unchanged.* When you apply estrogen, progesterone, DHEA, and testosterone topically, it's estrogen, progesterone, DHEA, and testosterone that circulate through your blood stream, not some liver-produced metabolite of the hormone. Admittedly, this may take a little more effort than popping a pill in the morning, but the health advantages are substantial!

Why Topical Dosing Is So Much Better than Oral Dosing

Topical hormone replacement has been the standard in many places in Europe for more than 30 years,[11] and with good reason. By by-passing first-pass liver metabolism, topically applying hormones does more than just promote normal hormone metabolism; it also helps smooth out the wide fluctuations in plasma hormone levels that occur following oral administration.

Only topical application of replacement hormones comes close to replicating the natural slow and gradual pattern of hormone secretion by endocrine glands. By contrast, one of the many problems with oral hormone dosing is that by swallowing them, the entire dose tends to reach the bloodstream at around the same time, resulting in a sharp, *unnatural* "spike" in "hormone" concentrations.

One group of European researchers studied the serum levels of estradiol and estrone in a group of 32 healthy postmenopausal women; half the women took an estradiol oral pill daily for 3 weeks; the other half used an estradiol skin patch. Topical application resulted in relatively constant concentrations of estradiol and estrone that remained within the range normally encountered in women during the early follicular phase (first few days) of the menstrual cycle. By contrast, oral dosing led to large pulses of estradiol and estrone shortly after administration and average daily plasma concentrations that were *12 times* and *9.4 times higher*, respectively, than those typically seen following topical application.[12]

Normally, in premenopausal women, roughly equal amounts of estradiol and estrone circulate through the bloodstream, ie, the circulating ratio of the two estrogens is about 1:1. In postmenopausal women using hormone replacement, however, that ratio can vary widely, depending on the dose and type of "estrogen" and especially, on the route of administration. One investigator compared the relative serum levels of estradiol and estrone reported in four different studies in which postmenopausal women used transdermal estradiol, oral estradiol, or oral Premarin®.[11] In the women using **transdermal estradiol** (at doses ranging from 50 micrograms to 3 milligrams per day), the circulating estradiol:estrone ratios were as follows for each of the women (a-g):

a.   1:1.2
b.   1:1.3
c.   1:1.1
d.   1:0.8
e.   1:0.7
f.   1:1.5
g.   1:0.9

In other words, regardless of dose, following transdermal administration of estradiol, all circulating levels of estradiol and estrone remained very close to the 1:1 ratio of free estradiol and free estrone found during the menstrual cycles of normal premenopausal women.

However, when women took their estrogen *orally*, the estradiol:estrone ratios were abnormally high. For oral estradiol (2 milligrams per day), the ratio was 1:5 in one study and 1:6.7 in another. That means that estrone levels were 5 to 7 times higher than estradiol levels. In women taking oral Premarin® (0.625 milligrams per day), the ratio was 1:3.2; estrone levels were 3 times higher than estradiol levels. Thus, again we see that taking estradiol or horse estrogens by mouth yields excessively high levels of estrone, the estrogen most closely linked to breast cancer.

The high concentrations of circulating estrogens caused by the very high doses of estradiol or horse estrogens typically prescribed for oral administration have other unhealthy consequences, as well. For example, side effects, such as *breast tenderness, headache,* and *breakthrough bleeding*, all common signs of too much estrogen, are much more frequent after oral dosing compared with topical dosing.[13]

Cardiovascular Benefits of Topical Estrogen Dosing

Numerous studies have demonstrated that topical application of estrogens is more beneficial for your cardiovascular system than oral dosing. These benefits include:

- *Reduced plasma triglyceride levels*. Topical, but not oral, administration of estrogen reduces serum concentrations of triglyceride, a fatty substance related to cholesterol. Elevated triglycerides levels are an important risk factor for coronary heart disease.[14, 15]

- *Less LDL-cholesterol oxidation.* Both topical and oral estrogen administration can reduce the levels of low-density lipoprotein (LDL) cholesterol (the "bad" cholesterol). However, LDL *levels* are only part of the story. LDL becomes a much greater danger after it has been *oxidized.** *Ovarian* estrogen has natural *antioxidant* effects, which help protect LDL from oxidation. This may be one of the reasons premenopausal women have such a low risk of heart disease.[16-18] However, only topical administration of replacement estrogen preserves, or even improves, this valuable antioxidant effect in women after postmenopause. When you take estrogen orally, even bio-identical estrogens do not prevent LDL oxidation.†

- *Normalized blood coagulation and clotting.* Blood clotting, a perfectly normal and healthy reaction when we have a cut or scrape, can also occur inside blood vessels, and contribute to the formation of plaque and eventually a dangerous *thrombus* (blood clot) at sites of minor irritation or inflammation. If one of these thrombi should break loose, it can travel through the bloodstream until it blocks a small artery, possibly causing a heart attack or stroke.

To keep thrombus formation under control, women's bodies before menopause produce a variety of *anti-clotting* substances, *including estradiol*, another reason why premenopausal women are less likely to suffer coronary heart disease. After menopause, though, the route by which women take replacement estrogen makes a huge difference. *Topical* estradiol reduces the tendency of clots to form (*antithrombotic effect*), decreasing the risk of heart attacks and strokes. On the other hand, *oral* estrogens tend to be *prothrombotic,* increasing the risk of intravascular clot formation.[19-24]

---

* Oxidation refers to the interaction of a substance with oxygen. Among the best known examples of this extremely common chemical reaction are iron rusting and browning of apples exposed to air. Oxidation of LDL-cholesterol is an important step in the formation of atherogenic plaque that can lead to heart attacks and strokes.
† One reason is that not all LDL particles are created equal. Topical estrogen administration results in the formation of larger particles of LDL, which resist oxidation. By contrast, the LDL particles formed in the liver after taking oral estrogen are smaller and more subject to oxidation, thus increasing the risk of cardiovascular disease.

- **Lower levels of C-reactive protein.** C-reactive protein (CRP) has been identified as a sensitive sign of underlying inflammation and is now recognized as a direct promoter of the growth and progression of atherogenic plaques. This makes high levels of CRP an important independent risk factor for heart attacks, strokes, and related cardiovascular events – just like fatty diets, obesity, and smoking.[25-27]

When women take estrogen replacement (either estradiol or Premarin®) orally, their CRP levels rise sharply and remain elevated for an extended period, suggesting the hormone has triggered a potentially dangerous inflammatory process and possibly increasing their cardiovascular risks. At first, this finding seemed strange, because estrogen normally tends to exert *anti-inflammatory effects*.[25]

How could this be? The reason seems to lie in the hormone's first-pass through the liver, since CRP levels rise only after estrogen is metabolized in the liver. Elevated levels of CRP were noted in the WHI study after women took Premarin® by mouth, and where they were also associated with a *200% increase* in the risk of coronary heart disease.[28]

Since topically applied estrogens avoid first-pass metabolism in the liver and pass directly into the general body circulation, just as Mother Nature intended, it should come as no surprise that they do not cause an increase in CRP. Consequently, as research consistently shows, this is one more reason why *topical bio-identical estrogen does not increase the risk of cardiovascular disease*.[24, 25, 29]

- **Less risk of venous thromboembolism (VTE).** A VTE is a blood clot that forms in the large veins. When these clots form in the deep veins in the legs, thighs, or pelvis, the condition is known as *deep vein thrombosis*. VTEs are most common after surgery, during or right after pregnancy, and in other situations where the lower limbs may be immobilized for extended periods, such as travel in confined circumstances ("coach-class syndrome"). By obstructing blood flow through an affected vein, VTE causes swelling and pain. More seriously, if a part or all of a clot in a deep vein breaks off from its site of formation, it can travel through the venous system, which returns blood to the heart, and could come to lodge in an artery connecting the heart to the lungs, forming a potentially life-threatening *pulmonary embolism.*

Because estrogen taken orally readily activates abnormal blood coagulation and clotting, it increases the risk of VTE in postmenopausal women. In the WHI study, oral Premarin® doubled the risk of VTE compared with placebo.[30] A compilation of results from many randomized long-term trials of oral ERT taken by otherwise healthy postmenopausal women found that pulmonary emboli accounted for about one-third of the potentially fatal cardiovascular events.[31]

By contrast, *topically applied estrogen causes no increase in VTE risk.*[17] A French study compared the risk of VTE in postmenopausal women taking oral estrogen vs. transdermal estrogen. The VTE risk in the transdermal estrogen group was one-fourth as high as that in the oral estrogen group.[32]

- ***Reduced risk of insulin resistance and diabetes.*** Diabetes is one of the principal risk factors for coronary heart disease and strokes, as well as blindness, kidney failure, and other serious conditions. The most common form of diabetes is known as *type 2 diabetes.* In the better known type 1 diabetes, the pancreas stops producing the hormone insulin so that insulin replacement injections are required. In type 2 diabetes, insulin becomes increasingly less efficient at doing its primary job, controlling blood glucose levels. As a result, the pancreas produces excessive amounts of relatively ineffective insulin, especially in the disease's early stages. This is due largely to a defect in body cells' ability to respond to, or process, the insulin, a condition termed *increased insulin resistance* or *reduced insulin sensitivity.* Untreated, type 2 diabetes can lead to the same severe complications as type 1.

What does estrogen replacement have to do with diabetes in postmenopausal women? Again, it depends largely on how you take the estrogen. Taking estrogen orally, whether it's estradiol or Premarin®, increases insulin resistance, reducing blood sugar control, and consequently, elevating the risk of cardiovascular disease and other serious diabetes complications.

By contrast, topical administration of estrogen (usually estradiol in these studies, but BHRT should work equally well) has the exact opposite – and healthier – effects: *decreasing insulin resistance, improving blood sugar control*, and *decreasing the risk of cardiovascular disease* and other adverse consequences of diabetes.[15, 25, 33-41]

"Aye, There's the Rub!" Applying Topical Hormones for Maximum Benefit and Safety

Many knowledgeable doctors who prescribe BHRT write their prescriptions for transdermal (or percutaneous, ie, "through the skin,") preparations. They instruct their patients to measure out a small amount of the hormone cream or gel and rub it into areas of skin that tend to be relatively thin, like their inner wrists or thighs, usually on a monthly cyclic schedule.

While this procedure certainly yields better results than taking hormones by mouth, and it often works quite well, we have found that women can approach the hormone balance Mother Nature had in mind much more closely by applying the hormone creams to the mucous/epithelial membranes that line their labia and vagina. Not only is absorption through these membranes more complete than through the skin, but hormones absorbed through the vaginal membranes enter the very same pelvic plexus of veins that the ovaries drain into. From here, the hormones are carried to the heart and lungs and then distributed all over the body.

Intravaginal Dosing Avoids "Dermal Absorption Fatigue"

At the Tahoma Clinic, we monitor the 24-hour urinary hormone levels of women using BHRT at regular intervals to make certain their levels are within their individual physiologic "target range." Over several years, this monitoring has shown us that, in many women using transdermal estrogen preparations, urinary estrogen levels begin to decline progressively, suggesting that they are absorbing less and less estrogen through their skin as time goes by.

Sometimes these lower levels result in a return of symptoms (eg, hot flushes), but not always (particularly in women who have been using BHRT for longer periods). Nevertheless, the possibility remains that, even though they may still be symptom-free, they may not be getting enough estrogen to provide them with the cardiovascular, bone, cognitive, genitourinary, and other benefits normally afforded by long-term BHRT.

However, we have found that when we switch the route of administration from transdermal to transvaginal – without altering the dose – their urinary levels rise right back up to their target range, and any symptoms of low estrogen they might have been experiencing quickly disappear.

We have attributed this loss of effect of transdermal administration to a factor we term *"dermal absorption fatigue:"* repeated transdermal applications over many months seem to cause the skin to lose some of its ability to transport the hormones into the blood stream. Why this happens remains a mystery, but we know it happens, and we know that switching to intravaginal dosing avoids it or reverses it.

Improving Progesterone Absorption

Not only does transvaginal application prevent dermal absorption fatigue for estrogens, but it also facilitates progesterone absorption. We have long known that progesterone absorption through the skin is not very efficient. This has led some critics of BHRT to argue that topical progesterone administration is useless, and might even be dangerous, since progesterone might not be available to "oppose" the potentially carcinogenic effects of potent estrogens in the uterus. However, when progesterone cream is applied to the vaginal tissue, its rate of absorption is much higher, quite enough to elevate serum progesterone levels higher and keep them elevated longer, compared with oral administration. Vaginal administration also minimizes drowsiness, the primary side effect of excessive doses of oral progesterone.[1]

Because of all these factors, we now routinely recommend transvaginal administration as the best method for using BHRT.

How about "The Patch"?

Pharmaceutical companies, quietly recognizing the superiority of topical administration of bio-identical estrogens, have developed various estradiol (and estradiol + progestin) skin patches as a means of patenting the otherwise unpatentable. By embedding estradiol in a high-tech, patented patch, they have created a product that can "deliver" the bio-identical hormone topically at a steady rate for up to several days at a time. In addition to affording topical (albeit transdermal but not transvaginal) administration, patches have the apparent advantage of convenience – you need only apply them once every couple of days; no need to bother with rubbing in a cream once or twice a day. And because these products are patented and FDA-"approved," mainstream doctors tend to be more comfortable with them and are usually quite willing to prescribe them in place of oral Prempro® or genuine, but "unproven" BHRT– "unproven" except by their presence in human bodies for hundreds of thousands of years!

The Illusion of "Convenience"

While the companies market patches for their convenience, when you look closely, this convenience often turns out to be an illusion:

- Constant delivery of a steady amount of estradiol (or estradiol + a progestin), while a definite improvement over oral administration of Premarin® or estradiol + progestin, still does not reproduce the natural daily ebb and flow of sex steroids the body is used to.

- The only bio-identical estrogen available in a commercial patch is 100% estradiol. What about estriol? Does any patent medicine company make an estriol patch to counter the potentially carcinogenic effects of estradiol and the estrone which also forms? Do we really need to answer that question?

- Patches are limited to a few standard doses, but what if those doses are not suited to an individual's specific hormonal needs?

- Patches are notorious for causing local skin reactions, such as itching, rashes, eczema, blisters, and burning. In order to minimize these reactions, manufacturers urge users to place the patch in a different place each time. This may help for a while, but sooner or later, as many as half the women who use hormonal skin patches develop some sort of skin reaction.

Such skin reactions are virtually unheard of with creams or gels personally formulated by compounding pharmacists. In the rare case where a woman develops a reaction to a specific compounded formulation, it is a simple matter for the pharmacist to compound the next dose using a different, and more "friendly," cream or gel base. In addition, unlike patches, creams and gels can be compounded using *any dose of hormone* your doctor determines is ideal for your unique system.

In a study conducted in Finland, postmenopausal women were divided into two groups: 60 women in one group used a daily estradiol gel, while 60 women in the other group used a commercial estradiol patch (2 per week). After 12 months, 28 women (47%) in the patch group complained of skin irritation, compared with only 2 women (3%) using the estradiol gel.[42]

Despite the apparent "convenience" of oral pills and estrogen patch systems, research indicates that, given a choice, women overwhelmingly prefer topical gels or creams. In one study of more than 300 postmenopausal women, only 54% of those using oral HRT continued treatment for more than 1 year, compared with 79% of those using a transdermal formulation.[43]

In yet another study, 80 postmenopausal women used either an estradiol patch or a gel for 25 days, and then were switched to the opposite treatment for another 25 days. More than 90% of the women judged both methods convenient in terms of their visual aspects. However, the gel was rated as far superior in terms of skin problems and "discomfort during intimacy." Furthermore, 80% of the women found the gel to be "more feminine"; over all, 61% preferred the gel compared to 32% who preferred the patch; 100% of the women rated the gel "not annoying," but none of the women rated the patch as "not annoying."[44] So much for the "convenience" of skin patches!

Topical Dosing: How Much? How Often?

One of the key advantages of BHRT is that the doses of each hormone can be adjusted to suit each woman's unique needs. This is in contrast to pharmaceutical brand hormones – whether pills, creams/gels, or patches – which are usually limited to a small number of *"approved"* dosages (eg, estradiol creams, 1 or 2 milligrams per day), which may be 4- or 5-times too high for most women.

Estrogens: Getting the Ratio Right

When I first began prescribing BHRT in 1982 using the 80:10:10 ratio, the average overall estrogen daily *starting* dose was a total of 2.5 milligrams of these three estrogens combined, which worked quite well for hundreds of women. We emphasize *starting* dose, because all women are different, and often their dosage needs to be modified after comprehensive testing to produce the optimal results. Like most doctors, I prefer to stay on the conservative side when prescribing. All compounding pharmacies can formulate Tri-Est or Bi-Est in these (or any other) proportions.

Occasionally the routine prescription isn't strong enough, even at higher doses, so that perimenopausal or menopausal symptoms persist. When this happens, I first increase the total dose of the combined estrogens. If even this isn't helpful, I then increase the proportion of estradiol (the strongest estrogen) to 20 or 25%. In situations like these, your doctor can ask your compounding pharmacist to alter the proportions of each estrogen to best suit your individual needs. (Try doing that with Premarin® or a patented estradiol patch or cream!) In a small percentage of women, even increasing the quantity of BHRT repeatedly doesn't relieve symptoms. This situation (and its remedy) is discussed below.

Progesterone: Never Take Estrogen without It

As we've mentioned before, conventional medicine is wedded to the absurd belief that postmenopausal women, who've had their uterus surgically removed (hysterectomy), do not need to take progesterone (or a progestin), because there's no risk of the estrogen replacement causing endometrial cancer. As we've also pointed out, progesterone does a lot more important things in the body than just "oppose" the carcinogenic properties of estrogen in the uterus. Therefore, if any physician insists on prescribing any form of estrogen without also an adequate amount of progesterone – whether you still have a uterus or not – we recommend that you insist that he/she do some basic research (perhaps by reading this book!) or that you find yourself another, better informed doctor.

Quantities of topical progesterone can vary from 25 to 50 milligrams (after menopause) and up to 50 to 100 milligrams (during the menopausal transition), depending on each woman's age and response. Progesterone is typically started on days 10 to 15 of each simulated cycle and continued through day 25, as noted below.

While progesterone creams are easily available without a prescription in over-the-counter (OTC) form, accurate dosing may often be difficult with these preparations (although this situation appears to be slowly improving). To be certain, though, we recommend getting your progesterone from a compounding pharmacist. There's likely to be little difference in cost and a potentially big difference in quality of product and accuracy of dosing.

DHEA: Help Restore Testosterone Levels

DHEA (dehydroepiandrosterone) is an androgen secreted by the adrenal glands. Like testosterone, DHEA levels decline with age, so the large majority of women of menopausal age (and even some younger women) would do well to replace this hormone, too. It is my observation that DHEA replacement is essential for maintaining optimum immune function and for helping to reduce the risk of cancer.* Some women report that DHEA does more for libido than testosterone, usually thought to be the major libido-enhancer in both sexes.

A daily schedule is recommended when replacing DHEA, because the adrenals secrete DHEA daily (not cyclically, like estrogen and progesterone). Since women's bodies metabolize DHEA into testosterone, I sometimes delay testosterone replacement until tests show whether DHEA is restoring their testosterone levels to normal. A reasonable, conservative starting dose of DHEA for most women is 15 milligrams per day, although for a few women, follow-up testing may indicate that the daily dose needs to be raised to 30 milligrams.

---

*   DHEA inhibits the enzyme glucose-6-phosphate dehydrogenase (G6PD), which is very important in the process of "anaerobic glycolysis" – "burning" sugar for energy without oxygen – a major source of energy for cancers.

Like progesterone, OTC versions of DHEA are also available. However, these are nearly all oral capsules. Continuing clinical observation is persuading me that the transdermal or transmucosal route is best for *all steroid hormones,* including DHEA. As with the other hormones, I write prescriptions for topical DHEA, because I have a greater trust in the standard material available through compounding pharmacists.

Testosterone: Women Need It, too, but at Much Lower Doses

If testing shows that a woman's DHEA is not getting metabolized to produce sufficient testosterone, she can also take testosterone (at an average dose of 2.5 to 5 milligrams daily). It's very important to remember that women require a fraction of the testosterone that men do. Thus, patented products containing bio-identical testosterone – patches or gels – designed for men are completely inappropriate – and dangerous – for women. The only option for women at the present time is testosterone formulated by a compounding pharmacist.

A woman's body will metabolize most testosterone into estrogens, so follow-up testing is mandatory to be sure that levels of both hormones are "just right" – neither too high nor too low.

As is the case with bio-identical estrogens vs. patent medicine "estrogens," bio-identical testosterone (in the right amounts at the right time) is safe, whereas patented "testosterones," sometimes called *anabolic steroids*, can be extremely dangerous and are sometimes even illegal. The only FDA-"approved" "testosterone" medication given to women is an anabolic steroid patent medicine called *methyltestosterone.* As discussed in Chapter 5, this "alien molecule," which is combined with a patented "estrogen" in the drug *Estratest*®, can have severe side effects, especially in the liver. Needless to say, this very dangerous patent medicine has no place in hormone replacement therapy, or any other human therapy of any kind.

---

* Methyltestosterone was patented in the past, but since the patent ran out years ago, numerous generic commercial versions are available.

Timing Hormone Replacement According to Nature's Clock

Women who use conventional HRT are given all sorts of misinformation about the "hormones" they are taking, including *when* to take them. Here are a few examples I've heard over the years:

- "My doctor told me to take Premarin® and Provera® on weekdays and not on weekends."

- "I just take Premarin® every day, no pauses."
- "I've used the 'estrogen patch' every few days for the last year or more."

- "My doctor says my uterus is gone [surgically removed], so cycling hormones isn't important any more."

We all know that Nature works in cycles. Ovaries don't secrete estrogens, progesterone, and testosterone on weekdays, but take weekends off; nor do they secrete hormones continuously for months or years without ever pausing.

Every woman knows her sex hormones come and go in cycles, because those cycles drove her monthly periods during her reproductive years, and when her regular hormone secretion went awry, she likely felt "different." Even doctors are taught about hormone cycling in medical school, although many seem to forget how important this is when it comes time to prescribe hormone replacement therapy for their menopausal patients. One fact that often gets ignored is that your sex hormones are not only *secreted* by the ovaries in a cyclic pattern, they are also *received* by your body's hormone receptors in the same cyclic pattern. After 40 years of receiving hormones in the same cycle, it is likely that these hormone receptors have become attuned to this pattern. Cells with estrogen receptors all over the body come to "*expect*" to be stimulated by a certain amount of estrogen at a predictable time for a predictable duration. The same is true for progesterone, testosterone, and others.

When this hormone receptor timing pattern is disrupted, especially over an extended period, it's quite likely something will go wrong, or at the very least, not function as well as it should. If you feel "funny" or "uncomfortable" when your estrogen cycle is "off," it's only indirectly because your ovaries are "out of whack"; it's really because estrogen receptors everywhere, from your uterus to your blood vessels to your brain, are missing their expected hormonal "fix." By replacing hormones in a way that closely approximates your lifelong natural cycle, your receptors receive their hormones on a schedule close to the one they've become accustomed to.

Surprisingly, there's been very little research on optimal hormonal timing, especially from the point of view of the hormone receptors. We might imagine that if the patent medicine companies can sell patented "estrogens" to millions of women for years at a time, they might fund a few studies to determine the best timing of these "hormones."

But since this hasn't happened – nor is it likely to happen – it's best to fall back on Mother Nature's schedule. Figure 9-5 shows the dosing pattern I usually recommend starting out with for the average woman, who had a "typical" 26 to 30 day cycle during her menstruating years. Remember, this is not my plan; it's the one designed by Mother Nature.

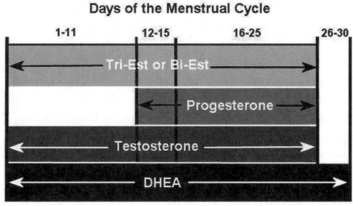

Basic BHRT Schedule
Days of the Menstrual Cycle

Figure 9-5. Schematic of a basic "start-up" BHRT schedule. The timing of the various hormones may have to be modified to suit individual women's needs.

As you read in Chapter 3, the ovaries secrete estrogen beginning on Day 1 of each menstrual cycle and continue secreting it until around Day 25. The ovaries – via the corpus luteum – produce the most progesterone around mid-cycle, at which time ovulation occurs. Like estradiol, ovarian progesterone secretion also ceases around Day 25. Days 26 through 30 – during which menstruation occurs – are largely hormone free (except for DHEA), which allows the respective hormone receptors to have their accustomed "rest," after which the cycle starts all over again.

When a woman starts on BHRT, we try to mimic as closely as possible the timing of the full menstrual cycles she experienced during her earlier years. Of course, as every woman knows, "period" length varies from one woman to another; for some the typical period may be 26 days, for others 32. We ask her to think back to her early 30s, when her periods were still regular, and tell us approximately how long they were. We then use that number of days as a starting point to modify the schedule shown in Figure 9-5. However, many women find it simpler and more practical to work with a "regular" *average* 30-day calendar.

Since she is no longer menstruating, the date she chooses to start her BHRT cycle is arbitrary. Her job is to keep track of the days she starts and stops each hormone. She can do this by crossing off days on a calendar or any other method she might find convenient. The exact pattern should always be specified by the pharmacist right on the prescription.

While estrogen cycling is pretty straightforward, the pattern for progesterone can be a bit more complicated. This is because progesterone's functions (despite what conventional medicine preaches) go beyond merely "opposing" estrogen activities. In addition to its role in the menstrual cycle, the body uses some progesterone as the basis for making a whole other class of steroids that include *cortisone, aldosterone,* and many others. So when progesterone production drops, so does the production of these other important hormones.

Although our basic schedule calls for adding progesterone midway through the "cycle," some women find they feel much better with continuous progesterone. For these women, we have found that we can modify their regimen by adding a small amount of progesterone (eg, 10-20 milligrams per day), depending on whether she is having a "bleeding cycle" or not. The highest daily dose of progesterone – about 25 to 50 milligrams – should be used during the "luteal phase" (Days 12-25 in Fig. 9-5). If she needs to use it the rest of the month, a "step-down" dose of about 10 milligrams per day should be adequate.

Fine Tuning Hormone Dosing

Variable Dosing

Some physicians recommend, and some women prefer, copying Nature even more closely by varying the amounts of estrogens, progesterone, and testosterone on a day-to-day basis throughout the month to more closely approximate the variations seen in a normal premenstrual woman's menstrual cycle. Although one prominent advocate of this position recommends doses so high they routinely exceed the amounts found even in premenstrual women's bodies (which I cannot recommend), another has a more reasonable "physiologic-dose" approach. If you are interested in the variable-dose approach, see *Menopause and Natural Hormones* by Daved Rosensweet, MD (Life Medicine and Healing P.A., 2002).

Filling the Gap

Let us re-emphasize, these guidelines are merely a starting point; they may work well for some women, but others may need fine tuning. For example, if hot flushes, sweating, or other menopausal symptoms occur during the 3 to 5-day "rest" period between cycles, many women benefit by taking a half-dose of Tri-Est or Bi-Est each day during that interval. If that is not sufficient to eliminate the symptoms, they can try a full dose, but it's likely best not to do that for a prolonged period of time.

Splitting the Dose

For most women, a single daily application of bio-identical hormones is sufficient. However, because the half-life of these hormones (ie, the rate at which the body metabolizes them) is relatively short, some women find that they get more satisfactory results by splitting the daily dose in two (eg, take half in the morning and half in the evening). If you apply hormones in the morning, but begin to feel symptoms later in the day, splitting the dose in two should solve this problem.

Avoiding Possible Side Effects

Most side effects associated with bio-identical hormones are a result of too high a dose, ie, excess hormonal activity. Reducing the dose almost always eliminates them. Here are the most common side effects that are associated with sex steroids:

Estrogen	Headache
	Breast tenderness
	Bleeding
Progesterone	Drowsiness
Testosterone or DHEA	Acne
	Body or facial hair growth
	Voice change (deepening)
	Aggression

Should you experience any of these or other side effects, please work with your doctor to modify your dosing regimen until they disappear.

Overcoming "Treatment Failure" with Low-Dose Cobalt Supplements

Doctors who've prescribed bio-identical hormones for menopausal or postmenopausal women for any period have experienced "treatment failures" or "nonresponders" in a small percentage of patients. Despite carefully escalating doses of bio-identical estrogens (and other accompanying steroids), the women still experience hot flushes and other symptoms.

In most cases, we've found that these treatment failures occur in women who have previously taken Premarin® or other non-bio-identical "hormone" replacements. In frustration, many of these women may want to return to Premarin®, since "at least it took care of my symptoms."

Over the years, it became obvious to us that nearly all BHRT "nonresponders" had a common "biochemical signature": When taking an "average treatment dose" of bio-identical estrogens, women prone to "treatment failure" tended to *hyperexcrete* estrogens. In other words, compared to women who responded normally to the same dose, these women were metabolizing estrogen at a very rapid rate and excreting most of it in their urine before it could exert its beneficial estrogenic effects.

Since estrogens are metabolized and "detoxified" by certain enzymes in the liver (during *second pass* metabolism), we hypothesized that in nonresponding women, these liver enzymes might have become "hyperactive" or "up-regulated." If they could be "down-regulated," estrogen metabolism might return to normal. A number of minerals are known to affect the function of these enzymes. Among these, **cobalt** had been shown to be safe and effective for "down-regulating" the overactive enzymes,[45] which should put the brakes on estrogen metabolism.

Sure enough, we found that daily *microdoses* of *cobalt chloride* are usually quite effective in arresting estrogen hyperexcretion and restoring the efficacy of BHRT. Although many women need only about 500 micrograms of cobalt chloride per day to "reset" their estrogen metabolism and help normalize their menopausal symptoms, some have occasionally needed up to 1,000 micrograms. (These doses of cobalt are quite harmless and are no greater than those found in the daily diets in some areas of the world.) In nearly all cases, cobalt supplementation can be discontinued without need for resumption once 24-hour urine tests show that estrogen metabolism has returned to normal, which usually takes about 10 to 20 weeks.

Tri-Est or Bi-Est?

As we've mentioned in passing, instead of Tri-Est, some natural medicine practitioners prefer to leave out the estrone component, due to its reputation for causing breast cancer, and to recommend a combination of estriol (80%) and estradiol (20%), commonly called "Bi-Est." I also follow this practice when follow-up testing of women taking Tri-Est indicates an apparent excess of estrone.

Following the venerable *"observe-and-copy-Nature"* principle, my starting recommendation remains: use two or three principal estrogens, always balanced in "anticarcinogenic" proportions and then *always* test and monitor hormone levels in the interests of safety. Actually, this is only one safety observation to be made after starting BHRT. Others are discussed below.

Are Monthly Menstrual Periods Necessary? Is There Really a Need to Bleed?

An important principle of natural medicine is to *prescribe the least amount of a substance necessary to do the job*. Following this principle, many practitioners of natural medicine (including myself) recommend sufficient hormones to eliminate menopausal symptoms and to provide protection against osteoporosis, heart and blood vessel disease, senile dementia, and Alzheimer's disease, but *not enough to induce a monthly menstrual period*.

On the other hand, some "experts" in BHRT advocate taking excessively high doses of estradiol (1-2 milligrams per day), in order to induce a monthly "menstrual period" (with no ovulation, of course). They claim that this assures that the body is getting enough estrogen to provide its other benefits, that it is advantageous to "flush" the uterus on a regular basis, that it may also help women feel more "youthful," and that it might even prevent uterine cancer.

Despite the contention of these few self-proclaimed "experts," research has so far failed to support any health value of inducing a monthly period in postmenopausal women.[46] In fact, at least one study by a team of French and American researchers, using both endometrial biopsies and hysteroscopies ("scopes" that peer inside the uterus), failed to find any evidence of endometrial hyperplasia (the tissue overgrowth that could lead to cancer) during 5 years of treatment with bio-identical estradiol (with progesterone, of course). It didn't matter whether the doses were low – producing no bleeding – or high enough to induce artificial monthly "periods." Noting the importance of using a "relatively low dose" of progesterone with every cycle, they concluded, in part, "Induction of withdrawal bleeding and endometrial secretory transformation, which require larger doses of progesterone, *do not provide additional benefit for prevention of hyperplasia.*[46]

In our more than 25 years of experience at the Tahoma Clinic, we've found that most women, when provided with all the options, choose not continue to continue having menstrual periods into their 60s, 70s, 80s, and 90s. In fact, most are relieved to hear they can obtain the benefits of BHRT without monthly menstrual cycles. Since lower doses of hormone provide an optimal spectrum of benefits, usually without inducing menstruation, we don't see any advantage either.

As a general rule, unless you and your doctor are following the "enough-hormones-to-induce-periods-every-month-indefinitely" theory, if bleeding should occur while taking bio-identical hormones, it's best to check with your doctor. Typically, bleeding is caused by too much estrogen, but paradoxically, for some women, the cause can be too little estrogen. If bleeding persists after dose adjustment, usually there is no problem, but rarely, it may indicate a precancerous or cancerous condition and should be checked.

Monitoring Hormone Levels for Safety

Hardly any doctors who prescribe non-BHRT "hormone" replacement bother to measure their patients' estrogen, progesterone, testosterone, or DHEA levels afterwards. How do they know their patients are getting appropriate quantities of hormone? It's simple: they don't!

Of course, if they're prescribing Premarin®, Provera®, or some other pseudohormone patent medicine, it's really pointless to measure "hormone" levels in the body anyway, because there are no *natural* levels of horse estrogens or progestins in the human body. It's no different than testing for the *natural* levels of any other patent medicine: there are no "natural" levels!

When it's estradiol they're prescribing – at the FDA-"approved" dose of 1 or 2 milligrams per day – if they did bother to measure estradiol levels, they might find them to be as much as 5 times higher than those of a normal premenopausal woman, not a good sign, as we pointed out earlier in this chapter.

Many studies referenced throughout this book show that horse estrogens, patented progestin drugs, and excessively high levels of estradiol (especially oral doses) can all increase a woman's risk of heart disease, cancer, diabetes, and other serious disorders, especially if taken by mouth. That's why the official "guidance" on *all patented estrogen* prescriptions these days is "the lowest dose for the shortest time possible."

Instead of worrying about a woman's estradiol levels, conventional doctors are taught to look out for serious trouble, such as signs of heart disease, strokes, blood clots in the legs and lungs, and cancer in the breast and uterus – and those are just the one's that can kill her. There's a whole other list of common side effects, like nausea, swollen breasts, and depression, that might be annoying and unpleasant, but are probably not deadly, yet still signal that something is not right.

It's not that we shouldn't be looking for these side effects; of course, we should always look for them, but that should be just the beginning of safety monitoring. If doctors prescribing BHRT, or even estradiol + a progestin, were to try measuring their patients' estradiol levels, they might actually find the *underlying cause* of most of these problems – *excessive estrogenic stimulation*. Also, if doctors were to measure the relative levels of estrone, estradiol, and estriol and then calculate an ***estrogen quotient*** (EQ) and the relative levels of *2-hydroxyestrone* and *16α-hydroxyestrone (2/16 ratio),* in addition to levels of 2-methoxyestradiol (an estrogen naturally synthesized by every woman's body), they might find important clues to their risk of breast cancer. (*See Chapter 7.*)

Unfortunately, conventional medical practice largely ignores the importance of estradiol (and other hormone) levels as a primary indicator of serious health risks. How else to explain the fact that the standard FDA-"approved" dose of estradiol leads to excessively high levels of two carcinogenic hormones, estradiol and estrone?

Careful practice of BHRT demands that, in addition to all the standard safety screens (*See box.*), women's hormone levels should also be measured every 3 to 6 months, especially early in therapy, not only to make sure they are within safe and effective limits, but also to make sure that these hormones are not being metabolized in a way that increases hormone-related cancer risk. Changes in hormone absorption during dosing or distorted hormone metabolism afterward can alter the relative levels of the major estrogens. Sometimes these disruptions cause side effects, but often they are "silent."

Not only is it important to measure levels of hormones prescribed as part of BHRT (ie, estradiol, estriol, estrone, progesterone, testosterone, and DHEA), it is equally essential that we measure their "downstream metabolites," including – but not limited to – the important "procarcinogens" 16α-hydroxyestrone, 4-hydroxyestrone, and dihydrotestosterone (DHT), as well as the even more important "anticarcinogen" metabolites, 2-methoxyestradiol, 2-hydroxyestrone, and androstanediol. Relatively high levels of procarcinogenic metabolites and/or low levels of anticarcinogenic metabolites *do not cause overt symptoms,* but their effects can be profound and, best of all, they can almost always be favorably altered with diet and supplementation.

Standard Tests and Recommended Exams for Women on BHRT

More than Once a Year

* Breast self-exam once a month.

* Hormone levels (in 24-hour urine samples) every 3 - 6 months after starting BHRT; once a year thereafter, as long as levels stay in the normal range.

Every Year

* Gynecologic exam and manual breast exam.

* Pap smear for women at high risk for gynecologic cancers.

* Fecal occult blood test for colorectal cancer.

* Fasting complete blood count (CBC) with differential and serum lipid panel.

Every 3 to 10 Years

* Pap smear every 3 years in low-risk women.

* Mammogram every 1 to 3 years (or mammogram every 5 years and thermograms yearly).

* DEXA (aka DXA), a widely used bone density scan for diagnosing osteoporosis, every 18 to 24 months after age 65.

* Colonoscopy every 10 years after age 50 for colon or rectal cancer.

Saliva, Blood, or Urine Testing?

Saliva Testing: Inexpensive, Convenient, and Highly Unreliable

Saliva tests are commonly available by mail order, through some compounding pharmacies, or some physicians. In the basic saliva test, you fill a small bottle with saliva, seal it and send it off to a laboratory for testing, and the results are sent to your doctor. The primary advantage of saliva tests for hormone levels is that they are relatively inexpensive, noninvasive, and convenient, because they can be performed at home without having to go to a doctor's office or lab.

On the other hand, you get what you pay for. Saliva testing may provide some useful information about sex steroid levels for younger women who are *not* using BHRT, but of the three major test modalities, it is certainly the least reliable.

Let's get one important point about saliva testing out of the way right now. **Saliva testing is not useful and not recommended for women on BHRT,** because it is very likely to indicate "sky high" hormone levels that bear no relation to their actual physiologic levels and may falsely suggest a hormone overdose. Nor can saliva testing show the wide range of procarcinogenic and anticarcinogenic metabolites of estrogens and testosterone.

Yet, BHRT critics love to set up the unreliability of saliva testing as a "straw man" in an attempt to discredit the entire practice of BHRT. They argue – *falsely* – that BHRT *requires* saliva testing and that all physicians who prescribe BHRT use it to test hormone levels in their patients.

Nothing could be farther from the truth.

It is a fact that saliva testing is widely promoted by labs, and that some doctors and compounding pharmacists, who could use a little more education in BHRT, may recommend them. However, doctors and pharmacists who are skilled and knowledgeable in BHRT are well aware of the limits of saliva testing and rarely if ever use it.

How unreliable are mail-order saliva tests of hormone levels? There's been almost no good research on this, but in one very small study, saliva samples from 2 women and 1 man were sent to 2 different labs. The labs advertised that, according to their standards, if they were to test the same sample (eg, for estradiol) more than once, the results should vary by less than 8% to 12%. If that were true, it would be reasonable.

However, the actual results of this small study showed a striking degree of variation, which severely limited their usefulness. The actual rates of variation were 35 to 73% for estradiol; 8 to 103% for progesterone; and 13 to 40% for testosterone.[47] With that much variation, it's safe to say the results from these tests were virtually meaningless.

It's true this was a tiny study and that a definitive conclusion requires a much larger, better controlled study on a wide range of labs. Nevertheless, these results are in accord with my own experience and that of many other colleagues who prescribe BHRT.

On the whole, it's best to avoid saliva tests altogether, especially if you're on BHRT.

Blood Testing: Sometimes Useful but Difficult to Interpret

We've all had blood tests, and the procedure for hormone blood tests is no different. Blood tests can measure levels of *total* estradiol, estrone, progesterone, testosterone, and DHEA in *serum* (the liquid portion of blood); the results can be relatively accurate for women whether or not they are on BHRT. However, interpretation of hormone levels based on blood tests must be done carefully, because levels may vary depending on the timing of the test.

Keep in mind that a blood test provides a kind of "snapshot" of what's going on in your body at the moment blood is drawn. In premenopausal women, the ovaries secrete their hormones in "pulses" (bursts and pauses). After menopause, women usually take their replacement hormones once or twice a day. Either way, the hormones do not circulate throughout your body at steady levels (unless you're using a "patch").

Thus, the results of a blood test will vary depending on when your ovaries secreted their hormones or when you took your replacement hormones relative to the time your blood was drawn; whether you took your hormones orally or topically; and whether you ate anything after taking your *oral* hormones.

Nor are blood tests ideal for monitoring the levels of estriol, one of the most important protective estrogens. In fact, estriol is practically unmeasurable in serum by most labs. The reason for this is not completely understood, but according to one research study,[48] estriol gets "cleared" from the blood rapidly due to its very short half-life (rapid metabolism).

Free, Bound, and Total Hormone Levels

When interpreting the results of standard hormone tests, doctors must be aware that most sex hormones present in the body will have undergone at least a degree of metabolism, even if they avoided first-pass metabolism in the liver. As a result, serum hormone levels as usually measured represent the total of *free* and *bound* hormone in the blood stream. What does this mean?

The vast majority of estradiol and testosterone molecules in the bloodstream attach either to a glycoprotein molecule called *sex hormone binding globulin (SHBG)* or to the protein *albumin*. Similarly, progesterone attaches to the protein *transcortin*. These hormones are said to be "bound." Estradiol and testosterone molecules bound to SHBG are inactive, "out of the game," and cannot bind to hormone receptors anywhere. Albumin-bound hormones are also inactive, but can be freed up under certain circumstances.

What's left after all this binding is a very small percentage of *free* hormone (eg, as low as 0.1% of *total* circulating testosterone). However, the tiny remaining amount of free hormone is the only portion that is available to carry out its normal functions in the body.

Nevertheless, the blood tests physicians order do not necessarily distinguish "total" (bound + free) estrogens or progesterone from the "free" (active) levels." (Fortunately, some physicians – including a few "conventional" ones – have learned to measure "total" and "free" testosterone.) Total hormone levels, as measured by the large majority of blood hormone tests, tell only part of the story.

Serum levels also differ depending on whether you take a hormone orally or topically. Estradiol taken via a lozenge (partially topical, partially oral) reaches its peak blood level about 1 hour after dosing and then declines rapidly, suggesting rapid metabolism. By contrast, estriol taken orally causes a peak blood level about 3 to 4 hours after dosing (slower metabolism). However, a second peak occurs if you consume a meal about 4 hours after taking an oral dose. If you apply estriol topically, though, food consumption does not affect serum levels.

Another disadvantage of blood/serum testing is that no assays are currently available to practicing physicians for measuring the many steroid metabolites that have recently been shown to influence the risk for cancer, such as *2-methoxyestradiol* (a "good" estrogen), *4-methoxyestrone* (one of the "worst" estrogens), androstanediol, and others. As noted below, 24-hour urine testing is far superior for detecting, not only these metabolites, but also for measuring estriol levels.

24-Hour Urine Testing: The "Gold Standard"

Because sex steroids are excreted in the urine, urine collection is without doubt the oldest and most reliable method of accumulating steroid hormones, dating back thousands of years to Chinese emperors, not to mention still serving as the source for Premarin®. Although conventional doctors rarely use urine assays for measuring steroid hormones, they have known about their advantages for decades. According to one standard medical textbook, "Urinary assays are considered to reflect the secretory activity of the endocrine glands … [and] to provide clinical information that can reflect the production rates of these steroids."[49]

Unlike the small urine sample most of us are used to giving for a typical urinalysis, urine collected to measure hormone levels is collected over 24 consecutive hours in a large bottle. In other words, for one full day, you are asked to urinate into a bottle. Not only does this method even out all the peaks and valleys that complicate analysis of blood test results, it also facilitates the measurement of "unbound" (ie, "free") levels of estradiol, estrone, estriol, progesterone, testosterone, and DHEA. Urine testing does not measure protein-bound hormones, which comprise the largest portion of "total" hormone production but are functionally irrelevant.*

Without a doubt, 24-hour urinary collection is the preferred method of measuring sex steroid hormone levels, the "gold standard." Moreover, this method is accurate for all women, whether or not they are on BHRT, unlike saliva testing. In women just starting BHRT, we usually recommend a 24-hour urine test every 3 to 6 months, until acceptable, stable levels of all hormones are achieved.

24-hour urine collections are also preferable for two other reasons. First, they give the careful physician so much more information, including whether the hormones taken as BHRT are getting metabolized to mostly "safe" metabolites, or excessively to "unsafe," possibly procarcinogenic metabolites. Second, the expense for capturing a 24-hour urine "picture" of 25 to 30 metabolites of the hormones administered as BHRT is very much lower than checking for all these metabolites in blood. In fact, as noted above, many of these metabolites can't even be measured with standard blood tests.

---

* 24-hour urine testing actually measures the sum of free and "conjugated" hormonal steroids. Conjugated steroids (as in "conjugated equine estrogens") are those molecules that have combined with other simple molecules, such as acids. Since conjugated steroids can be active, although usually not as active as the free molecules, it's always a good idea to measure them as well.

References

1. Kuhl H. Pharmacology of estrogens and progestogens: influence of different routes of administration. *Climacteric.* 2005;8 Suppl 1:3-63.

2. Friel P. Laboratory evaluation of estrogen metabolism. *Townsend Letter for Doctors & Patients.* 2003;245:62-66.

3. Tepper R, Goldberger S, Cohen I, et al. Estrogen replacement in postmenopausal women: are we currently overdosing our patients? *Gynecol Obstet Invest.* 1994;38:113-116.

4. Friel P, Hinchcliffe C, Wright J. Hormone replacement with estradiol: conventional oral doses result in excessive exposure to estrone. *Altern Med Rev.* 2005;10:36-41.

5. Onland-Moret NC, Kaaks R, van Noord PA, et al. Urinary endogenous sex hormone levels and the risk of postmenopausal breast cancer. *Br J Cancer.* 2003;88:1394-1399.

6. Activella® (estradiol/norethindrone acetate) Tablets. *Prescribing Information.* 2006;Novo Nordisk, Princeton, NJ.

7. Prestwood KM, Kenny AM, Kleppinger A, Kulldorff M. Ultralow-dose micronized 17β-estradiol and bone density and bone metabolism in older women: a randomized controlled trial. *JAMA.* 2003;290:1042-1048.

8. Melamed M, Castano E, Notides AC, Sasson S. Molecular and kinetic basis for the mixed agonist/antagonist activity of estriol. *Mol Endocrinol.* 1997;11:1868-1878.

9. Siiteri PK, Sholtz RI, Cirillo PM, et al. Prospective study of estrogens during pregnancy and risk of breast cancer. *Department of Defense Breast Cancer Research Meeting.* 2002;http://cdmrp.army.mil/bcrp/era/abstracts2002/p13%5Fc hemoprevention/9919358%5Fabs.pdf:DAMD17-99-9358.

10. Barnes R, Lobo R. Pharmacology of Estrogens. In: Mishell D, Jr, ed. *Menopause: Physiology and Pharmacology.* Chicago: Year Book Medical Publishers, Inc.; 1987.

11. Archer D. Estradiol gel: a new option in hormone replacement therapy. *OBG Management.* http://www.obgmanagement.com/article_pages.asp?AID=3384& UID=38469;September 2004:Accessed October 31, 2006.

12. Setnikar I, Rovati LC, Vens-Cappell B, Hilgenstock C. Pharmacokinetics of estradiol and of estrone during repeated transdermal or oral administration of estradiol. *Arzneimittelforschung.* 1996;46:766-773.

13. Hirvonen E, Lamberg-Allardt C, Lankinen KS, Geurts P, Wilen-Rosenqvist G. Transdermal oestradiol gel in the treatment of the climacterium: a comparison with oral therapy. *Br J Obstet Gynaecol.* 1997;104 Suppl 16:19-25.

14. Crook D, Cust MP, Gangar KF, et al. Comparison of transdermal and oral estrogen-progestin replacement therapy: effects on serum lipids and lipoproteins. *Am J Obstet Gynecol.* 1992;166:950-955.

15. Stevenson JC, Crook D, Godsland IF, Lees B, Whitehead MI. Oral versus transdermal hormone replacement therapy. *Int J Fertil Menopausal Stud.* 1993;38 Suppl 1:30-35.

16. Samsioe G. Transdermal hormone therapy: gels and patches. *Climacteric.* 2004;7:347-356.

17. Modena MG, Sismondi P, Mueck AO, et al. New evidence regarding hormone replacement therapies is urgently required transdermal postmenopausal hormone therapy differs from oral hormone therapy in risks and benefits. *Maturitas.* 2005;52:1-10.

18. Vehkavaara S, Hakala-Ala-Pietila T, Virkamaki A, et al. Differential effects of oral and transdermal estrogen replacement therapy on endothelial function in postmenopausal women. *Circulation.* 2000;102:2687-2693.

19. Koh KK, Bui MN, Mincemoyer R, Cannon RO, 3rd. Effects of hormone therapy on inflammatory cell adhesion molecules in postmenopausal healthy women. *Am J Cardiol.* 1997;80:1505-1507.

20. Kroon UB, Silfverstolpe G, Tengborn L. The effects of transdermal estradiol and oral conjugated estrogens on haemostasis variables. *Thromb Haemost.* 1994;71:420-423.

21. Oger E, Alhenc-Gelas M, Plu-Bureau G, et al. Association of circulating cellular adhesion molecules with menopausal status and hormone replacement therapy. Time-dependent change in transdermal, but not oral estrogen users. *Thromb Res.* 2001;101:35-43.

22. Scarabin PY, Alhenc-Gelas M, Plu-Bureau G, Taisne P, Agher R, Aiach M. Effects of oral and transdermal estrogen/progesterone regimens on blood coagulation and fibrinolysis in postmenopausal women. A randomized controlled trial. *Arterioscler Thromb Vasc Biol.* 1997;17:3071-3078.

23. Sumino H, Ichikawa S, Ohyama Y, et al. Effect of transdermal hormone replacement therapy on the monocyte chemoattractant protein-1 concentrations and other vascular inflammatory markers and on endothelial function in postmenopausal women. *Am J Cardiol.* 2005;96:148-153.

24. Vehkavaara S, Silveira A, Hakala-Ala-Pietila T, et al. Effects of oral and transdermal estrogen replacement therapy on markers of coagulation, fibrinolysis, inflammation and serum lipids and lipoproteins in postmenopausal women. *Thromb Haemost.* 2001;85:619-625.

25. Vongpatanasin W, Tuncel M, Wang Z, Arbique D, Mehrad B, Jialal I. Differential effects of oral versus transdermal estrogen replacement therapy on C-reactive protein in postmenopausal women. *J Am Coll Cardiol.* 2003;41:1358-1363.

26. Verma S. C-reactive protein incites atherosclerosis. *Can J Cardiol.* 2004;20 Suppl B:29B-31B.

27. Ridker PM, Hennekens CH, Buring JE, Rifai N. C-reactive protein and other markers of inflammation in the prediction of cardiovascular disease in women. *N Engl J Med.* 2000;342:836-843.

28. Pradhan AD, Manson JE, Rossouw JE, et al. Inflammatory biomarkers, hormone replacement therapy, and incident coronary heart disease: prospective analysis from the Women's Health Initiative observational study. *JAMA.* 2002;288:980-987.

29. Abbas A, Fadel PJ, Wang Z, Arbique D, Jialal I, Vongpatanasin W. Contrasting effects of oral versus transdermal estrogen on serum amyloid A (SAA) and high-density lipoprotein-SAA in postmenopausal women. *Arterioscler Thromb Vasc Biol.* 2004;24:e164-167.

30. Cushman M, Kuller LH, Prentice R, et al. Estrogen plus progestin and risk of venous thrombosis. *JAMA.* 2004;292:1573-1580.

31. Beral V, Banks E, Reeves G. Evidence from randomised trials on the long-term effects of hormone replacement therapy. *Lancet.* 2002;360:942-944.

32. Scarabin PY, Oger E, Plu-Bureau G. Differential association of oral and transdermal oestrogen-replacement therapy with venous thromboembolism risk. *Lancet.* 2003;362:428-432.

33. Chu MC, Cosper P, Nakhuda GS, Lobo RA. A comparison of oral and transdermal short-term estrogen therapy in postmenopausal women with metabolic syndrome. *Fertil Steril.* 2006;86:1669-1675.

34. Mueck AO, Seeger H, Lippert TH. [Effect of transdermal versus oral estradiol administration on the excretion of vasoactive markers in postmenopausal women]. *Gynakol Geburtshilfliche Rundsch.* 2000;40:61-67.

35. Os I, Os A, Abdelnoor M, Larsen A, Birkeland K, Westheim A. Insulin sensitivity in women with coronary heart disease during hormone replacement therapy. *J Womens Health (Larchmt).* 2005;14:137-145.

36. O'Sullivan AJ, Ho KK. A comparison of the effects of oral and transdermal estrogen replacement on insulin sensitivity in postmenopausal women. *J Clin Endocrinol Metab.* 1995;80:1783-1788.

37. Sztefko K, Rogatko I, Milewicz T, Jozef K, Tomasik PJ, Szafran Z. Effect of hormone therapy on the enteroinsular axis. *Menopause.* 2005;12:630-638.

38. Vehkavaara S, Westerbacka J, Hakala-Ala-Pietila T, Virkamaki A, Hovatta O, Yki-Jarvinen H. Effect of estrogen replacement therapy on insulin sensitivity of glucose metabolism and preresistance and resistance vessel function in healthy postmenopausal women. *J Clin Endocrinol Metab.* 2000;85:4663-4670.

39. Weissberger AJ, Ho KK, Lazarus L. Contrasting effects of oral and transdermal routes of estrogen replacement therapy on 24-hour growth hormone (GH) secretion, insulin-like growth factor I, and GH-binding protein in postmenopausal women. *J Clin Endocrinol Metab.* 1991;72:374-381.

40. Basurto L, Saucedo R, Ochoa R, Hernandez M, Zarate A. [Hormone replacement therapy with transdermal estradiol lowers insulin-cortisol and lipoproteins levels in postmenopausal women]. *Ginecol Obstet Mex.* 2002;70:491-495.

41. Saucedo R, Basurto L, Zarate A, Martinez C, Hernandez M, Galvan R. Effect of Estrogen Therapy on Insulin Resistance and Plasminogen Activator Inhibitor Type 1 Concentrations in Postmenopausal Women. *Gynecol Obstet Invest.* 2007;64:61-64.

42. Hirvonen E, Cacciatore B, Wahlstrom T, Rita H, Wilen-Rosenqvist G. Effects of transdermal oestrogen therapy in postmenopausal women: a comparative study of an oestradiol gel and an oestradiol delivering patch. *Br J Obstet Gynaecol.* 1997;104 Suppl 16:26-31.

43. Cano A. Compliance to hormone replacement therapy in menopausal women controlled in a third level academic centre. *Maturitas.* 1994;20:91-99.

44. Gelas B, Thebault J, Roux I, Herbrecht F, Zartarian M. [Comparative study of the acceptability of a new estradiol Tx 11323 (A) gel and a transdermal matrix system]. *Contracept Fertil Sex.* 1997;25:470-474.

45. Maines MD, Kappas A. Metals as regulators of heme metabolism. *Science.* 1977;198:1215-1221.

46. Moyer DL, de Lignieres B, Driguez P, Pez JP. Prevention of endometrial hyperplasia by progesterone during long-term estradiol replacement: influence of bleeding pattern and secretory changes. *Fertil Steril.* 1993;59:992-997.

47. Hagen J, Gott N, Miller DR. Reliability of saliva hormone tests. *J Am Pharm Assoc (Wash DC).* 2003;43:724-726.

48. Longcope C. Estriol production and metabolism in normal women. *J Steroid Biochem.* 1984;20:959-962.

49. Burtis C, Ashwood E, eds. *Tietz Textbook of Clinical Chemistry, Third Edition.* Philadelphia, PA: WB Saunders; 1998.

CHAPTER 10

HORMONES FOR HIM: WHY MEN NEED BHRT, TOO

BHRT isn't just for women. As we discuss in this chapter, male menopause (increasingly termed "andropause") is just as real as the female variety, and the steps men can take to improve or eliminate their symptoms and prevent the destructive long-term effects of low hormones are not all that different from those that women can take. Only the hormones are different. If you have a male partner who's 40 or older, he may be dealing with many of the same issues that you are and not even know it. It's vital that he look into the possibility of BHRT too, because conventional medicine being what it is, he's not likely to hear anything from his doctor.

We've written a lot about the Women's Health Initiative (WHI) in this book. One of the reasons doctors skilled and knowledgeable in BHRT were not exactly surprised to learn that Premarin® + Provera® increased the risk of breast cancer, heart disease, senility, and other disorders was that this was not the first time "hormone experts" had made a deadly miscalculation. In fact, it was at least the *fifth* time.

From the 1940s to 1960s, there was the DES (diethylstilbestrol) disaster. DES is a patented alien-molecule with some estrogen-like activity that was found to cause breast cancer in the women who took it while they were pregnant. Problems caused by DES arose years after it's use, and not just in their own bodies: their daughters were at increased risk for cervical and breast cancer, and also otherwise almost unheard of vaginal cancer (among other serious problems). Their sons had a higher rate of testicular cancer; and now, hints of certain genitourinary abnormalities in their grandsons and granddaughters! (*See Chapter 4.*)

In the mid-1970s, there was the realization that "unopposed" horse estrogens were causing uterine (endometrial) cancer in postmenopausal women. And, while the patented alien-molecule "progestin" (Provera®) helped solve that immediate problem, it opened the door to scores of other serious side effects, including increased risks of heart disease and breast cancer.

But one of the first times our conventional-medicine hormone "experts" got it really, really wrong was in the 1940s and 1950s, and that time it was in *men*! It's not well known in medical circles today, but hormone replacement for andropausal men preceded female HRT by several decades, and like the subsequent attempts at female "hormone replacement," early male HRT was also an unmitigated disaster.

In a very near parallel to the WHI debacle, drug companies sold hundreds of thousands of men FDA-"approved" doses of a patented alien-molecule, pseudohormone named *methyltestosterone*, pawning it off as real testosterone. After a few years of taking this "anabolic steroid" drug, which, of course, had never before seen the inside of a human body, many of the men who took it developed liver diseases, including cancer, and heart disease, among others. Many of them died as a result.

Sound familiar? In their new-found wisdom, the "experts" of the day proclaimed that these unfortunate results *proved* that what they called "testosterone therapy" was dangerous, even deadly. (Exactly as FDA and other conventional "experts" are proclaiming bio-identical estrogens to be dangerous based on "evidence" from patented, alien-to-the-human body pseudoestrogens!) As a consequence, research on actual – bio-identical – testosterone, which was looking very promising until patented methyltestosterone and other patented anabolic steroids came along, went into eclipse and didn't begin to reappear until nearly a half century later.

Among many of those who practice conventional medicine today, the old prejudices against testosterone replacement are very much alive and kicking. A couple of years ago, a group of modern-day "experts," convened by the Institute of Medicine (IOM), an offshoot of the National Academy of Sciences, picked up where the old "experts" had left off, declaring that men should not consider testosterone replacement as preventive medicine against symptoms of aging and andropause. An IOM advisory committee concluded that "...*existing scientific evidence does not justify claims that testosterone treatments can relieve or prevent certain age-related problems in men.*"[1]

We could hardly disagree more. A normal, physiologic level of *natural* or *bio-identical testosterone*, sustained for a lifetime, may be one of the most important antiaging and health-maintenance tools a man can use. And, again, manmade, alien, testosterone-like patent medicines just don't cut it!

For over 25 years, I (JVW) have worked with men aged 40 and older, whose symptoms and tests indicated they had a deficiency in endogenous (internally produced and secreted by the testicles) testosterone. The wives and families of many of these men have observed that, since Grandpa started using testosterone, "He's a lot less grumpy," "remembers things better," and that "he laughs and smiles a lot more often." Contrary to what the IOM and other mainstream "experts" would have us believe, bio-identical testosterone replacement in these men has been gratifying for everyone involved, with results such as:

- Improved mood, memory, and cognitive function

- Enhanced libido and sexual/erectile performance

- Improved muscle mass and strength

- Stronger bones

- Healthier heart and blood vessels

- Lower total cholesterol

- Higher HDL ("good") cholesterol

- Lower blood pressure

- Lower risks of dangerous blood clots that can cause heart attacks and strokes

- Improved tissue oxygenation and blood sugar levels

- Improved prostate gland health

So what's all the fuss about? Again it's evident that these "experts" do not "get" the difference between bio-identical hormones and, alien-to-the-human-body hormone-like patent medicines. As the chairman of the IOM panel pointed out, "Recent experience with the Women's Health Initiative – which studied *hormone therapy* in postmenopausal women for many years – underscores the importance of approaching future studies of testosterone therapy thoughtfully and carefully." (Emphasis added.) Of course, the WHI did not study "hormone therapy" at all; it studied Premarin® and Provera®.

No one contests that testosterone replacement therapy should be done "thoughtfully and carefully," but the IOM committee, like most other conventional medicine "authorities," is apparently more than a little confused about the meaning of the WHI. They take the bad results from a horse-hormone-and-patented-progestin study and baselessly extend them to natural, bio-identical hormones, branding the latter as

The Three Faces of Testosterone

In men, testosterone is produced primarily in endocrine glands called the testes, from which it spills directly into the local blood supply. (A small amount of testosterone is also produced in the adrenal glands.) Like estrogens in women, testosterone (or its primary metabolite, *dihydrotestosterone, or DHT*) in men is carried by the blood stream to specific target cells all over the body, where it binds and exerts a variety of vital effects, depending on the target tissue. These effects fall into three broad categories:

- *Masculinization*: body and facial hair, deep voice

- *Anabolism*: building muscle mass and bone strength

- *Sexual arousal*: libido and erectile function

Although testosterone is generally considered to be a "male hormone," it can and does produce these same effects (except for penile erections, of course) in both men and women.

potentially dangerous and of questionable efficacy. They ignore positive results from quality research on bio-identical testosterone, published in mainstream journals as far back as 1935. They ignore the perfectly obvious: bio-identical hormones are precisely identical to the hormones present in human bodies for hundreds of thousands of years! Patented pseudohormones are alien to the human body and have no business being there.

And to top it all off, they somehow manage to forget all the glaring failures of patent medicine "hormones" and hormone manipulating drugs over the last century, as they look forward with great anticipation to yet another new, still untested class of patentable, alien drugs – *selective androgen receptor modulators* (*SARMs*) – as a potentially *safer* alternative to natural/bio-identical testosterone.[1, 2] But then, we've come to expect such arrogant and oblivious nonsense from mainstream "experts," who look exclusively to the labs of Big Pharma – not to Mother Nature – for all their medical advances.

So instead of relying on the half-truths such "experts" continue to pass off as fact, let's take a brief look at some of the evidence published over the last few years, which definitively demonstrates that bio-identical testosterone can be extraordinarily beneficial – and quite safe – for men who need it.

The "Andropause" Syndrome

Everybody knows that menopause is a major event in each woman's life. But in men, too? Yes, men undergo their own version of menopause (*andropause*), and while the hormones may be different, the effects on their lives are remarkably similar. If your male partner is over 40, he should pay close attention to the information in this chapter, because he isn't likely to hear it from his regular doctor.

It's no longer a secret that an adult man's testosterone level declines with age. Even the IOM won't deny that. Menopause in women is easy to recognize, with its well-known symptoms, and relatively rapid and predictable time course, reflecting the decline in estrogen and progesterone as the ovaries shut down around age 50.

By contrast, andropause is a much more gradual, almost imperceptible process, usually beginning during men's 40s and following the slow but steady decline in testosterone secretion by the testes. Each man follows his own unique pattern, of course, but sooner or later, the results are pretty much the same for all.

As shown in Table 10-1, andropausal men experience many of the same symptoms as menopausal women, and like women, these can profoundly affect their health and happiness. Like women, men often suffer subtle declines in physical, mental, and emotional acuity. And also like women, men face a growing risk of serious "age-related" chronic disorders and diseases, including heart attacks, strokes, high cholesterol, high blood pressure, depression, loss of cognitive function, and even osteoporosis. Although breast cancer is rare in men, prostate cancer is extremely common, and benign (noncancerous) prostate enlargement is almost universal if men live long enough. Although low testosterone is probably not the only cause of these conditions, it can be an important factor in each of them.

Eventually, nearly every man reaches a point where his testosterone no longer drives his sex life as well as he (*and you!*) might like. So far, impaired sexual function is about the only disorder that conventional medicine will acknowledge as being related to low testosterone levels. As we shall see, though, it's only one of many, and perhaps the least important disorder, from an anti-aging perspective.

It's simply common sense. Although conventional medical wisdom hasn't caught up yet, more and more scientific evidence suggests that, like estrogen and progesterone replacement in women, bio-identical testosterone, applied topically by men at physiologic doses and on a schedule closely approximating Nature's own timing, can help prevent and even *reverse* virtually all of the symptoms and disorders listed on the male side of Table 10-1.

The various patent medicine chemical cousins of testosterone (*anabolic steroids*) commonly used as substitutes for bio-identical testosterone for the last 50 to 60 years are finally on their way out. These man-made, patented pseudohormones are alien molecules based on the structure of bio-identical testosterone but modified to make them more active after

Menopause vs. Andropause: More Alike than Different

Menopause	Andropause
Reduced estrogen & progesterone	Reduced testosterone
Reduced libido	Reduced libido
Hot flushes	Hot flushes
Vaginal thinning/dryness	Erectile dysfunction
Painful intercourse	Ejaculatory dysfunction
Disturbed sleep	Disturbed sleep
Anxiety/depression	Anxiety/depression
Heart disease & atherosclerosis	Heart disease & atherosclerosis
Osteoporosis	Osteoporosis
Breast cancer	Prostate enlargement/cancer
Endometrial (uterine) cancer	Muscle weakness
Fatigue	Fatigue
Irritability	Irritability
Thinning/sagging skin	Thinning/sagging skin
Slow wound healing	Slow wound healing
Poor concentration/memory lapses	Poor concentration/memory lapses
Irregular menstruation	
Urinary incontinence	
Urinary tract infections	

Table 10-1.

oral dosing, longer-lasting than bio-identical testosterone and, of course, more profitable because they're patentable. In no way are they better or safer. (*This should be a familiar refrain by now.*)

Like Premarin® and Provera® in women, these drugs produce a grossly unnatural hormonal environment in men's bodies that can be associated with wild mood swings along with other serious and sometimes even deadly side effects.

Testosterone Restores Sexual Function *and* Desire for Men

We all know about the "Viagra® revolution" that started about 10 years ago. Viagra® was the first patent medicine "approved" by the FDA for helping men enhance and maintain their erections, and it brought millions of men out of the impotence (erectile dysfunction or ED – in polite company) closet.

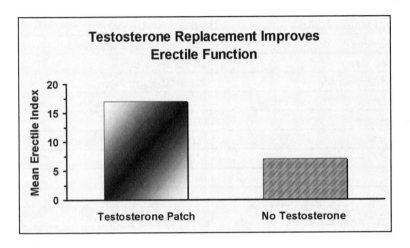

Figure 10-1. In a double-blind, placebo-controlled trial, testosterone-deficient men using a testosterone patch reported higher levels of sexual arousal and desire over 12 months.

Source: Arver et al, 1996

While Viagra® and other similar drugs can be effective in some men for their limited erection-building function, it's quite common for andropausal men with a normal age-related decline in testosterone to also suffer a loss of sexual desire – *low libido*. Viagra-like all patent medicines, designed only to boost erections, does nothing to enhance a low libido. If the sexual fires aren't already burning, these patent medicines won't ignite them.

Both a sagging libido and poor erections are often at least partly a result of declining testosterone levels,[*] known in medicalese as *hypogonadism*.

---

[*]   Erectile dysfunction in men of andropausal age is also likely related to progressing atherosclerosis in the arteries that deliver blood to the penis. Viagra-like drugs may help these men by temporarily dilating those arteries, whereas testosterone may actually help open the arteries by preventing or reversing the atherosclerotic process. This effect of testosterone takes a lot longer to work, but it is much longer-lasting and may even reflect a general improvement in cardiovascular health in other vital arteries, such as those that serve the heart and brain.

There's no doubt that replacing testosterone in hypogonadal men can relight the fires of sexual desire and also restore erectile ability. It is for these reasons that the FDA has "approved" several products, including skin patches and gels made with bio-identical testosterone (*Finally, they got that right!*). Figures 10-1 and 10-2 show results from a study using one of these products (a skin patch) in which testosterone replacement resulted in improved erections and enhanced sexual arousal and desire (libido) in hypogonadal men.[3]

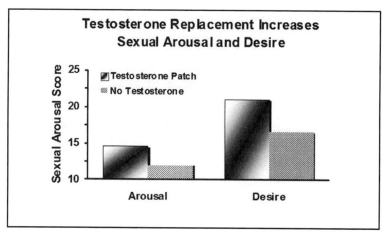

Figure 10-2. In a double-blind, placebo-controlled trial, testosterone-deficient men using a testosterone patch reported higher levels of sexual arousal and desire over 12 months.

Source: Arver et al, 1996

Although testosterone replacement products are currently FDA-"approved" only for enhancing men's sexual function, they can be extremely helpful for lots more than just keeping a man's sexual organs alive and kicking. As we discuss below, testosterone is important for the continuing health of his heart, his bones, his muscles, his mind, and yes, even his prostate gland. Unfortunately, most mainstream physicians are completely unaware of these benefits, and given what they've been taught in medical school and beyond, some may recoil in horror at the thought of prescribing testosterone for anything other than poor libido and ED, believing it to be dangerous. As such, these physicians are depriving their male patients of an extremely valuable – and safe – resource for keeping them youthful and active long into old age.

Testosterone Protects Men's Hearts

Testosterone's role in the health of the male heart is still mired in the myths and misconceptions of the 1950s, which said that testosterone replacement could actually *cause* heart disease. In fact, if one bothers to study the scientific evidence, *low testosterone levels* have been repeatedly linked to a long list of heart disease risk factors (Table 10-2). Replacement using *bio-identical testosterone*, and *not patented anabolic steroids*, can be beneficial for the heart and blood vessels and quite safe.

If you think about it, it makes no sense physiologically that testosterone should be bad for men's hearts. If high endogenous testosterone levels promoted heart disease, why are young men, who have by far the highest testosterone levels, virtually immune to heart disease, while older men, whose testosterone levels are in decline, are the most vulnerable? By the late 1980s, it had become undeniable that instances of heart disease that had long been blamed on testosterone replacement were really caused by use of patented *anabolic steroids,** like *methyltestosterone,* which came into vogue in the late 1940s and '50s.

When research on testosterone replacement first began in the 1930s and '40s – using bio-identical testosterone (which was very costly and difficult to produce in those days) – one of the first targets those scientists focused on was heart disease, and their results were nearly uniformly positive. It wasn't until cheaper, easier-to-make methyltestosterone and other patented anabolic steroids came along and pushed real testosterone aside did "hormone-related" heart (and liver) diseases begin to appear. Only then did real, bio-identical testosterone get its undeserved reputation, because, thanks to patent medicine company marketing practices, most doctors at the time didn't understand that anabolic steroids and testosterone were not the same thing.

Believe it or not, testosterone's undeserved unsavory reputation exists to this day, more than 50 years later. Ask almost any conventional

---

* These drugs are the testosterone-like "steroids" that athletes are often accused of taking to help them "bulk up" in order to improve their performance. They are related to testosterone in the same way that Provera® is related to progesterone.

Low Testosterone Levels Increase Men's Heart Disease Risk

Men with low testosterone tend to have these heart disease risk factors:

- Angina pectoris

- Atherosclerosis

- Insulin resistance/diabetes

- High blood glucose levels

- High LDL-cholesterol

- Low HDL-cholesterol

- High triglycerides

- High blood pressure

- High body mass index (obesity)

- High waist-to-hip ratio (obesity)

- High levels of blood clotting factors

Table 10-2.

doctor about using testosterone replacement to prevent or treat heart disease, and they'll likely give you one of those puzzled, patronizing looks and then write you out a prescription for Lipitor®.

Most doctors today have been taught that testosterone makes heart disease worse. What they don't realize is that the so-called "testosterone" they're referring to isn't testosterone at all, but rather the patented anabolic steroids of yesteryear. Without a doubt, those drugs can cause heart disease, not to mention liver disease, but, of course, *they're not* *testosterone.* In over 70 years of research, there has not been a single piece of quality scientific evidence proving that bio-identical testosterone causes or worsens heart disease in men, quite the contrary.*

Diseases of the heart and blood vessels kill about half a million men in the United States each year. Everyone recognizes that the risk of developing heart disease grows with age, but the fact that that risk may be tied to andropause and the age-related decline in testosterone has not yet penetrated the walls of mainstream medicine. This is very sad, because an ample and ever-growing body of scientific evidence indicates that:

- Testosterone is vital for the health of the heart and blood vessels.

- Testosterone levels decline with age.

- Restoring testosterone (and the androgen DHEA) to youthful levels can provide significant protection against the various manifestations of coronary artery disease and heart failure.

We're can't go through all the evidence here, but let's glance at a few key illustrative studies:

- In 2007, 119 men with proven coronary artery disease in one or more arteries were found to have significantly lower endogenous testosterone levels compared to a group of healthy men. Moreover, men with the lowest levels of testosterone had the most severe disease, including the most clogged arteries.[4]

- One of the clearest examples of testosterone replacement's benefits for the heart is a reduction in *angina* symptoms.† English researchers, analyzing the results of 10 well-controlled studies, found that testosterone replacement significantly reduced the frequency and severity of angina attacks, and increased the amount of exercise required to trigger them.[5]

---

* That's not necessarily true in women, where too much testosterone can contribute to heart disease, just as too much estrogen can in men. Believe it or not, some doctors do not understand that distinction, thinking that because too much testosterone is dangerous in women, so it must also be in men.

† Angina pectoris is transient chest pain caused by partial blockage of one or more coronary arteries. It is an important danger sign that a heart attack may be imminent.

- In one randomized, double-blind, placebo-controlled study, 50 men with electrocardiographic (ECG) evidence of angina received weekly injections of either a long-acting form of testosterone or placebo. While attached to an ECG recorder, the men took a standard exercise stress test before starting treatment and again after 4 weeks and 8 weeks of treatment. Normally, such exercise can trigger an angina attack in men with coronary atherosclerosis, if their disease is severe enough and their exertion is intense enough. Angina scores were calculated as a function of the amount of time the men could exercise before pain and/or ECG signs of angina appeared.

  Testosterone replacement had an unmistakable benefit. As shown in Figure 10-3, testosterone resulted in a 32% improvement in angina score (ie, longer exercise time until angina or ECG irregularities appeared) after 4 weeks and a 51% improvement after 8 weeks. By contrast, the placebo had no effect on the men's angina scores.[6]

- Other recent research has shown that testosterone replacement could mitigate a different, but quite dangerous ECG abnormality – *QT dispersion* – which occurs in men suffering from congestive heart failure.[7]* Endogenous testosterone levels were found to be abnormally low in men with chronic heart failure and QT dispersion, but topical testosterone replacement significantly increased their cardiac output[8] and exercise capacity.[9] In a review of heart failure in men, the researchers concluded that androgen replacement (testosterone and DHEA) might be "a natural tonic for the failing heart" and that it could "potentially ameliorate symptoms by improving cardiac and vascular function and increasing strength and endurance."[5]

For Men, Testosterone Reduces Blood's Abnormal Clotting Tendency

Heart attacks and strokes are a direct result of the formation of intra-arterial blood clots, or *thrombi*. An increased tendency of blood to clot as men age may be due at least in part to declining testosterone

---

* Congestive heart failure (or simply "heart failure") is a common condition in which the ability of the heart to fill with or pump a sufficient amount of blood through the body is impaired. Heart failure has an annual mortality rate of 10% and is one of the leading causes of hospitalization in people aged 65 and older.

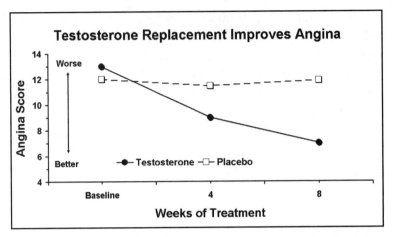

Figure 10-3. Men with angina showed significant improvement when treated with "testosterone" over a period of 8 weeks, compared to those treated with a placebo.

Adapted from Jaffe, 1977

levels. One reason is that testosterone favorably affects the balance between blood factors that promote clotting and others that inhibit clotting. In a highly oversimplified sketch of the extremely complex clotting process, blood clots form when an insoluble protein – *fibrin* – is formed from *fibrinogen*. Fibrin forms the essential portion of all blood clots. Factors that inhibit fibrin formation are said to be *fibrinolytic*.

In men, *testosterone replacement enhances the fibrinolytic* side of the equation in a manner that resembles how estrogens work in women.[10] In one study in normal, healthy men, 16 weeks of treatment with high doses of testosterone (injections), caused their fibrinogen levels (ie, blood clotting tendency) to decline by about 15%.[11]

Other research suggests that testosterone may have an anti-inflammatory effect that protects against the progression (worsening) of atherosclerosis in coronary arteries and that this effect may be important for inhibiting clot formation and progression to angina and/or heart attack.[12]

Testosterone Normalizes a Man's Cholesterol Levels

For decades it has been the conventional medical wisdom that testosterone replacement *increases* a man's risk of heart disease, in part by disturbing the normal lipid balance [ie, by increasing the dangerous LDL ("bad") cholesterol and triglycerides and by decreasing beneficial HDL ("good") cholesterol].

While many doctors still believe this, it has since become apparent to anyone paying attention to the scientific literature that it is nonsense. Most recent research has confirmed that high endogenous (internally produced and secreted) testosterone levels are associated with normal-to-high HDL-cholesterol levels and low LDL and triglyceride levels.[13-19] In a review of studies on the androgen-lipid relationship, one of the leading American medical "authorities" on this subject, Dr. Elizabeth Barrett-Connor, of the University of California, San Diego, reported that *every study that included 100 or more men had found a positive association between testosterone and HDL-cholesterol.* She concluded, "Adult men with high normal concentrations of endogenous testosterone have more favorable levels of several major heart disease risk factors, including HDL-cholesterol, a more suitable fat pattern, and lower glucose and insulin levels than do men with low testosterone concentrations." She added that "physiologic testosterone levels in the high normal range appear to be conducive to optimal cardiovascular health for adult men."[20]

Only a few small studies have prospectively examined the effects of testosterone replacement on cholesterol levels.[21-24] In one such study, 22 men with low testosterone levels were given biweekly testosterone injections for a year. As shown in Figure 10-4, their total cholesterol levels fell from a mean of 225 mg/dL ("borderline high"*) at the start of treatment to 198 mg/dL ("optimal") after 12 months. LDL-cholesterol levels dropped from 139 mg/dL ("borderline high") to 118 mg/dL ("near or above optimal"). There was no significant decrease in HDL-cholesterol.[25]

---

* According to American Heart Association (AMA) standards.

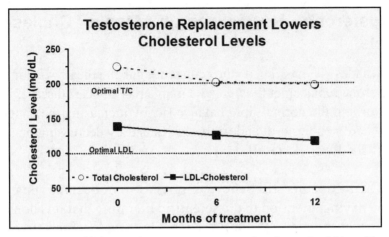

Figure 10-4. Men with low endogenous testosterone levels received biweekly testosterone injections for 12 months. During this time, their total cholesterol (T/C) and LDL-cholesterol levels declined from "borderline high" to "optimal" or "near optimal" (according to American Heart Association standards. Their HDL-cholesterol levels remained normal. (mg/dL = milligrams per deciliter)

Source: Zgliczynski et al, 1996

In reviewing testosterone trials, Dr. Barrett-Connor noted that, "Exogenous testosterone given parenterally [administered in a way that avoids the digestive tract, eg, via injection or topical cream/gel] in physiologic doses to middle-aged men does not lower HDL-cholesterol and may reduce visceral adiposity ["spare tire" or "love handle" syndrome], glycemia [elevated blood sugar], and insulin resistance [a sign of diabetes and precursor to coronary heart disease]."[20]

Hormonal Heresy

We should perhaps point out the obvious, that treating heart disease by replacing testosterone comes pretty close to heresy as far as conventional medicine is concerned. The cardiology community in the United States and other Western countries is married to the "clogged plumbing" model of cardiovascular disease, which involves symptomatic treatment with patent medicines (eg, to lower cholesterol and control blood pressure) and surgery, angioplasty, and other risky interventions to ream open or replace blocked arteries.

Measures such as bio-identical testosterone replacement, which can prevent or reverse the major pathologies of cardiovascular disease, are a clear threat to the lucrative axis of Big Pharma, wealthy heart surgeons and the hospitals where they operate, government regulatory agencies, and disease advocacy groups, all of which are highly invested in – and in many circumstances are financially dependent on – the conventional heart disease paradigm. Although study after study supports a role for *unpatentable, bio-identical* testosterone in preventing and treating heart disease, it will likely be a very long time – if ever – before we see a significant paradigm shift, such that testosterone replacement becomes an accepted preventive or treatment modality rather than just another "quack" remedy.

We believe there is more than enough data now to support the careful application of testosterone replacement in men who are vulnerable to cardiovascular disease and even in those who are already showing early signs of it. Ideally, we would like to see large, long-term, placebo-controlled studies to verify testosterone's benefits, but the eternal question then arises: Since testosterone isn't patentable, who will sponsor these studies?

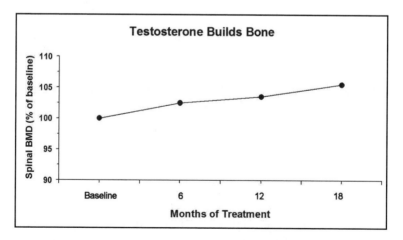

Figure 10-5. In men with low testosterone levels, testosterone replacement for 18 months resulted in a 5% increase in spinal bone mineral density.

Adapted from Katznelson et al, 1995

If a man has been diagnosed with heart disease, we recommend that he raise the testosterone option with his physician. If the physician is open to the use of testosterone replacement and is knowledgeable in using it, fine. If not, we recommend he find a physician who is. (*See Chapter 11 for more about finding physicians who are skilled and knowledgeable in treating men with bio-identical hormones.*)

Testosterone Helps Keep Bones and Muscles Strong

In addition to its masculinizing properties (eg, facial and body hair, a deeper voice, an enlarged penis, etc), testosterone has long been recognized for its essential *anabolic* (tissue-building) role in building strong bones and muscles. A flood of testosterone (along with good diet, exercise, and conditioning) is the primary reason why a boy can enter puberty as a frail, skinny, 98-pound weakling and leave a few years later as a linebacker. The fact that men have lots of testosterone while women have much less is why, for the most part, men are also generally much larger in stature than women and have greater muscle strength.

But what testosterone giveth, the decline in testosterone can taketh away. As men age, the gradual downslide in testosterone levels that usually begins in their 40s, slows the rate at which their bodies can rebuild and restore muscles and bones. For example, people are often surprised to learn that the bone wasting disease, *osteoporosis*, is not just one of those "female diseases" but is common in men, too, especially if they live long enough. In fact, about one hip fracture in three occurs in a man, and when men do break a hip, they have a much greater risk than women of ending up permanently disabled or dead.[26-28] However, in men, osteoporosis is tied to a decline in testosterone, not to estrogen, as it is women.

Another important difference between men and women who get osteoporosis is that women begin experiencing fractures long before men do. Still, by the time men reach their late 70s, they usually catch up with women.[29-31] This latency is due in large part to the fact that men generally start out with bones that are thicker and denser than women's. Therefore, they need to lose more bone tissue before their bones become fragile enough that they easily fracture, which can take a few more years.

Can replacing missing testosterone resurrect lost bone and muscle in men like these? According to my own (JVW) clinical experience and that of many colleagues, the answer is, most assuredly "Yes, it can."

Our clinical observations are supported by lots of research confirming the ability of supplemental testosterone to help build stronger bones and muscles.[22, 32-36] One typical study from the Harvard Medical School measured the effects of testosterone injections on bone mineral density (BMD) and other measures of bone health in 29 men (mean age, 58 years) with low testosterone levels. A group of age-matched healthy men with normal testosterone served as placebo controls. Over a period of 18 months, compared to pretreatment (baseline) levels, testosterone treatment led to a *5% increase in BMD* (Fig. 10-5), a *14% decrease in body fat* (Fig. 10-6), and a *7% increase in lean muscle mass*.[34]

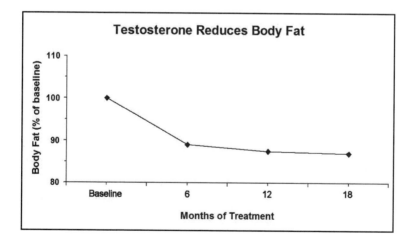

Figure 10-6. In middle-aged men with low testosterone levels, "testosterone" replacement therapy for 18 months resulted in a 14% decrease in body fat.

Adapted from Katznelson et al, 1995

Much of this early research employed old-fashioned injectable forms of testosterone, which are not truly bio-identical (although much closer to bio-identical than alien, patented anabolic steroids) and are used less commonly these days. However, to prove that these benefits are not flukes, recent studies using testosterone topical gels and patches have been showing comparable results. For example, two 12-month studies in 371 men using a topical bio-identical testosterone gel (marketed as Testim®) found significant increases in BMD, as well as significant improvements in body composition – increased muscle mass, decreased fat mass, and decreased percentage of fat. Not only did testosterone replacement make the men stronger and leaner, it also helped improve their mood and sexual function – sexual performance, motivation, and desire, as well as an increase in spontaneous erections.[37]

Testosterone Sharpens a Man's Brain Function and Improves His Mood

One of the most consistent findings on the role of testosterone over the years has been the claim that it enhances feelings of well-being and mental "sharpness." More than 1,000 years ago, Chinese doctors in the Imperial Court employed an early form of "hormone replacement therapy" – hormone-rich urine (collected from young men and dried) – as a treatment for disturbances of the "psyche," including what has since been described as the "neuroses and psychoses of aging." (*See Chapter 4.*)[38]

Since the 1940s, numerous studies have demonstrated improvements in mood and cognitive abilities in men treated with testosterone. For example, a landmark 1944 study found that 17 of 20 men with low endogenous testosterone and symptoms of "male menopause" responded to testosterone injections with "complete abolition" of such symptoms as *depression, impaired memory, nervousness,* and *inability to concentrate.*[39]

Although this and other early studies lacked some important experimental controls, more recent "gold-standard" studies have reinforced the conclusions of their earlier, less well-controlled predecessors. Here is a small sample of some of the most encouraging new findings:

- *Testosterone may act as an antidepressant* in men with low or borderline testosterone levels and refractory (difficult-to-treat) depression. Application of a testosterone topical gel in 56 men, aged 30 to 65 years, for 8 weeks resulted in *significantly greater improvement in depression scores* compared with placebo on a standard measure of depression. The authors concluded that "testosterone gel may produce antidepressant effects in the large and probably under-recognized population of depressed men with low testosterone levels."[40]

- *Testosterone replacement significantly improved cognitive function* in a group of 25 healthy men, aged 50 to 80. Cognitive function was measured by tests of spatial memory (recall of a walking route), spatial ability (block construction), and verbal memory (recall of a short story).[41]

- *Testosterone replacement significantly improved verbal memory* in older men with low testosterone levels. Those men who used a gel containing only dihydrotestosterone (DHT), testosterone's primary active metabolite, showed *significant improvements in spatial memory.*[42]

- *Lowering testosterone levels in normal, healthy young men caused a significant decrement in verbal memory.* In this unusual study, 32 *young* men with normal testosterone levels were treated for 8 weeks with either testosterone injections, which raised their testosterone levels; or levonorgestrel (a patented progestin), which lowered their testosterone levels. *Lowering testosterone resulted in a significant decline in the men's verbal memory.* The fact that raising testosterone in these men had no effects on their cognitive abilities comes as no surprise. Testosterone can have a wide variety of beneficial effects but only in men who have low endogenous testosterone levels to begin with, such as older men or younger men who are "hypogonadal" due to disease, trauma, or genetics.[43] As demonstrated in this study, the effects of testosterone supplementation in young men with normal testosterone levels is typically negligible.

- *Chemical castration can impair memory in older men.* Based on the questionable assumption that testosterone fuels abnormal prostate growth, castration, either surgical or chemical (using powerful testosterone-suppressing drugs), has long been a common treatment for men with advanced prostate cancer. Unfortunately, castration may also impair memory in these men, possibly by affecting activity in a region of the brain known as the hippocampus, which is known to be involved in memory consolidation.[44] Castration can also contribute to loss of bone and muscle mass in these men, making them increasingly frail. In one study, castration resulted in the acceleration of osteoporosis in 14% of treated men, compared to just 1% of noncastrated controls.[45]

- *Testosterone supplementation improved working memory in older men.* Working memory improved when the testosterone:estradiol ratio was high (ie, more testosterone relative to estradiol). So, as with heart and prostate disease, it appears to be the *balance between testosterone and estrogen* that is a crucial factor in the preservation of cognitive function in men. The authors concluded that "sex steroids can modulate working memory in men and can act as modulators of cognition throughout life."[46]

Other exciting recent research is beginning to demonstrate that testosterone replacement can help men slow the progress of Alzheimer's disease and other forms of age-related dementia. The conclusions of these studies include the following:

- Based on a literature review, testosterone loss may be a risk factor for cognitive decline and possibly for dementia in elderly men.[47] Data from a lab animal study has shown that androgen depletion accelerates the development of neuropathology similar to that found in the brains of people with Alzheimer's disease. Treating men with the testosterone metabolite DHT prevented this neuropathology.[48]

- Testosterone replacement for 6 weeks in men, aged 63 to 85, who had mildly impaired cognitive functions due to Alzheimer's disease resulted in significant improvements in spatial memory, constructional abilities, and verbal memory.[49]

- Testosterone replacement for 12 months in 36 aging men with mild-to-moderate Alzheimer's disease improved cognition, including visual-spatial skills.[50]

Testosterone and the Prostate: Anything to Fear?

A largely unfounded fear of prostate cancer has been perhaps the major stumbling block to the therapeutic use of testosterone replacement by men. There's no doubt that prostate cancer is among the most common malignancies affecting American men. According to the American Cancer Society, 234,460 men in the United States were diagnosed with prostate cancer in 2006, and 27,350 will die as a result. The risk of prostate cancer increases with age, ranging from 3% for men aged 60 to 64 to 15% for men aged 80 and older.[51]

Far more common is a condition known as benign prostatic hypertrophy (BPH), an enlargement of the prostate, which can have the same symptoms as prostate cancer, except that the excess growth (*hypertrophy*) is nonmalignant. BPH is almost as common a part of aging as gray hair. As life expectancy rises, so does the occurrence of BPH. Nearly 75% of men in their 60s have symptoms of BPH, and by the time they reach their 70s or older, BPH affects more than 80%.[52]

Testosterone can stimulate the growth of prostate tissue, especially when low testosterone levels have caused the gland to shrink. However, whether testosterone *causes* BPH or prostate cancer, as goes the gospel of conventional medicine, is becoming increasingly debatable.

As might be expected, the Institute of Medicine's testosterone review committee along with much of the rest of the conventional medicine establishment discourages testosterone replacement therapy by playing on the fear of prostate cancer. "There is still much we don't know about whether testosterone therapy might increase the risk of prostate cancer," the committee chairman wrote. Yet, according to the IOM report, "The committee found *no compelling evidence of major adverse side effects resulting from testosterone therapy.*" But that didn't stop them from concluding that *current evidence is "inadequate to document safety."* (Emphasis added.) In fact, dozens of studies show just how safe testosterone therapy really is.[53] The evidence is only "inadequate" if you refuse to acknowledge it.

A good deal of recent evidence suggests that abnormal prostate growth may actually be related to an imbalance between testosterone and estradiol, ie, too much estradiol relative to testosterone, which commonly occurs as men age. If that turns out to be the case, low testosterone levels may be a greater danger to the prostate than high levels, and testosterone replacement – and/or estrogen suppression – may be a good way to *prevent* or even *treat* prostate hypertrophy.

Recent studies show that prostate cancers that arise in men who have low serum testosterone levels (hypogonadism) are more malignant and less responsive to hormone treatments than those that arise in men with normal levels.[54] In a study in male military veterans, low serum testosterone levels were associated with increased mortality (although not necessarily from prostate disease).[55]

In 2002, a study evaluated 207 men, aged 40 to 83 years, with low or low-normal testosterone levels, after 1, 3, and 6 months of testosterone replacement. Overall, 90% of the men responded favorably to testosterone treatment with significant *decreases in prostate volume, PSA* (prostate-specific androgen, a standard blood test for prostate cancer), and *common symptoms of prostate enlargement*, such as urinary frequency, urgency, "dribbling," and getting up often at night to urinate.[56]

Most recently, a well-controlled Swedish study measured testosterone and other hormones in 392 men with prostate cancer, comparing them with 392 healthy controls.[57] The researchers found no significant associations between androgen levels and the risk of prostate cancer. Similarly, a smaller study from the UCLA School of Medicine found that 6 months of testosterone injections in men with declining testosterone levels had little effect on prostate volume or functions.[58]

There is still much to be learned about the causes of and treatments for prostate diseases. Nevertheless, one thing seems abundantly clear: currently "approved" treatments – drugs that basically inhibit androgenic activity (to try to shrink enlarged prostates) or dilate the ureters (to facilitate urine flow *despite* prostate enlargement) – act merely as *symptom suppressors* with limited efficacy, no effect on the course of the disease, and lots of potential side effects. On the other hand, they do earn patent medicine companies billions of dollars.

Far from causing prostate trouble, many studies suggest that testosterone replacement may actually benefit the prostate. However, there remains a remote possibility that it *might* fuel the growth of an already established malignancy (although this also is far from certain). *Due to this small amount of uncertainty, just to be on the safe side, I continue to recommend that men, who choose to undertake testosterone replacement therapy, always have their prostate carefully checked (both with a physical exam and blood tests – either the total or free PSA, or the newly "approved" HAAH prostate cancer test) – before starting treatment and again at regular intervals during treatment.*

Want to Know More about Bio-Identical Male Hormone Replacement?

Although we've only scratched the surface about BHRT for men, we hope we've whetted your appetite enough to learn more about this important, but badly under-exploited area of medicine. Even though there is a huge amount of research on the subject, some of it going back many decades and much of it quite current, conventional medicine seems loathe to recognize it, preferring to stick with its misguided, patent medicine-oriented paradigms. It would not surprise us in the least if you found that your regular doctor knows less about the real benefits and risks of BHRT in men than you do, except perhaps for all its alleged "dangers."

BHRT is just as important for men as it is for women for living to a ripe old age in optimal heath. Despite what we may hear from the IOM and other so-called "experts," when used appropriately, bio-identical testosterone replacement in men is just as safe as bio-identical estrogens and progesterone are in women. Nevertheless, it seems most doctors would rather write prescriptions for Viagra®, Lipitor®, Proscar® (a prostate shrinker), antihypertensives, antidepressants, and countless other expensive, dangerous, patented symptom-suppressing drugs and not be bothered with treating the real causes of andropause properly.

Wouldn't you like your partner to live a long, healthy life, just like you? But if he's waiting for his doctor to ask him about starting testosterone replacement and other aspects of BHRT for men, he's likely to be a very old man before the subject ever comes up, if it ever does.

Want to learn more about male BHRT? We recommend you and your partner get started by reading our book on the subject: *Maximize Your Vitality & Potency for Men Over 40* (Smart Publications). In that book, we go into much greater depth on the subjects we could only skim in this chapter and lots more. You'll learn all about the value of BHRT for men and many other valuable natural treatments for andropause, so that when you and he go to see his doctor for a testosterone prescription, you'll be fully informed to discuss the possibilities.

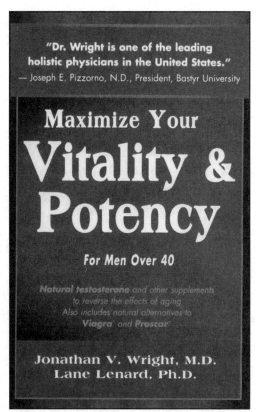

"Dr. Wright is one of the leading holistic physicians in the United States."
— Joseph E. Pizzorno, N.D., President, Bastyr University

Maximize Your
Vitality & Potency
For Men Over 40

Natural testosterone and other supplements to reverse the effects of aging
Also includes natural alternatives to Viagra® and Proscar®

Jonathan V. Wright, M.D.
Lane Lenard, Ph.D.

References

1. Liverman C, Blazer D, eds. *Testosterone and Aging: Clinical Research Directions*. Washington, DC: The National Academies Press; 2004.

2. Miner JN, Chang W, Chapman MS, et al. An orally active selective androgen receptor modulator is efficacious on bone, muscle, and sex function with reduced impact on prostate. *Endocrinology.* 2007;148:363-373.

3. Arver S, Dobs AS, Meikle AW, Allen RP, Sanders SW, Mazer NA. Improvement of sexual function in testosterone deficient men treated for 1 year with a permeation enhanced testosterone transdermal system. *J Urol.* 1996;155:1604-1608.

4. Rosano GM, Sheiban I, Massaro R, et al. Low testosterone levels are associated with coronary artery disease in male patients with angina. *Int J Impot Res.* 2007;19:176-182.

5. Pugh PJ, English KM, Jones TH, Channer KS. Testosterone: a natural tonic for the failing heart? *QJM.* 2000;93:689-694.

6. Jaffe MD. Effect of testosterone cypionate on postexercise ST segment depression. *Br Heart J.* 1977;39:1217-1222.

7. Malkin CJ, Morris PD, Pugh PJ, English KM, Channer KS. Effect of testosterone therapy on QT dispersion in men with heart failure. *Am J Cardiol.* 2003;92:1241-1243.

8. Pugh PJ, Jones TH, Channer KS. Acute haemodynamic effects of testosterone in men with chronic heart failure. *Eur Heart J.* 2003;24:909-915.

9. Malkin CJ, Pugh PJ, West JN, van Beek EJ, Jones TH, Channer KS. Testosterone therapy in men with moderate severity heart failure: a double-blind randomized placebo controlled trial. *Eur Heart J.* 2006;27:57-64.

10. Bennet A, Sie P, Caron P, et al. Plasma fibrinolytic activity in a group of hypogonadic men. *Scand J Clin Lab Invest.* 1987;47:23-27.

11. Winkler U. Effects of androgens on haemostasis. *Maturitas.* 1996;24:147-155.

12. Malkin CJ, Pugh PJ, Jones RD, Jones TH, Channer KS. Testosterone as a protective factor against atherosclerosis--immunomodulation and influence upon plaque development and stability. *J Endocrinol.* 2003;178:373-380.

13. Dai WS, Gutai JP, Kuller LH, Laporte RE, Falvo-Gerard L, Caggiula A. Relation between plasma high-density lipoprotein cholesterol and sex hormone concentrations in men. *Am J Cardiol.* 1984;53:1259-1263.

14. Dai WS, Kuller LH, LaPorte RE, Gutai JP, Falvo-Gerard L, Caggiula A. The epidemiology of plasma testosterone levels in middle-aged men. *Am J Epidemiol.* 1981;114:804-816.

15. Gutai J, LaPorte R, Kuller L, Dai W, Falvo-Gerard L, Caggiula A. Plasma testosterone, high density lipoprotein cholesterol and other lipoprotein fractions. *Am J Cardiol.* 1981;48:897-902.

16. Hamalainen E, Adlercreutz H, Ehnholm C, Puska P. Relationships of serum lipoproteins and apoproteins to sex hormones and to the binding capacity of sex hormone binding globulin in healthy Finnish men. *Metabolism.* 1986;35:535-541.

17. Heller RF, Wheeler MJ, Micallef J, Miller NE, Lewis B. Relationship of high density lipoprotein cholesterol with total and free testosterone and sex hormone binding globulin. *Acta Endocrinol (Copenh).* 1983;104:253-256.

18. Khaw KT, Barrett-Connor E. Endogenous sex hormones, high density lipoprotein cholesterol, and other lipoprotein fractions in men. *Arterioscler Thromb.* 1991;11:489-494.

19. Lichtenstein MJ, Yarnell JW, Elwood PC, et al. Sex hormones, insulin, lipids, and prevalent ischemic heart disease. *Am J Epidemiol.* 1987;126:647-657.

20. Barrett-Connor EL. Testosterone and risk factors for cardiovascular disease in men. *Diabete Metab.* 1995;21:156-161.

21. Marin P, Holmang S, Jonsson L, et al. The effects of testosterone treatment on body composition and metabolism in middle-aged obese men. *Int J Obes Relat Metab Disord.* 1992;16:991-997.

22. Morley JE, Perry HMD, Kaiser FE, et al. Effects of testosterone replacement therapy in old hypogonadal males: a preliminary study. *J Am Geriatr Soc.* 1993;41:149-152.

23. Tenover JL. Testosterone and the aging male. *J Androl.* 1997;18:103-106.

24. Urban RJ, Bodenburg YH, Gilkison C, et al. Testosterone administration to elderly men increases skeletal muscle strength and protein synthesis. *Am J Physiol.* 1995;269:E820-E826.

25. Zgliczynski S, Ossowski M, Slowinska-Srzednicka J, et al. Effect of testosterone replacement therapy on lipids and lipoproteins in hypogonadal and elderly men. *Atherosclerosis.* 1996;121:35-43.

26. Poor G, Atkinson EJ, Lewallen DG, O'Fallon WM, Melton LJ, 3rd. Age-related hip fractures in men: clinical spectrum and short-term outcomes. *Osteoporos Int.* 1995;5:419-426.

27. Poor G, Atkinson EJ, O'Fallon WM, Melton LJ, 3rd. Predictors of hip fractures in elderly men. *J Bone Miner Res.* 1995;10:1900-1907.

28. Poor G, Atkinson EJ, O'Fallon WM, Melton LJ, 3rd. Determinants of reduced survival following hip fractures in men. *Clin Orthop.* 1995:260-265.

29. Cooper C, Atkinson EJ, O'Fallon WM, Melton LJD. Incidence of clinically diagnosed vertebral fractures: a population- based study in Rochester, Minnesota, 1985-1989. *J Bone Miner Res.* 1992;7:221-227.

30. Seeman E. The dilemma of osteoporosis in men. *Am J Med.* 1995;98:76S-88S.

31. Seeman E. Osteoporosis in men. *Baillieres Clin Rheumatol.* 1997;11:613-629.

32. Anderson FH, Francis RM, Peaston RT, Wastell HJ. Androgen supplementation in eugonadal men with osteoporosis: effects of 6 months' treatment on markers of bone formation and resorption. *J Bone Miner Res.* 1997;12:472-478.

33. Griggs RC, Kingston W, Jozefowicz RF, Herr BE, Forbes G, Halliday D. Effect of testosterone on muscle mass and muscle protein synthesis. *J Appl Physiol.* 1989;66:498-503.

34. Katznelson L, Finkelstein JS, Schoenfeld DA, Rosenthal DI, Anderson EJ, Klibanski A. Increase in bone density and lean body mass during testosterone administration in men with acquired hypogonadism. *J Clin Endocrinol Metab.* 1996;81:4358-4365.

35. Seidell JC, Bjorntorp P, Sjostrom L, Kvist H, Sannerstedt R. Visceral fat accumulation in men is positively associated with insulin, glucose, and C-peptide levels, but negatively with testosterone levels. *Metabolism.* 1990;39:897-901.

36. Wang C, Eyre DR, Clark R, et al. Sublingual testosterone replacement improves muscle mass and strength, decreases bone resorption, and increases bone formation markers in hypogonadal men--a clinical research center study. *J Clin Endocrinol Metab.* 1996;81:3654-3662.

37. Dean JD, Carnegie C, Rodzvilla J, Smith T. Long-term effects of Testim® 1% testosterone gel in hypogonadal men. *Rev Urol.* 2005;6 Suppl 6:S22-29.

38. Needham J. *Science and Civilization in China, Vol. 5, Part 5*. Cambridge, UK: Cambridge University Press; 1983.

39. Heller C, Myers G. The male climacteric and its symptomatology, diagnosis and treatment. *JAMA.* 1944;126:472-477.

40. Pope HG, Jr., Cohane GH, Kanayama G, Siegel AJ, Hudson JI. Testosterone gel supplementation for men with refractory depression: a randomized, placebo-controlled trial. *Am J Psychiatry.* 2003;160:105-111.

41. Cherrier MM, Asthana S, Plymate S, et al. Testosterone supplementation improves spatial and verbal memory in healthy older men. *Neurology.* 2001;57:80-88.

42. Cherrier MM, Craft S, Matsumoto AH. Cognitive changes associated with supplementation of testosterone or dihydrotestosterone in mildly hypogonadal men: a preliminary report. *J Androl.* 2003;24:568-576.

43. Cherrier MM, Anawalt BD, Herbst KL, et al. Cognitive effects of short-term manipulation of serum sex steroids in healthy young men. *J Clin Endocrinol Metab.* 2002;87:3090-3096.

44. Bussiere JR, Beer TM, Neiss MB, Janowsky JS. Androgen deprivation impairs memory in older men. *Behav Neurosci.* 2005;119:1429-1437.

45. Daniell HW. Osteoporosis after orchiectomy for prostate cancer [see comments]. *J Urol.* 1997;157:439-444.

46. Janowsky JS, Chavez B, Orwoll E. Sex steroids modify working memory. *J Cogn Neurosci.* 2000;12:407-414.

47. Moffat SD. Effects of testosterone on cognitive and brain aging in elderly men. *Ann N Y Acad Sci.* 2005;1055:80-92.

48. Rosario ER, Carroll JC, Oddo S, LaFerla FM, Pike CJ. Androgens regulate the development of neuropathology in a triple transgenic mouse model of Alzheimer's disease. *J Neurosci.* 2006;26:13384-13389.

49. Cherrier MM, Matsumoto AM, Amory JK, et al. Testosterone improves spatial memory in men with Alzheimer disease and mild cognitive impairment. *Neurology.* 2005;64:2063-2068.

50. Tan RS, Pu SJ. A pilot study on the effects of testosterone in hypogonadal aging male patients with Alzheimer's disease. *Aging Male.* 2003;6:13-17.

51. Penson D, Chan J. Prostate Cancer. *http://kidney.niddk.nih.gov/statistics/uda/Prostate_Cancer-Chapter03.pdf.* National Institute of Diabetes and Digestive and Kidney Diseases: Accessed March 11, 2007.

52. Wei J, Calhoun E, Jacobsen S. Benign Prostatic Hyperplasia. In: Litwin M, Saigal C, eds. *Urologic Diseases in America: Interim Compendium.* Washington, DC: US Department of Health and Human Services, Public Health Service, National Institutes of Health, National Institute of Diabetes and Digestive and Kidney Diseases.; 2004:43-67.

53. Heikkila R, Aho K, Heliovaara M, et al. Serum testosterone and sex hormone-binding globulin concentrations and the risk of prostate carcinoma: a longitudinal study. *Cancer.* 1999;86:312-315.

54. Schatzl G, Madersbacher S, Thurridl T, et al. High-grade prostate cancer is associated with low serum testosterone levels. *Prostate.* 2001;47:52-58.

55. Shores MM, Matsumoto AM, Sloan KL, Kivlahan DR. Low serum testosterone and mortality in male veterans. *Arch Intern Med.* 2006;166:1660-1665.

56. Pechersky AV, Mazurov VI, Semiglazov VF, Karpischenko AI, Mikhailichenko VV, Udintsev AV. Androgen administration in middle-aged and ageing men: effects of oral testosterone undecanoate on dihydrotestosterone, oestradiol and prostate volume. *Int J Androl.* 2002;25:119-125.

57. Wiren S, Stocks T, Rinaldi S, et al. Androgens and prostate cancer risk: a prospective study. *Prostate.* 2007;67:1230-1237.

58. Marks LS, Mazer NA, Mostaghel E, et al. Effect of testosterone replacement therapy on prostate tissue in men with late-onset hypogonadism: A randomized controlled trial. *JAMA.* 2006;296:2351-2361.

CHAPTER 11

COMPOUNDED BIO-IDENTICAL HORMONES: JUST WHAT THE DOCTOR ORDERED

The Triad

We don't often think about it, but when we fill a prescription at a pharmacy, we enter into a three-way relationship, or "Triad" that includes 1) the *doctor*, who determines the patient's needs and writes the prescription; 2) the *pharmacist,* who fills the prescription; and 3) us, the *person* who uses the medication (Fig. 11-1).

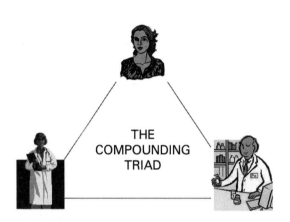

THE COMPOUNDING TRIAD

Figure 11-1.

As we explain in this chapter, the Triad relationship is most significant for women (and men) who are using BHRT. However, for women who elect conventional "hormone replacement" therapy (HRT) – or most other patent medicines – it is virtually invisible.

You know the drill: Once your gynecologist or family physician diagnoses menopause or perimenopause, he or she writes you a "script," which you take to your local CVS or Walgreen's, where the pharmacist – often anonymous and interchangeable – grabs a bottle of PremPro® off the shelf and counts out a month's worth of pills, which you bring home and take one a day, as instructed.

This is a classic example of an extremely bad characteristic of conventional medicine: instead of recognizing that each woman is a unique individual, it treats all woman exactly the same. (To be "fair," conventional medicine does the same thing to men!) It matters little who your doctor is or who your pharmacist is; your drug dose is standardized at the factory, regardless of your age, estrogen levels, stage of menopause, or other health conditions you might have. (*But it's a perfect system for a species of identical living robots!*)

If your HRT prescription winds up causing you unpleasant or dangerous side effects at the recommended doses – 0.3 milligrams of Premarin® and 1.5 milligrams of Provera® these days – your doctor can't lower the dose any farther, because Wyeth – the drug's manufacturer – doesn't make lower doses. Besides, there's no solid clinical evidence that lower doses would be any better.

After a few months, you may go back to your doctor for a check-up to see how you're doing and what side effects you might be experiencing. There's no point in having your hormone levels checked, because there are no *normal* levels of horse estrogens or pseudoprogesterone patent medicines in the human body. *All levels of these substances are abnormal!* If you are experiencing side effects, your only real options are to endure them, switch to a different regimen (preferably BHRT) or give up on hormone replacement altogether.

By contrast, women who elect BHRT find the "Triad" relationship profoundly important. While any doctor can write a prescription for PremPro®, doctors who prescribe BHRT need to have special knowledge and training to do so properly. They understand that they are treating you, not merely to suppress your hot flushes and other annoying symptoms, but rather to restore your sex steroid hormone balance as closely as possible to your premenopausal levels. They take the extra time to get to know your menstrual history. In coordination with your compounding pharmacist, they carefully instruct you in their proper use and have you return to the office periodically to monitor your hormone levels, as well as the treatment's effectiveness and possible side effects. Based on this information, they can fine tune your doses to achieve the optimal outcome.

It is not uncommon for your doctor and compounding pharmacist to consult with each other, and for doctors with less experience prescribing bio-identical hormones, to rely on an experienced compounding pharmacist for advice about proper dosing strategies.

Compounding Pharmacies: Back to the Future

More now than ever before, people are becoming dissatisfied with conventional medicine's "nothing-but-standardized-patent-medicines" approach and have been aggressively seeking out nonstandard medical alternatives. The public demand for more *natural and individualized health care*, as well for the economic and human benefits of *small, traditional, personal service pharmacies,* have combined to stimulate the rebirth of the compounding pharmacy.

Bio-identical hormones, which have been leading the return to compounding, can be obtained with a prescription only from one of the growing number of *compounding pharmacies* in the United States. Compounding pharmacists, most of whom also dispense ordinary pharmaceuticals, are able to custom prepare hormones for each patient in the form (eg, cream, gel, lozenge, oral capsule, etc) that is best suited to her/his individual needs and preferences, as directed by their doctor's prescription.

In the centuries before the patent medicine industry took over the manufacturing of nearly all medications, every pharmacist was a compounding pharmacist. As recently as the 1930s and early '40s, about 60% of all prescriptions were compounded locally in the neighborhood pharmacy. Today, though, most ordinary pharmacists have been relegated to little more than over-educated pill counters. In fact, in some locations, vending machines that dispense prescription drugs like candy or soda have started appearing. "I liken it to a Coke machine," remarked an official at a Rhode Island clinic that uses these machines. "You put the order in, and plop, it comes out."[1]

Many small, traditional, personal-service pharmacies are being driven out of business by cost-cutting insurance companies, "managed care" organizations, HMOs, and Medicaid that contract with giant "big-box" drugstore chains to offer massive quantities of deeply discounted manufactured patent medicines. Some insurance companies and managed care organizations even have their own mail-in patent medicine warehouse operations, by-passing ordinary pharmacies altogether. Against this kind of competition, the local, privately owned pharmacy doesn't stand a chance.[2]

However, with consumer demand rising rapidly, and with modern technology and innovative techniques and research available, compounding is becoming a valuable path to economic survival for an increasing number of smaller, personal-service pharmacies. And for pharmacists who want to use their education for more than pill counting, compounding offers a professionally satisfying return to their roots.

Most compounding pharmacists belong to professional organizations, such as the *International Academy of Compounding Pharmacists (IACP)*, the *Professional Compounding Centers of America (PCCA)*, the *National Community Pharmacists Association (NCPA)*, and the *American Pharmacists Association (APhA)*, which perform such vital functions as continuing education; updating practice standards; advocacy in courts, Congress, and the public arena to raise awareness of the value of compounding; supplying pharmacists with FDA-approved unformulated chemicals, compounding equipment, and other supplies; and pharmacy locating and referral services.

Today, independent compounding pharmacies, most which tend to be relatively small "neighborhood" businesses, are literally our only sources for prescription bio-identical hormones and other individualized prescription items. Run by dedicated, well-trained compounding pharmacists, they are a welcome change from huge chain "drugstores," which tend to be little more than convenience stores with a patent medicine department in the back.

Most physicians graduate from medical school completely ignorant about BHRT. Since the patent medicine model of medicine has been the only one taught in American medical schools for several generations, chances are that anything a young doctor does happen to learn about bio-identical hormones (and it's probably not very much) is going to be off-putting, misleading, and wrong.

This is where compounding pharmacists can often serve an important educational function in their community by providing doctors (and patients) with valuable information about bio-identical hormone dosing and prescribing. Some compounding pharmacists even run seminars on BHRT for local physicians and also for the community at large.

Customized Dosing

Compounding pharmacists can produce literally whatever the doctor orders, usually in a variety of forms that best suit each patient's individual needs. They have access to bulk quantities of high-quality, (including some *FDA-"approved")* bio-identical hormones, and other bio-identical hormones, including estriol, which are "approved" by Mother Nature if not by the FDA, as well as the specialized equipment they need to process them. They measure out appropriate doses and add them to whichever medium (eg, cream, gel) the physician has prescribed and the patient is most comfortable with. In order to facilitate accurate dosing, they usually put hormone formulations into a set of small syringes (without needles, of course) for precise measurement of dosages.

Most pharmacies are able to do simple compounding, like combining two ointments into one or adding a flavoring to liquid medication to make it easier for a child to consume. However, only specialized pharmacies can perform more complex compounding, such as that required to produce bio-identical hormone preparations, which may account for half of the prescriptions the compounding a pharmacy fills. The equipment needed for complicated compounding can be quite costly. For example, if a compounded preparation must be sterile – not typically required for BHRT – an entire "clean room" might be needed.

The medications and hormones that compounding pharmacists produce are indistinguishable in chemical structure from the mass-produced variety, except that they're thankfully missing the usual chemical dyes, flavorings, fillers, and preservatives that may cause allergic or sensitivity reactions in some people; nor do they come in the range of shapes, colors, and designs patent drug companies often use to distinguish their products from the competition – Remember "*The Purple Pill?*" – and to discourage drug "counterfeiting." They can also adjust the dose to fit each person's unique physiology. This is especially important, as we have pointed out, for bio-identical hormones. Were it not for this service, bio-identical hormones would not be available.

Even if patent medicine companies truly appreciated the benefits of bio-identical hormones, they would still not market them, not only because they are unpatentable, but also because they're impractical from a mass production perspective. For both reasons, they're not nearly as profitable as a one- (or in some cases, two- or three-) size-fits-all mass marketed patent medicine. Compounding pharmacists, on the other hand, are in a good position to produce high-quality, individualized bio-identical hormone preparations without having to worry about mass production, packaging, distribution, and marketing, not to mention the nonmedical demands of Boards of Directors, and stockholders. While it's true they're not nearly as profitable, compounding pharmacists – most of whom are philosophically convinced that individual treatment for each individual is best – can still make a living.

Despite the slanders we hear in the media from BHRT opponents, the quality of individually prepared bio-identical hormones or drugs produced by compounding pharmacists is typically excellent for several reasons:

- The materials used by compounding pharmacies are the same pure-grade, high- quality chemicals used by the major patent medicine companies. All materials are subject to FDA inspection and the agency's Good Manufacturing Procedures code.

- While all pharmacists receive a minimal amount of compounding training in pharmacy school, compounding pharmacists opt for more extensive postgraduate training in the most up-to-date compounding methods.

- Recently, the *Pharmacy Compounding Accreditation Board (PCAB)* has been set 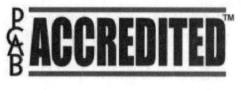 up to provide voluntary accreditation for all compounding pharmacies. The PCAB Seal assures physicians and customers that a compounding pharmacy meets the highest quality and safety standards.

- Like all other pharmacies, every compounding pharmacy is licensed and inspected by its State Pharmacy Board.

The FDA, urged on by the patent medicine industry, has tried in recent years to usurp the states' regulatory function over compounding pharmacies, and in the process to limit or even do away with compounding altogether. It's no surprise that Big Pharma would like to see competition from compounding pharmacists eliminated. So far, this effort has been stalled in the courts and Congress, thanks to the vigorous lobbying and legal efforts of representatives of the compounding pharmacists, knowledgeable medical professionals, hundreds of thousands of concerned consumers, and others fearful of losing their access to bio-identical hormones and other compounded medications. For the moment, at least, the compounding pharmacy, one of the last bastions of health care freedom remaining in the United States, seems safe, but things could change rapidly. (*See Chapter 12 for more about efforts to eliminate compounding pharmacies.*)

How to Find a Compounding Pharmacist

Compounding pharmacies are located all over the country, and finding one is not usually very difficult. If there is no compounding pharmacy nearby, you can almost always work with one anywhere in the country via mail, email, internet, phone, and/or fax.

The easiest way to locate a compounding pharmacist is to contact either the International Academy of Compounding Pharmacists (IACP) or the Professional Compounding Centers of America, Inc. (PCCA).

International Academy of Compounding Pharmacists (IACP)
4638 Riverstone Blvd.
Missouri City, TX 77459
Internet: www.iacprx.org
Tel: 281-933-8400
Compounding Pharmacist Referral: 800-927-4227
Fax: 281-495-0602

Professional Compounding Centers of America, Inc. (PCCA)
9901 South Wilcrest Drive
Houston, TX 77099
Internet: www.pccarx.com
Tel: 800-331-2498 or 281-933-6948
Fax: 800-874-5760 or 281-933-6627

PCCA (Canada)
744 Third Street
London, ON
Canada N5V 5J2
Internet: www.pccarx.ca
Tel: 800-668-9453 or 519-455-0690
Fax: 800-799-4537 or 519-455-0697

PCCA (Australia)
Unit 1, 73 Beauchamp Road
Matraville, NSW 2036 Australia
Tel: 02-9316-1500
Fax: 02-9316-7422

Compounding Costs and Insurance Coverage

The cost of compounded medications, including bio-identical hormones, tends to be competitive with ordinary patent medications, and this cost has usually been reimbursed by most health insurance plans. However, recently some major insurance companies have adopted a new policy of refusing to cover BHRT prescriptions, based on the bogus claim that compounded bio-identical hormones are *"experimental, investigational, and unproven"* and *"not medically necessary."*

The insurance companies claim to have based this action on the results of a biased, unscientific FDA survey of a few compounding pharmacies that has been thoroughly debunked. (*See Chapter 12 for more about this FDA survey.*) Nevertheless, it seems likely that they are using this "survey" merely as an excuse to succumb to pressure from their Big Pharma clients, who have been pulling out all stops to crush BHRT competition from compounding pharmacies.

Obtaining a Prescription for Bio-Identical Hormones

Bio-identical estrogens and testosterone are available only with a physician's prescription. Progesterone and DHEA can be purchased without a prescription, but, while some of these over-the-counter (OTC) products may be quite acceptable, some may not be. To avoid the uncertainty, we always recommend that you obtain your bio-identical hormones by doctor's prescription from a compounding pharmacist. Compounding pharmacies have access to the highest quality raw materials and can be trusted to prepare them at the proper dose. The same cannot always be said about nonprescription products sold in drug stores, health food stores, or over the internet.

Women desirous of something other than patented HRT formulations to relieve their menopausal symptoms often start by looking to their "regular" gynecologist or family physician. Unfortunately, more often than not, this strategy leads to disappointment. Because most of their hormone- and drug-related information comes from drug company "sales reps" and industry-sponsored medical journals, advertising, conventions, and continuing "medical education" (CME) programs, the average medical doctor knows lots about PremPro® and other alien patent medicines, but next to nothing about the benefits and proper use of bio-identical hormones (or other substances natural to the human body, for that matter. Sad, no?). In fact, because they are exposed to so much misinformation about BHRT, most of what mainstream doctors might *think* they know about bio-identical hormones is probably wrong.

Moreover, mainstream doctors are all too often intimidated by the FDA as well as by their state medical boards, medical societies, and other peer groups, all of which tend to reflexively disapprove of BHRT and other nonpatented "natural" remedies. It is not uncommon for these government agencies and regulatory and professional organizations to harass doctors who prescribe bio-identical hormones and other "unconventional" treatments, sometimes even to the point of revoking their licenses to practice medicine.

If your regular doctor has closed his or her mind to BHRT, though, rather than argue about it and try to convince him/her, it may be best to move on and find another doctor who is more knowledgeable, or at least more open-minded.

On the bright side, growing numbers of physicians are becoming dissatisfied with the "approved" methods available for treating menopausal women, because, in addition to well-known clinical studies like the WHI, they've also seen with their own eyes how unpleasant and dangerous these treatments can be. Open-minded enough to recognize that the patent medicine industry doesn't have all the answers, many physicians are happy to oblige women who ask for BHRT, because they're genuinely looking for better ways to help their patients. If your doctor fits this description, we suggest you recommend he/she read this book to help convince them that the FDA/conventional medicine claims that BHRT is unsafe and unproven are false and completely unfounded.

Beware of "False Prophets" of BHRT

However, not all physicians who are willing to prescribe BHRT know enough about it to do a proper job. Among those physicians who've been able to see through government/drug company lies, some may be paying too much attention to a few vocal advocates of BHRT, who promote themselves as BHRT "experts," but whose knowledge is often superficial, incomplete, and oversimplified at best.

How can you tell who these mistaken vocal advocates may be? A key indicator is a relative or total lack of emphasis on rigorous follow-up monitoring for safety and efficacy. Moreover, the excessively high doses of bio-identical hormones they may recommend (often just 100% estradiol and progesterone) tend to produce circulating levels of estradiol and estrone far in excess of that to which even a young woman's body is accustomed. They also often opt for oral dosing, overlooking the safest, most effective routes of administration (transdermal and transmucosal). These "variations" of BHRT may indeed reduce menopausal symptoms, probably with fewer unpleasant side effects than Prempro®, but evidence suggests they may also increase the risk of breast cancer, heart disease, and thromboembolism. (*See Chapter 9.*)

The Compounding Pharmacy Connection

Perhaps the easiest way to find a physician who's experienced in prescribing BHRT is to ask a nearby compounding pharmacist which doctors they work with and whom they would recommend.

An increasing number of "regular" doctors, though uninformed about BHRT, have nevertheless heard enough good things about it to pique their interest and may be willing to give it a try. However, they probably don't know enough to be comfortable prescribing it, and may not realize that prescribing BHRT is much more complicated than prescribing PremPro®.

If your doctor is willing but not necessarily able, you may be able to help make him/her more comfortable by putting him/her in touch with a local compounding pharmacist who is experienced in BHRT. Dealing with hundreds of BHRT prescriptions each month, compounding pharmacists can also be a veritable fount of experience and information for doctors just getting their prescribing feet wet. Compounding pharmacists are always eager to offer inexperienced doctors support, reassurance, and education in prescribing bio-identical hormones. Having such a consultation with a well-informed professional, who can explain the advantages of these products and provide some dosing guidelines, is often enough to convince most hesitant doctors to at least give them a try.

In addition to one-on-one consultations, compounding pharmacists working with physicians expert in BHRT (including the author – JVW) sometimes hold seminars for doctors (as well as for patients) interested in learning about the latest BHRT research and dosing guidelines. Your physician can find information about BHRT seminars for physicians and other health care professionals at www.tahomaclinic.com and/or www.bioidenticalhormonesociety.com

Finding a Doctor

Although the American Medical Association would probably like you to believe otherwise, there are qualified medical professionals who are not members and might even have letters other than MD after their name. Many of these doctors have a far better understanding of bio-identical hormones, and usually considerably more experience in using them than the average "regular" MD.

A quick and easy way to find a knowledgeable, open-minded doctor is to locate one who is a member of the American College for Advancement in Medicine (ACAM), the International College of Integrative Medicine (ICIM), the American Academy of Environmental Medicine (AAEM), and some members of the American Association of Naturopathic Physicians (AANP).

The American College for Advancement in Medicine

ACAM is a not-for-profit medical society dedicated to educating physicians and other health care professionals on the latest findings and emerging procedures in preventive/nutritional medicine, including BHRT. ACAM's goals are to improve doctors' skills, knowledge, and diagnostic procedures as they relate to complementary and alternative medicine; to support research; and to develop awareness of alternative methods of medical treatment.

The largest and oldest organization of its kind in the world dedicated exclusively to serving the educational needs of the health professions, ACAM represents more than 1,000 physicians in 30 countries. All ACAM members are skilled and experienced in the prescription and use of bio-identical hormones, as well as of various nutritional, herbal, and botanical products. ACAM members have studied and listened to discussions by dozens of experts [including the author (JVW) on occasion] concerning the biochemistry, effects, and uses of these substances.

For a referral to an ACAM doctor near you, contact the organization at:

<u>American College for Advancement in Medicine</u>
24411 Ridge Route Ste 115
Laguna Hills, CA 92653
Physician Referral Hotline: 888-439-6891
Internet: www.acamnet.org

The International College of Integrative Medicine

ICIM is a community of healthcare professionals dedicated to advancing emergent innovative therapies in integrative and preventive healthcare by conducting educational sessions, supporting research and publications and cooperating with other professional and scientific organizations, while always promoting the highest standards of practice. They offer advanced medical care, which combines the best of conventional, preventive, and innovative health care. Their goals are to dramatically improve the quality of life of their patients, prevent illness, extend lives, provide safe, effective treatments, and reduce costs. They believe that every patient has the right to receive and they have the responsibility to offer advanced, healing medicine, and they advocate a massive research and educational effort to explore the many variables and techniques that can be used together to promote healing and achieve high-level wellness.

For a referral to an ICIM doctor near you, contact the organization at:

<u>International College of Integrative Medicine</u>
122 Thurman St.
Box 271
Bluffton, OH 45817
Email: wendy@icimed.com
Telephone: (866) 464-5226, (419) 358-0273
Internet: www.icimed.com/

The American Academy of Environmental Medicine

AAEM was founded in 1965 by a group of clinicians from various specialties, who formed a medical society that has evolved into the American Academy of Environmental Medicine. Their mission is to promote optimal health through prevention and safe and effective treatment of the causes of illness by supporting physicians and other professionals in serving the public through education about the interaction between humans and their environment.

For a referral to an AAEM doctor near you, contact the organization at:

The American Academy of Environmental Medicine
6505 E. Central Avenue, #296
Wichita, KS 67206
Phone: (316) 684-5500
Fax: (316) 684-5709
Email: administrator@aaemonline.org
Internet: www.aaemonline.org/

American Association of Naturopathic Physicians

Naturopathic medicine is based on the belief and observation that when the human body is given the correct natural materials and energies, it possesses enormous power to heal itself. Unlike conventional MDs, naturopathic physicians strongly emphasize *disease prevention, lifestyle change,* and *optimizing wellness.*

After earning a standard undergraduate degree, including premedical requirements, such as chemistry, biochemistry, biology, and physics, future naturopathic physicians go on to a 4-year graduate level, accredited naturopathic school of medicine, where, upon graduation, they earn an ND degree. NDs receive training in all the same sciences as MDs, but with less emphasis on drugs, radiation, and surgery, and more emphasis on nutrition, bio-identical hormones, botanical remedies, manipulation, homeopathy, acupuncture, psychology, and other holistic and nontoxic therapies. Before licensure, naturopathic physicians must complete at least 4,000 hours of study in specified subject areas and then pass a series of rigorous professional board exams.

Although naturopathic physicians can be found in every US state and Canadian province, they're currently licensed by state boards only in Alaska, Arizona, California, Connecticut, Hawaii, Idaho, Kansas, Maine, Montana, New Hampshire, Oregon, Utah, Vermont, Washington, and the District of Columbia, as well as the US territories of Puerto Rico and the US Virgin Islands. In Canada, naturopaths are licensed in British Columbia, Manitoba, Ontario, and Saskatchewan. (Naturopathic physicians are allowed to prescribe BHRT in some states, but not all.)

To locate a naturopathic physician, contact the *American Association of Naturopathic Physicians (AANP)* at:

American Association of Naturopathic Physicians
4435 Wisconsin Avenue, NW
Suite 403
Washington, DC 20016
Tel: 866-538-2267
Fax: 202-237-8152
Internet: http://www.naturopathic.org

Osteopathic Physicians

After earning an undergraduate degree, doctors of osteopathic medicine graduate from a 4-year osteopathic medical school with a DO degree. Osteopaths' training and accreditation is also similar to that which medical doctors receive.

Most osteopaths are primary-care physicians, but many specialize in such areas as internal medicine, surgery, pediatrics, radiology, or pathology. Residencies in these areas typically require an additional 2 to 6 years of training beyond medical school.

Although many DOs are members of the AMA, generally they differ from MDs in their emphasis on the "whole person" as well as on a *preventive approach* to the practice of medicine. Rather than treating (ie, suppressing) specific symptoms, as most conventional "allopathic" MDs are usually taught to do, DOs are trained to focus on the body's various systems – particularly the musculoskeletal system – and how they interact with each other. Although DOs can and do prescribe conventional drugs, and many practice in a way that is indistinguishable from the average AMA member, in general they are more likely to be open to and knowledgeable about natural remedies, including BHRT.

Osteopaths are licensed to practice medicine and prescribe drugs and bio-identical hormones in all US states and Canadian provinces. To find an osteopath, a good starting point is the *American Osteopathic Association (AOA)* or the *Canadian Osteopathic Association (COA)*. The American Osteopathic Association can be contacted at:

American Osteopathic Association
142 E. Ontario Street
Chicago, IL 60611-2864
Tel: 800-621-1773
Fax: 312-202-8200
Internet: www.osteopathic.org/

Canadian Osteopathic Association
P.O. Box 24081
London, Ontario
N6H 5C4 Canada
Tel: 519-439-5521
Internet: www.osteopathic.ca/

Other Good Sources of Information about Bio-Identical Hormones

Several new medical organizations dedicated to furthering bio-identical hormone research and prescribing have recently formed:

International Hormone Society

The International Hormone Society (IHS) has two major goals: 1) to make the public aware of the importance and availability of doctors specializing in the medical science of hormone deficiencies or excesses and in the medicine of aging; and 2) to work within the medical community to bring the "medicine of aging" to a more prominent level of utilization in the various medical specialties.

IHS collects and summarizes significant data with respect to the safe use of hormone therapies. This includes the most recent advances in applied hormone therapies utilizing human growth hormone, DHEA, melatonin, thyroid, testosterone, estrogens, progesterone, and others.
The best way to contact the IHS is through their website: www. intlhormonesociety.org.

The Bio-Identical Hormone Society

An excellent source of high-level medical information about BHRT is the Bio-Identical Hormone Society. BHS was founded on the medical imperative to provide reliable and predictive body chemistry management centered on hormone analysis, quality interpretation, and bio-identical hormone management. BHS is devoted to administering bio-identical hormone science to the individual patient with the express goal of naturally optimizing body chemistry to age, lifestyle, and personal goals. Another goal is to provide physicians with the best testing methods, to equip them with the ability to prescribe bio-identical hormones with high specificity and confidence, and to understand the pros and cons of hormone therapy.

The BHS website is the most complete source of literature support for bio-identical hormone replacement therapy available anywhere. The BHS document archive is an easy-to-explore repository of current thought, published science, and clinical insights on BHRT. It includes the most extensive and up-to-date collection of relevant full-length articles and abstracts, many of which are contributed by BHS members.

BHS also sponsors regular seminars where doctors and pharmacists can learn about the latest BHRT dosing guidelines developed over the last 25 years. The seminar faculty includes the author (JVW) and other knowledgeable physicians.

Access the BHS at their website: www.bioidenticalhormonesociety.com.

American Association for Health Freedom

The AAHF is a division of the Health Freedom Foundation (HFF), a nonprofit organization that promotes access to integrative medicine, dietary supplements, and, of course, bio-identical hormones. AAHF has been particularly effective in the political realms of lobbying and litigating. Their website is an excellent source of news regarding the politics of BHRT and other areas of natural and natural/alternative/integrative medicine. They also provide a search engine for locating physicians who prescribe BHRT.

American Association for Health Freedom
4620 Lee Highway, Suite 210
Arlington, VA 22207
Phone: 800-230-2762 or 703-294-6244
Fax: 703-294-6380
Internet: www.healthfreedom.net/

Women in Balance

Women in Balance (WIB) is a national, nonprofit association of women, doctors, health care professionals and organizations dedicated to helping women achieve hormone balance. Women in Balance was founded to educate women and the health care community about hormone imbalance, and its impact on a woman's health and well-being as she ages. WIB was born out of the desire to be a trusted health resource for women over 40 who are experiencing the natural hormonal transitions of perimenopause and menopause.

They strongly believe that hormone balance is essential to a woman's overall health and well-being, greatly affecting her longevity and quality of life. The organization is dedicated to empowering women to take charge of their hormone health. They are dedicated to the proposition that the "one dose fits all" approach to achieving hormone balance and optimal health for women is wrong. Ideally, each woman should work with a qualified health professional to determine her unique health needs. If hormones are recommended, bioidentical hormones should be used only in physiological doses.

WIB also provides a physician-finder to help you locate physicians and healthcare providers in your area who practice in accord with their principles.

Women in Balance
PO Box 5517
Washington, DC 20016
Also: PO Box 12004, Overland Park, KS 66282
Email: info@womeninbalance.org
Internet: www.womeninbalance.org/

Bioidentical Hormone Initiative

A community of conventionally trained, practicing physicians who have successfully used bioidentical hormones for decades, the BHI is dedicated to prevention, patient advocacy and the practice of humanistic medicine through the use of bioidentical hormones, supplements, diet, exercise, lifestyle, sleep, and stress management.

Founded by a group of conventionally trained, practicing physicians who have successfully used bioidentical hormones for decades to treat hormone imbalances in men and women, the Bioidentical Hormone Initiative seeks to encourage the use of bioidentical hormone therapy as a key tool in the growing movement to promote true prevention with respect, compassion, and patient advocacy.

To make this possible, BHI seeks to inspire a community of concerned, like-minded caregivers by sharing the latest theories, science, and practical, clinical experience on their website and through an active program of online webinars, case reviews, and outreach. Members of their peer network have access to cutting-edge experts in bioidentical hormones, supplements, diet, exercise, lifestyle, sleep, and stress management, who focus on improving patients' lives through true prevention.

BHI also sponsors the *Bioidentical Hormone Institute*, America's first physician-led, fully-accredited continuing education (CE) and continuing medical education (CME) institute dedicated to the ongoing training of physicians and other caregivers in the clinical use of bioidentical hormones for aging, prevention, and overall health and wellness.

BHI's Guiding Principles include:

- Restoring humanity to a safer healthcare system by providing care, respect, hope, and empowerment to their patients.
- Recognizing the importance of the doctor-patient relationship and understanding that the patient comes first,
- Focusing on true prevention, rather than the diagnosis of disease.
- Incorporating the use of bioidentical hormones, supplements, diet, exercise, lifestyle, sleep, and stress management into a comprehensive new medicine based on humanism and compassion.

BHI is in the process of building a Patient Referral Network of accredited physicians to help you find physician who is trained in the use of BHRT and other BHI guiding principles.

Bioidentical Hormone Initiative
Internet: www.bioidenticalhormoneinitiative.org

References

1. Rowland C. Drug vending units worry pharmacists. *Boston Globe.* July 3, 2004; http://www.boston.com/news/nation/articles/2004/07/03/drug_vending_units_ worry_pharmacists/?page=2:Accessed April 13, 2007.

2. Russakoff D. The corner drugstore, barely clinging to health. *The Washington Post.* July 1, 2007;http://www.washingtonpost.com/wp-dyn/content/ article/2007/06/30/ AR2007063000309.html: Accessed October 31, 2007.

FREE Hormone Assessment!

www.stayyoungandsexy.com

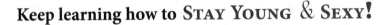

Keep learning how to STAY YOUNG & SEXY!

- Do you need bio-identical hormones? Take the on-line self assessment!
- Find a knowledgeable doctor and compounding pharmacy!
- Join the community forum and share your success!
- Sign up for FREE email updates regarding bio-identical hormones!

Plus:
Claim your FREE sex-enhancing product from one of our sponsors!

You can STAY YOUNG & SEXY! when you visit
www.stayyoungandsexy.com

CHAPTER 12

THE POLITICS OF BIO-IDENTICAL HORMONES: WHY AND HOW THEY'RE TRYING TO TAKE THEM AWAY

"First they ignore you, then they ridicule you, then they fight you, then you win."

— *Mahatma Gandhi*

In an ideal world, a menopausal therapy as promising as bio-identical hormone replacement (BHRT) would be happily welcomed by the medical establishment. This is especially so in light of recent findings confirming the dangers – including increased risks of heart disease and cancer – of the dominant conventional "hormone replacement" therapy (HRT) – Premarin® + Provera® (Prempro®).

But as we all know, the world of conventional medicine is far from ideal, in large part due to its domination by the global pharmaceutical (patent medicine) industry and its confederates in the federal Food and Drug Administration (FDA). Thanks to aggressive, multi-pronged, coordinated attacks by these entities, BHRT exists in the United States today in a legal/regulatory "twilight zone," forced to fight off constant, costly, attacks by government agencies, industry, and medical professional and advocacy groups, all of which are well-financed and encouraged by Big Pharma, especially Wyeth Pharmaceutical, the world's largest manufacturer of conventional "hormone replacement" products, including Premarin® and Prempro®.

"If the FDA Takes a Tougher Stand on Compounding, Wyeth Stands to Benefit."

Conventional medicine doesn't know what to make of a superior but *unpatentable* treatment like BHRT. Although they may doubt the value of the research that supports BHRT's safety and health benefits, one would think that they would at least recognize its *potential*. Ironically, they do recognize BHRT's potential: not it's potential as valuable treatment for menopausal women, but rather its potential as a *threat to their profits*.

An article in *BusinessWeek Online* spelled out the relationship between Wyeth Pharmaceuticals and the FDA quite simply: "If the FDA takes a tougher stand on compounding, Wyeth stands to benefit. Annual sales of the Premarin family of drugs shriveled in the wake of the Women's Health Initiative [WHI] study, falling from $2.1 billion in 2001 to $909 million… [in 2005]. Wyeth is now fighting 4,500 personal injury cases related to Premarin® and Prempro®."[1]

Let's try a little thought experiment. Imagine that bio-identical hormones were completely patentable, just like Premarin®, Provera®, and thousands of other drugs. Without a doubt, Big Pharma would be all over them; you can be sure of that. In their day, Premarin® and Provera® were among the largest selling drugs in the world, worth *billions* in profits for Wyeth, even though hundreds of studies conducted in laboratories and women all over the world have demonstrated that bio-identical hormones are safer and more efficacious.

As the Baby Boom generation floods into their menopausal years, the demand for safe, effective hormone replacement grows stronger every year. What if patentability were not an issue? Based on what scientific research currently tells us about HRT and BHRT, what woman in her right mind would freely choose estrogens designed for a horse over those designed for a human?

If bio-identical hormones were patentable, their existing scientific data base (*see Moskowitz,[2] Head,[3] Holtorf,[4] and previous chapters in this book for recent comprehensive reviews of these data*) would be more than sufficient for patent medicine companies to justify the requisite large-scale clinical trials required to get them FDA-approved and onto the market, where they could easily earn back their research costs. Bio-identical hormones currently have much, much more research support than Premarin® and Provera® did before their introduction. However, since bio-identical hormones are not patentable, Big Pharma's enthusiasm for spending hundreds of millions of dollars to get them FDA-"approved" tends to wane rather quickly.

Based on past performance, though, it doesn't take much of a leap to at least *wonder* whether BHRT might be a superior option. If drug companies would only run a couple of their typical large, long-term, well-controlled, *comparative* clinical trials to try to verify or disprove these nearly uniformly positive "preliminary" findings, we have every confidence that all doubt about the value of BHRT would quickly vanish and the FDA would "approve" their use.

A fair comparison of published clinical and nonclinical research on HRT and BHRT clearly shows BHRT to be far safer and more effective (*See Holtorf's recent review, in particular, in part because it was published in a peer-reviewed mainstream journal, Postgraduate Medicine[4], but mostly for all the excellent information to be found there!*) There can be no doubt about this. However, good scientists are not comfortable drawing comparative conclusions based on data from separate studies run on different populations under different conditions. This gives those with an anti-BHRT mindset an easy way to discount them. Nevertheless, such comparisons can certainly be suggestive.

What's really needed are head-to-head studies, where women from the same population use HRT or BHRT under the same conditions. Of course, there haven't been any such studies of HRT and BHRT *yet*, and we don't need to tell you why. However, a small, *independent* comparative trial is currently under way at the University of Kansas (*See Appendix.*).

[Actually, the above isn't merely a "thought experiment." As we discuss below, one patent medicine company is actively seeking FDA "approval" for exclusive use of "Trimesta®" (bio-identical estriol, re-named) in treating multiple sclerosis (MS), while at the same time trying to ban the use of unbranded estriol by everyone else, claiming it is untested and potentially dangerous. Another patent medicine company has already gained FDA "approval" for "Prasterone®" (a branded version of bio-identical DHEA); and a third patent medicine company is trying for FDA "approval" for the natural estrogen metabolite (and very potent *anti*carcinogen) 2-methoxyestradiol, which they've re-named "Panzem®." (*See Chapter 7.*) Despite the fact that these FDA-"approved" (or to-be-"approved") versions of these bio-identical hormones are no different chemically from their non-"approved" versions, we can be sure of one thing, once FDA-"approved," they will cost users (and their insurance companies) tens of millions of dollars more. Could these Big Pharma patented versions of bio-identical hormones be another incentive for the FDA's current efforts to stop pharmacy compounding of BHRT?]

Alas, as we depart Fantasyland and return to the real world, it becomes painfully obvious that, regardless of the two treatments' relative merits, patent medicine companies are never going to willingly sponsor studies comparing their products to bio-identical hormones. The risk that *nonpatentable* BHRT might show up their *patented* HRT cousins is way too high. Imagine Wyeth's embarrassment at having to publicly admit that their heavily marketed patented "hormone" products were patently (*pun intended*) inferior to nonpatentable bio-identical hormones. How to explain to you and millions of other women that Wyeth would much prefer that you use their demonstrably inferior and more dangerous "hormone replacement" products instead of BHRT, because Wyeth earns lots more money that way?

Buying Influence

Despite what their ads might say, never lose sight of the fact that drug (patent medicine) companies are not in the business of making people healthier and happier; their customers' health and happiness are only secondary goals. Like all other large corporations, their *raison d'être* is to earn money for their stockholders and executives, and over the last century, they've done very well at that, earning them hundreds of billions of dollars. The patent medicine industry continues to be one of the most profitable in the world, but only if they sell *patented*, (ie, *alien-to-the-human body*) medicines. Bio-identical hormone replacement, as described in this book, just doesn't fit their business plan (although, as noted above, that could be changing).

In the days before the WHI results became public in 2002, when Premarin® and Prempro® were still among the best selling patent medicines in the world, Wyeth and other companies didn't pay much attention to BHRT. As long as they could aggressively and successfully market HRT, it was easiest to simply ignore BHRT and avoid bringing unneeded attention to it. Leave it to those "quack" doctors who are foolish enough to prescribe it to their "health-nut" patients.

Since the WHI, though, millions of women have quit HRT, many of them flocking to BHRT. Unwilling to market BHRT themselves, patent medicine companies now see their best option as discrediting it and ultimately getting the FDA to eliminate it. How else to protect their bottom line as they watch BHRT grow from molehill to mountain?

Today BHRT faces hostility on a wide range of fronts: FDA regulations try to strangle it; "independent" medical organizations disparage it in their publications and position statements; and consumer media lap up anything the patent medicine companies feed them as "scientific gospel." Behind it all are Wyeth and the rest of Big Pharma, spreading disinformation via paid medical "opinion leaders," "reputable" professional medical organizations, and "disease advocacy" groups, all of which receive huge "grants" from Wyeth via "educational" programs, honoraria, "consulting" agreements, money for research, and many other avenues. (*See Appendix 1 for a list of these groups and their recent payments from Wyeth.*)

Few would dispute that Big Pharma is one of the most powerful "players" in the US government and economy today. Between January 2005 and June 2006, drug companies and industry trade groups spent $155 million trying to influence legislation, employing about 1,100 lobbyists – that's more than two lobbyists for each Senator and Member of Congress![5] In 2007, Washington's biggest lobby upped the ante by 32%, spending more than $189 million. Altogether, in the past decade, Big Pharma has spent more than $1 billion trying to influence legislation in Washington.[5]

Between 1998 and 2004, Wyeth alone dispersed more than $24 million among 26 different lobbying firms to look after their legislative interests.[6] Since 2002, a major portion of that cash has no doubt gone into shoring up its mortally wounded HRT franchise, while at the same time beating down the perceived threat from BHRT. In the wake of the WHI and other recent studies, it's a safe bet that the survival of Premarin® and Provera® can be attributed to many of those millions. Beyond lobbying the government, including the FDA, Big Pharma commands a vast advertising and public relations empire devoted to disparaging BHRT and convincing patients to ask for their patent medicines and for physicians to prescribe them.

In a *Washington Monthly* article entitled "Hot Flash, Cold Cash,"[7] author Alicia Mundy gives us a taste of the way things work in the influence peddling business, as she describes how Wyeth used its deep pockets to virtually take over a 12-year-old, once- independent, *nonprofit*, advocacy organization, the *Society for Women's Health Research (SWHR)*.

In April 2002, just 3 months before the WHI revelations (Did Wyeth know what was coming?), the SWHR threw a blue-ribbon dinner in Washington, DC, themed "Coming of Age." The affair's ostensible purpose was to celebrate "women in midlife and beyond," but Mundy noticed something about the evening that seemed different from the average DC black-tie happening. "The whole event had been underwritten by the pharmaceutical company Wyeth," she wrote. Wyeth's CEO Robert Essner gave a brief speech, which was followed by "menopause maven" Gail Sheehy reading from her book, *The Silent Passage.* Sheehy opined "… how women were enjoying better lives because of 'lifesaving preventative measures, including hormone-replacement therapy'" – ie, Premarin® + Provera®.

Reports Mundy, "Some participants were taken aback. 'Without mentioning Wyeth,' says one [attendee], 'it was like they [SWHR] were doing an ad for Wyeth.' The whole evening was, she recalls, 'a perfect way to ensure you'll keep one of your biggest benefactors happy: a dinner theme tied to one of their biggest selling products.'" And it worked like a charm; the following week, on the occasion of Premarin's 60th anniversary, Wyeth rewarded SWHR with a "donation" of a quarter of a million dollars.

A few months later, as the WHI revelations began to dominate the news, though, things started getting a little dicey for Wyeth. One *truly independent* women's advocacy group after another cautioned women about the newly confirmed potential dangers associated with conventional HRT. However, Mundy points out, SWHR "… did the opposite, *attacking the study, its authors, and its conclusions* on chat shows and in newspaper articles. Instead of taking the side of its constituents, the society seemingly took the side of its donors – and of Wyeth in particular …."

According to Mundy, Wyeth's "curious behavior" may represent "the latest innovation in the art of Washington influence peddling." Instead of trying to generate pro-business policy thinking and political momentum in Washington by *creating* and funding new independent-sounding but thinly disguised think tanks and advocacy groups – standard DC operating procedure for decades – Wyeth discovered that "…generosity no more expensive than an ordinary public relations campaign can enable corporations to *all but take over* an already existing and respected nonprofit, and *use its credibility to advance their own interests*. The tactic is so clever, it's a wonder other industries didn't think of it – though many will surely copy it," she wrote.

Guilt by Association

Although the WHI used only one "hormone" replacement regimen – Prempro® (or Premarin® alone in "women without a uterus") – the FDA has subsequently used the study's results to support its decree that, until proven otherwise, *all* "estrogens," *all* progestins, and *all* "estrogen"- progestin or estrogen-progesterone combinations should be considered to have a cancer- and heart disease-causing potential at least equivalent to that of Premarin® and Prempro®.

Following this thinking to its illogical conclusion, we are expected to believe that human estrogens and progesterone, which the body of every normal, healthy woman secretes naturally and safely for 40 or more years, are nevertheless potentially just as dangerous as Prempro® when taken as postmenopausal bio-identical hormone replacements. This "logic" also suggests that women's bodies have evolved over millions of years to produce and safely utilize the very hormones used in BHRT, but suddenly, around age 50, these hormones somehow turn toxic.

What's the FDA's primary evidence for this conclusion? It's simple; the body reacts to alien-to-the-human-body *horse estrogens* and *pseudohormone progestin drugs* this way; therefore, it should react to bio-identical hormones in exactly the same way. In other words, the only evidence available showing potential adverse effects of BHRT comes from studies using conventional, patented HRT. ***They have absolutely no other scientific basis to generalize these findings to bio-identical hormones***.

In defense of their "logic," skeptics point to the absence of any large, costly, double-blind, placebo-controlled clinical trials proving the safety of BHRT. It's true, of course; there are no such trials of bio-identical hormones, not because BHRT is inherently inferior, but because patent medicine companies have – for their own selfish interests – carefully avoided running them, and no one else can afford to.

As we have emphasized in this book, because it's vitally important to the story of bio-identical hormone replacement (*please forgive us if you're sick of hearing this refrain.*), the "approval" system in the US is loaded against bio-identical hormones and any other natural, unpatentable products. The prescribed trials are too costly to be run by anyone but Big Pharma and/or the Federal government. Thus, the FDA's decree becomes a "self-fulfilling prophesy: no "approved" studies ➔ no publications in "reputable" journals ➔ confirmation that bio-identical hormones have no *"proven"* clinical value and are therefore likely to be just as dangerous as alien, patented products."

At the same time, though, not a single valid study of bio-identical hormones – and there are literally hundreds of relevant published reports going back decades, despite protestations to the contrary from the FDA and the rest of conventional medicine – even hints at the possibility that bio-identical hormones, when properly used, are not superior in efficacy to Premarin®, Provera®, et al, or carry anywhere near the same risks. Even when mainstream medicine authorities do recognize the existence of these studies, they are quick to denigrate them and minimize their significance to suit their biases, as they did in the days before the WHI. (*See Chapter 8.*)

One typical patent medicine industry strategy is to exploit its considerable resources to propagate misinformation. They often do this by hiring/ co-opting apparently respectable medical "authorities," or "key opinion leaders," whom they pay to "consult" with the company, to "author"* articles for the medical literature and consumer media, to teach continuing "medical education" courses, and to act as "expert" spokespeople for media interviews.

For the most part, Big Pharma has the mainstream media all to itself, in part because the mainstream media is too lazy to look beyond the latest Big Pharma press release and partly because they receive millions in advertising revenue from them. There's no way BHRT can compete financially. In one all-too-typical article in *BusinessWeek Online*,[1]

---

* We use the verb "to author" rather than "to write," because most often the "authority" just puts his/her name on an article written by a company-hired ghostwriter. Such articles may well present accurate information, but they are usually also shaped and approved by company marketing experts to assure they contain their key marketing messages. Most well-paid "authors" have little trouble with this arrangement, given the often five- or six-figure "honoraria" they earn from the company, as well as the opportunity it provides to pad their résumés and enhance their professional reputations.

Michelle P. Warren, MD, director of a women's health center at Columbia University, is quoted as saying, "Many [compounding pharmacists] say bio-identicals mimic the body's own processes more accurately than the regulated products do. But that's hard to validate because *'these cocktails have never been studied.'*" (Italics added; also notice the disparaging use of the word *"cocktails"* to refer to doctor-prescribed, carefully measured, individualized mixtures of pharmaceutical quality compounded bio-identical hormones.)

Even more "disturbing," according to Dr. Warren, compounded estrogen mixtures typically contain *estriol*, which, she points out, is "a version of the hormone that has *not been approved by the FDA,*" completely ignoring the fact that, until very recently, Wyeth was marketing estriol in two different products in Europe (brand names "Cyclo-Menorette" and "Estriolsalbe"), billing estriol as the *"ideal therapy"* for the menopausal woman. (They recently ceased marketing these drugs, according to Wyeth, due to "lack of sales.") Indeed, Wyeth is correct for once: estriol has never been shown to cause serious problems in European women taking these drugs. They obviously want to have it both ways: estriol's a potentially dangerous, untested, unapproved "drug" in the US, and "ideal therapy" in Europe. Perhaps something's getting lost in the translation.

As noted above, estriol is currently undergoing clinical trials in the US for treating multiple sclerosis (MS) under the brand name Trimesta® and most likely *will be* declared FDA-"approved" within the next year or 2. According to the company's (Pipex Pharmaceuticals) website, *"Estriol has been approved and marketed throughout Europe and Asia as a mild estrogenic agent for over 40 years for the treatment of post-menopausal hot flashes."*[8] *BusinessWeek Online* somehow missed this point in their article. Moreover, Pipex couldn't say those words unless the FDA approved them.

Is Dr. Warren making these statements based on her own research, clinical experience, and impressive credentials, including her Ivy League academic appointment? Well, perhaps, but Dr. Warren also turns out to be a paid "consultant" to Wyeth and several other patent medicine companies. To give you some idea how Dr. Warren's bread is buttered (*maybe with even a little "jam" added, too!*), her official academic title includes *Wyeth-*

Ayerst Professor of Women's Health at Columbia University College of Physicians & Surgeons. In other words, it would certainly seem to be in her best financial interests to stick to the Wyeth party line and to disparage BHRT at every opportunity. Peel aside the curtain from nearly every "expert" anti-BHRT statement you come across in the mainstream media and you're almost guaranteed to find a similar arrangement.

So, what's so sinister about estriol? The way Dr. Warren dismisses estriol as *not FDA-approved* suggests she hasn't any idea what reputable scientists and physicians have been reporting about it for decades: that hundreds of clinical and nonclinical studies support it's safety and efficacy; and that estriol is widely recognized outside the US as a safe and probably *anticarcinogenic* alternative to horse estrogens. And back here in the good old USA, estriol has been recognized for just as long as safe by the United States Pharmacopoeia (USP). The USP is the official, *nongovernmental, not-for-profit* public standards-setting authority for all prescription and over-the-counter medicines and other health care products manufactured or sold in the United States.

Neither Wyeth nor FDA bureaucrats have ever gotten around to evaluating estriol or comparing it head-to-head to their dangerous-but-FDA-approved-and-astronomically-more-profitable horse estrogens. This anti-estriol strategy is built upon a healthy dose of hypocrisy and willful ignorance. It disregards a substantial body of scientific evidence – not to mention millions of woman-years of real-life "clinical" experience – supporting the use of estriol and the other hormones in BHRT. Among the hundreds of trials that have been reported in medical journals, *not one has ever convincingly shown that estriol, when used appropriately, increases the risk of cancer or any other serious chronic disease,* something the FDA itself has recently admitted, as we shall soon see. Nevertheless, as we discuss shortly, the FDA/Wyeth attack on estriol use may be the most serious one BHRT has yet faced.

Myths about BHRT and Compounding

Using tactics such as those described above, as well as other more ordinary means, Wyeth/mainstream medicine has propagated anti-BHRT myths such as these:

- ***Despite what the WHI and other studies have shown, HRT may not be as bad as first thought.*** Since the original publication of the WHI results, the medical literature and consumer media have been full of reviews and reconsiderations of the WHI conclusions emphasizing the study's weaknesses and limitations. The underlying message: Sure, HRT may have its faults, but used properly – ie, the lowest dose for the shortest possible time, in the ideal population (healthy, younger menopausal women), it still gets rid of hot flushes without raising the risks of heart disease and breast cancer.

  This strategy ignores the fact that low-dose, short-duration conventional HRT has yet to be demonstrated in a well-controlled WHI-like trial to be any safer than older, higher dose, longer duration regimens. It's just a convenient supposition that Wyeth got the FDA to agree to, based on a re-analysis of the WHI data, in order keep their franchise from being flushed down the toilet. Nor does conventional HRT – especially under the new supposedly *safer* prescription guidelines – do anything to prevent other long-term consequences of estrogen decline, such as heart disease, osteoporosis, senility, depression, and incontinence, long-espoused claims of HRT efficacy.

- ***The differences between patented pseudohormones and bio-identical hormones (if they exist at all) are minimal and of little or no clinical consequence.*** Many otherwise bright, and apparently well-informed doctors and researchers continue to refer to horse estrogens as "estrogen" and to Provera® and other progestins as "progesterone," apparently unwilling or unable to make these vital distinctions. If all "estrogens" and "progestogens" were equal, then the FDA's warnings about the potential dangers of BHRT might make some sense. In fact, though, the small, seemingly insignificant changes in the estrogen and progesterone molecules that are made to create patent medicine "hormone" products can mean the difference between a safe, naturally active bio-identical hormone and a toxic pseudohormone. There is no scientific justification for assuming that bio-identical hormone molecules carry the same high risks and low benefits as patent medicine horse estrogens and lab-created pseudohormone molecules, and every thinking scientist should know this.

- *No clinical research supports the efficacy and safety of BHRT.* Aside
from being an outright distortion of reality, this statement neglects
to acknowledge a vast literature – much of it in European and Asian
journals, but many in US journals, too – that shows bio-identical
hormones to be safe and efficacious. Throughout this book we have
cited hundreds of published research papers in support of the efficacy
and safety of bio-identical hormones in clinical and nonclinical
studies. As noted above, Wyeth itself has marketed estriol in Europe
as an "ideal therapy."

- *Women who use BHRT are taking unnecessary risks.* Because
conventional medicine parochially refuses to distinguish between
patented pseudohormones and bio-identical hormones, or to accept
the hundreds of clinical trials of bio-identical hormones in menopausal
women, we are asked to *assume* that they are just as dangerous as
Premarin® and Provera®. Falling back on the "devil-you-know-vs.-the
devil-you-don't-know" logic, they argue that, given a choice, HRT is
preferable, because at least you know what the risks are. Again, we cite
the considerable medical literature that disputes this assumption.

- *Doctors who prescribe BHRT are "offbeat quacks," who
are misleading or deceiving their patients.* Most doctors who
conscientiously prescribe BHRT have taken special training courses
and have become highly skilled in prescribing, dosing, and (most
importantly) monitoring their patients, both in office visits and with
appropriate laboratory tests. To assert that these doctors are outright
frauds and should not be allowed to practice is libelous name-calling
at its most despicable level, lacking even a shred of evidence to
support it.[9] If there are physicians who are prescribing what they
call "BHRT" but are not following the principles laid out in this
and other authoritative books and published papers, we urge them
to cease doing so immediately, get themselves a good education in
proper BHRT prescribing, and alter their ways, because they may be
doing more harm than good for the BHRT "cause," not to mention
to their patients.

- *BHRT dosing is uncertain because it <u>requires</u> unreliable saliva tests
to measure hormone levels.* In order to denigrate BHRT, critics have
unjustifiably made saliva testing into a convenient "straw man." As

we discussed in Chapter 9, saliva tests are *not* a good way to measure steroid hormones in menopausal women, especially those on BHRT. Saliva tests and lab analysis services are widely marketed, because they are easy to perform, relatively inexpensive, and profitable for those labs that market them, but *knowledgeable* doctors know that blood tests and especially 24-hour urine tests are far superior. *There's nothing inherent in BHRT that demands saliva analysis, but the friendly folks at Wyeth and the FDA would like us to think there is and that every doctor who prescribes BHRT relies on these tests.*

- ***Hormones compounded by a pharmacist may be unreliable and potentially dangerous.*** Wyeth and the FDA insist that compounded hormones may be contaminated, poorly formulated, misdosed, costly, not FDA-approved, and possibly even illegal. They present no valid evidence to support any of this; it is pure misdirection. Compounding has been an important part of pharmacy practice since the beginning of modern medicine and was recognized as legal at the founding of the FDA in 1938 and reaffirmed as recently as 1997. Moreover, it is regulated by State Pharmacy Boards in all 50 States.

Over the years, compounding skills and techniques have improved significantly, as especially evidenced by the recent inauguration of the Pharmacy Compounding Accreditation Board (PCAB). (*See Chapter 11.*) The FDA's recent campaign – at the behest of Wyeth and other patent medicine companies – to discredit compounding is transparently dishonest, political, and lacking in objective validity. It is based primarily on a widely discredited, unscientific FDA "limited survey" discussed later in this chapter.

- ***Compounding pharmacists promote and sell their products directly to consumers.*** According to *BusinessWeek Online*, which has on occasion flagrantly spouted Wyeth talking points, "Compounding pharmacies ... sell [their] compounds *in brochures and on the Internet.*[1] (As if Big Pharma doesn't?)

The article conveniently overlooks the fact that compounding pharmacists *never* dispense estrogens, testosterone, or any other FDA-"approved" medication without a doctor's prescription. While many pharmacists do promote their services to patients and physicians in the community [as do Big Pharma companies, using slick, expensive media campaigns: *"Ask your doctor whether (fill in the blank) is right for you."*], no one can obtain a compounded medication without first presenting a valid doctor's prescription.

Making the point that some compounding pharmacies fill prescriptions over the Internet is an attempt to cast a sinister pall over the entire profession. However, the article neglects to indicate that most compounding pharmacies are small, independent, community-based businesses staffed by well-trained, State-regulated professionals. If they use the internet as a marketing tool – and who doesn't these days? – they still require a valid prescription before dispensing any hormone or drug, and like all pharmacies, are subject to State regulations and inspections.

The article snarkily remarks, compounding pharmacies "...form a *shadow industry* that has largely dodged the scrutiny of the US Food & Drug Administration. They *market their concoctions* without subjecting them to the rigorous trials normally requested for prescription medicines."[1] If compounding pharmacies have "dodged" FDA scrutiny, it's because 1) they are adequately regulated by State pharmacy boards; and most importantly, 2) *the FDA has no legal authority over them.* (Italics added.) As for their "concoctions," we again point out that compounding pharmacists are highly trained professionals, who use FDA-approved bulk ingredients and carefully measure and mix them according to a physician's prescription and approved compounding procedures. Not a single valid scientific study has ever shown otherwise.

- *Compounding pharmacists are really __drug manufacturers__ and should therefore be subject to the same FDA regulations as Big Pharma companies.* Raising the alarm about the growing compounding "threat," one Washington lawyer on the Big Pharma payroll was quoted by *BusinessWeek Online* saying that compounders "... are *running drug companies* under the guise of pharmacies. *It's a serious public health problem.*"[1]

This claim is another hyperbolic fabrication with no basis in fact. Equating compounding with manufacturing is ludicrous and self-serving. The whole point of compounding is to produce individualized prescriptions according to a doctor's prescription. Mass production by pharmacists would be wasteful and counterproductive. Moreover, no valid scientific study has ever shown that compounded prescriptions are any more dangerous than conventional prescriptions for patented medications. Like all pharmacists, compounding pharmacists are regulated and monitored by pharmacy boards in every state, a system that has worked well for decades.

- ***There's something sinister about "plant-derived hormones."*** A common, but subtle, avenue of attack against BHRT is that it employs "plant-derived hormones," as if there's something wrong with that. First, emphasizing the plant derivation of bio-identical hormones blurs the distinction between human bio-identical steroids and plant estrogens, or *phytoestrogens** (eg, isoflavones and lignins), which are *natural,* sometimes useful, and usually safe sources of estrogens, but they are *no more bio-identical for humans than are horse estrogens.* For some peri- or postmenopausal women, phytoestrogens may be helpful for reducing common symptoms of declining estrogen levels, but they are *not a substitute for true bio-identical hormones.*

Next, as we've noted several times in this book, except for phytoestrogens and Premarin®, virtually all sex steroids in use today – both bio-identical and patented – whether for menopausal hormone replacement, contraception, or other uses, are synthesized from the same plant chemical, *diosgenin.* The often unspoken message is that Premarin® is somehow better and more "natural" because it is animal-based; never mind that it is made from horse urine and its mixture of estrogens is unsuited for the human body. The important point, again, is not where the hormones come from but how closely the final molecules resemble natural human hormone molecules. The hormones used in BHRT are *exact replicas*, whereas horse estrogens, patented estrogens, progestins, and phytoestrogens are significantly different.

---

* **Phytoestrogens are estrogens produced by certain plants (eg, soy, flax) that may act like estrogens in animal cells and human bodies and may mimic and/or supplement the actions of the body's own estrogens.**

Compounding or Manufacturing?

"The fundamental difference between compounding and manufacturing, and the key element in making any such distinction, is the existence of a pharmacist/prescriber/patient 'triad' relationship. This triad should control the preparation of a drug product. Furthermore, compounded drugs are not for resale, but rather, are personal and responsive to a patient's immediate needs.

"Conversely, drug manufacturers produce batches consisting of millions of tablets or capsules at a time for resale, while utilizing many personnel and large scale manufacturing equipment, without knowledge of the specific patient who will ultimately consume them."

American Pharmacists Association
Statement to the US Senate Special Committee on Aging
April 19, 2007

Still, we have to put up with flagrant ignorance, such as that displayed by Stephen Barrett, MD, a self-appointed "quack buster." On his website, "Pharmwatch," under the heading *"Steer Clear of 'Bioidentical' Hormone Therapy,"* Barrett states the following:

"Compounded 'bioidentical hormones' are plant-derived hormones that pharmacists prepare and label as drugs. The products are claimed to be biochemically similar or identical to those produced by the ovaries or body. However, the relevant chemicals (steroids) in plants are not identical to those in humans. To make products that work in humans, raw materials from the plants must be converted to human hormones synthetically. Thus, to the extent that they are potent, the 'bioidentical' products would pose the same risks as those of standard hormones – plus whatever problems might be introduced during compounding."[10]

If you're having trouble understanding what Dr. Barrett is saying here, you no doubt understand more about BHRT than he does. He points out that, to make plant-derived steroids work in humans, the raw materials must be converted to human hormones synthetically. True enough, and there's nothing wrong with this; as noted, virtually all steroid hormones in use today, except for Premarin®, are made this way. But then he makes a breathtaking leap in logic, to argue that the mere fact of this synthesis somehow suggests that bioidentical products pose the same risks as those of "*standard* hormones." First, we must ask, What are "*standard* hormones?" Presumably he means some sort of patented hormone products, since those are the only ones he recognizes as having any clinical validity. Second, how does synthesizing bio-identical hormones from plant steroids automatically make them equivalent to "standard" hormones in terms of risk? There is no evidence to support this point; it is uninformed nonsense.

Finally, he takes a cheap shot at compounding, by suggesting the compounding process somehow introduces unspecified "problems." What's his evidence for these "problems?" Well, in a previous paragraph, he does refer to an unscientific, flawed, and widely discredited 2001 FDA "limited survey," which we discuss in detail below.

As a general rule, it's safe to assume that anything Stephen Barrett says about BHRT (or in fact nearly anything else) is utter claptrap, based not on objective fact, but on an undisguised bias against any and all aspects of complementary and alternative medicine. Still, mainstream medicine and media – in their laziness and ignorance – often look upon him and others like him as valuable "truth tellers."

- *If women really want BHRT, they can use FDA-approved formulations of estradiol and progesterone.* This attitude represents a fundamental misunderstanding of BHRT, the purpose of which is not simply to suppress menopausal symptoms, which "approved" formulations can do, but rather to restore a close-to-premenopausal hormonal environment. To accomplish this latter function, individualized preparations – preferably topical – of bio-identical estrogens, progesterone, and possibly testosterone and DHEA are all required to copy Nature as closely as possible. Also to copy Nature, these hormones all need to be used at physiologic doses (which may not be available in "approved" formulations) and on a physiologic timetable (which is not recommended by "official" labeling of these products). True bio-identical hormone preparations are available only from a compounding pharmacist.

FDA-"approved" bio-identical hormones, which include only 100% estradiol (creams, gels, patches, and pills), progesterone (mostly oral capsules), and testosterone (creams, gels, patches – approved for men only) are limited as to dose and formulation. These "approved" hormones are used in ways which do not closely copy Nature at all:

  o 100% estradiol creams, gels, and pills are formulated at dangerously high doses (1-2 milligrams per day). Estradiol skin patches deliver their hormone at lower doses but on a constant, nonphysiologic schedule. (*See Chapter 9.*)

  o Estriol, which is essential to buffer the procarcinogenic effects of estradiol and estrone, may be ultimately FDA-"approved" (although at Wyeth's urging, the FDA is currently trying very hard to ban it) but not marketed in replacement doses by any US manufacturer. Virtually no advocates of "FDA-approved BHRT" recommend using estriol, despite its widespread successful use in Europe and Asia.

  o Progesterone is often recommended in high-dose oral capsules as micronized progesterone (which may contain peanut oil, and would thus be problematic for women with peanut allergies). But "oral" progesterone doesn't copy Nature's route through the body, at all. Topical progesterone, which is superior to oral (as it follows Nature's route) and requires lower doses, is not FDA-"approved" but is available from compounding pharmacists.

o Testosterone is FDA-approved only in doses suitable for men. The only available sources of testosterone for women are compounding pharmacists.

Thus, there is no such thing as FDA-"approved" bio-identical hormones. The only hormones suitable for BHRT are available solely from compounding pharmacists.

If You Can't Beat Them with Facts, Beat Them with *Fear*: The FDA "Surveys" Compounding Pharmacists

A substantial portion of the anti-BHRT heat these days gets aimed directly at compounding pharmacists. This strategy makes perfect sense: curtail or eliminate pharmacists' ability to compound bio-identical hormones and BHRT simply goes away. You can't get rid of the patients, and it's hard (but not impossible, as demonstrated by the current legal confrontation over estriol) to control what doctors prescribe, but compounding pharmacies make an inviting regulatory target.

A choice anti-compounding weapon recently has been an FDA-run "limited survey" of compounded drugs and hormones, which found that 34% of the samples, gathered from 12 different "community" compounding pharmacies, failed one or more of the agency's quality tests.[11] On its face – and that's about all you ever hear in the media – this sounds very disturbing, suggesting that women who elect to use BHRT can expect that as many as one in three of their hormone prescriptions may be of substandard quality, perhaps even dangerous; obviously another good reason to avoid BHRT.

However, it would be a big mistake to take these results on their face value. The FDA itself readily acknowledges their so-called *survey* is "limited" (Title: "Report: Limited FDA Survey of Compounded Drug Products"); they just don't tell us *how limited*. In fact, this very small, informal, uncontrolled survey was never peer-reviewed or published in a medical journal, and with good reason; no legitimate journal would ever publish it. A brief summary of the study appears only on the FDA's website. When finally confronted about the survey's shortcomings by a Congressional committee, the FDA official in charge of the survey confessed that *it lacked any scientific validity.*

The survey was conducted between June and December 2001, with FDA "researchers" ordering 29 different compounded medications from 12 different compounding pharmacies. No information is provided on how these pharmacies were selected, except that their sole qualification seems to have been that they were advertising on the internet and were willing to 1) fill prescriptions without one-on-one consultation with the prescribing doctor or patient; and 2) mail the compounded medications to the "patient," no questions asked. There does not seem to have been any effort to investigate the quality of the pharmacies in any way. (*We can also presume that the products were obtained under false pretenses, using prescriptions written by FDA "doctors" for fictitious "patients."*)

The 29 sampled preparations were ordered in 5 different dosage forms: 13 sterile injections, 9 ophthalmic liquids or ointments, 2 pellet implants, 1 inhalation product, and 4 oral dosage forms (capsules or tablets). They included reproductive steroid hormones (estradiol and progesterone), antibiotics, corticosteroids, anesthetics, and drugs for treating glaucoma, asthma, iron deficiency anemia, and erectile dysfunction. The reproductive hormone samples included 2 progesterone *injectables*; 2 estradiol *pellets for implanting under the skin*; 3 progesterone *oral capsules*; and 1 estradiol *oral tablet.*

The FDA analytical labs rated the products in terms of their quality, purity, and potency. Overall, they found that 10 of the 29 samples (34%) did not meet the FDA's standards; 9 of these 10 failed because their potency was lower than the label promised. Of these preparations, 2 of the progesterone products – 1 injectable and 1 capsule – were found to have a lower potency than was stated on the label; the dose-deficient progesterone capsule also failed due to problems with "content uniformity." **The 7 other deficient products were not sex hormones at all but standard, FDA-"approved" drugs.**

Now, once we hear in the media that an FDA survey has found a *34% error rate* in a study of compounding pharmacies, wouldn't we be crazy not to think twice before using a compounded medication? This is especially so when we're reminded by the FDA that another, unrelated, agency-sponsored study of more than 3,000 *commercial patented drug products* (the kind you buy at your average drugstore) found only a *2% error rate*. Which would you prefer, 1 error in every third prescription, or 1 in every 200? There's simply no *comparison*.

Well, that's true, there *is* simply no comparison. That's why the FDA makes this comparison with the help of lots of smoke and mirrors. There's no valid way to compare the results of these two "studies." In the simplest terms, here's why: the populations were completely different; the two studies' methods were completely different; the medications/hormones were completely different, and the sample sizes differed by a factor of 100 – and that just scratches the surface of the differences.

All by itself, the miniscule size of the compounded medicine survey renders its results meaningless. Apparently, the pharmacies were not chosen randomly and there were only 12 of them. Are we to believe these 12 were representative of the more than 1,000 competent compounding pharmacies in the US today, many of which have been recently certified by the PCAB? Are we to believe the 29 products obtained by the FDA 10 or 11 years ago are representative of the millions of prescriptions compounded each year today?

Moreover, if the FDA-"prescribed" hormones had really been intended for use in BHRT, especially today, the formulations were entirely wrong. There is no place in BHRT for progesterone *injections* or estradiol *pellet implants*. (Neither one can "copy Nature" by being "cycled.") Oral estradiol and progesterone are prescribed by some practitioners, but knowledgeable physicians today find topical creams and gels to be far more effective, safer, and better tolerated. However, no topical cream or gel hormone formulations were "prescribed" or evaluated by the FDA (*must have been an oversight*). Taken together, these design flaws make generalizing these findings to all compounding pharmacies and BHRT prescriptions totally meaningless.

In 2003, before a hearing of the US Senate Health, Education, Labor, and Pensions Committee, the FDA was severely reprimanded for using this spurious survey to try to discredit compounding pharmacies.[12] In a dialogue with Sen. John Ensign (R-NV), Dr. Steven Galson, the Director of the FDA's Center for Drug Evaluation and Research, which performed the "survey," stated defensively, "*I want to emphasize that this was **not a comprehensive scientific survey**. It was a small sample size.*"

"I don't normally take witnesses to task," Sen. Ensign shot back. "But I do want to take you to task for something. You're a scientist, and to present *nonscientific data studies* … is problematic … you presented that in a fashion that is *misleading*."

To which Dr. Galson impotently replied, "***I wasn't trying to present these as scientific data***."

So, Dr. Galson, if they weren't scientific data, what were they? Ah yes, propaganda, of course.

Unscientific as they were, we continue to find the results of this survey cited as scientific data almost every time BHRT/compounding critics put words to paper, usually with the unstated implication that *all the deficient samples were bio-identical hormones*, which they were not. In fact, for what it's worth, 7 of the 9 deficient products were *not* bio-identical hormones, but compounded versions of FDA-"approved" patent medicines, which are perfectly legal and which they FDA claims to have no interest in restricting. Moreover, while the FDA tested a wide range of medications in its "survey," virtually the only time the "survey" results ever get cited is by someone trying to discredit compounded bio-identical hormones, not compounded antibiotics, not compounded corticosteroids, not compounded anesthetics, nor other compounded medications. The implication – always unstated – is that all the compounded products were bio-identical hormones.

The sole evidence against compounded bio-identical hormones in the "survey" consisted of 2 out of 8 hormone products found to be low in potency. There's certainly no excuse for miscalculating the dose of progesterone or any other hormone or drug, and we would hope that today's well-trained, well-equipped, PCAB-*certified* pharmacists practicing "state-of-the-art" compounding would have a better record than the anonymous internet-savvy pharmacists of a decade or more ago, whose compounding skills and training are unknown. On the bright side, though, none of the samples was contaminated with impurities or dangerous in any other way.

Nevertheless, here's the subliminal message – what they want us to believe, but won't come right out and say because they know it's a lie: If 3,000 *compounded* prescription samples were analyzed in the same way the 3,000 patent medicine samples were analyzed in the older study cited above, we should expect 1,000 or more to show up as substandard. This is an extremely invalid and dishonest way to present data, especially data they *know* will be widely disseminated to women looking for a way to ease the discomforts of menopause.

Had the results turned out differently and *supported* the value of pharmaceutical compounding, we can be certain that the FDA and other mainstream medicine authorities would have either buried them altogether or else ripped them to shreds – "Just another one of those small, poorly controlled studies; can't tell anything from those. Only large, double-blind, placebo-controlled studies provide meaningful data." Sound familiar?

But since these bogus results can be twisted to bolster the anti-BHRT/anti-compounding position, they've become a valuable, widely quoted piece of "scientific" evidence, part of the "gospel" that is regularly cited as proof of the inherent inferiority of pharmacy compounding and bio-identical hormones. (*See Wyeth's "Citizen Petition" below.*) If truth be told, when Wyeth, the FDA, and other BHRT opponents argue that bio-identical hormones and other compounded products should either be more closely regulated or banned altogether, this laughable survey is, in fact, the *only* piece of "hard" evidence they seem to be able to dig up in support of their claim.

To take these results at face value, which admittedly is quite a stretch, and use them as part of a wholesale condemnation of compounding and BHRT, is beyond shameless.

Disseminating Misinformation

Misinformation about bio-identical hormones is routinely disseminated by Wyeth and other patent medicine companies. As we described earlier, these companies are not shy about opening their wallets to co-opt otherwise "independent" researchers and medical professional and advocacy organizations like the Society for Women's Health Research.

Among the many professional organizations, the American College of Obstetricians and Gynecologists (ACOG) turns out to be one of the most aggressive and regressive with regard to BHRT. ACOG, which receives considerable financial support from Wyeth and other drug companies (*See Appendix.*), never seems to miss an opportunity to impugn BHRT. For example, in an October 2005 press release headlined "*No Scientific Evidence Supporting Effectiveness or Safety of Compounded Bioidentical Hormone Therapy,*" ACOG acclaimed the results of the FDA's unscientific compounding survey just cited above.[13] (*Purely by coincidence, no doubt, the press release came out just about the same time as Wyeth's notorious "Citizen Petition" to the FDA, discussed below.*)

A year earlier, ACOG had posted on its website a series of "New Recommendations" based on its "Task Force Report on Hormone Therapy." A verbatim quotation from a small section entitled "*Topical Progesterone, Testosterone, and Other 'Natural' Hormones*" is shown in the accompanying box. This single paragraph is so chock full of misinformation as to make one wonder whether the authors did any research at all or just made things up to suit their biases: (*We have numbered the ACOG statements in the excerpt to make it easier to reference them in the deconstruction that follows.*)

1. Clearly, the first statement is nonsense. A casual perusal of the references used in this book reveals hundreds of "formal" studies conducted over several decades that validate the safety and effectiveness of bio-identical hormones.

2. Natural progesterone creams (and other formulations) prepared by specially trained, professional compounding pharmacists contain carefully measured amounts of the hormone. No one has ever presented any valid evidence to suggest otherwise. It is certainly

> ## *Topical Progesterone, Testosterone and other "Natural" Hormones*
>
> 1) At this point, no formal studies have been conducted to determine the safety and/or effectiveness of these products. 2) Many so-called "natural" progesterone creams do not contain substances that the human body can use as progesterone. 3) These products are often derived from wild yam extracts and contain a substance, diosgenin, that only plants can metabolize into active progesterone. 4) Other such products contain these plant extracts plus chemically synthesized progesterone, which is added to the plant extract in the cream. 5) It is not always possible for a woman to tell exactly how much progesterone is available to her body by using these creams. 6) And there's no evidence to date that progesterone creams can prevent the overstimulation of the uterine lining by estrogen or reduce the risk of endometrial cancer. 7) There's even less information about the safety and effectiveness of testosterone creams, which have been studied only in men.
>
> *www.acog.org/from_home/publications/press_releases/nr10-01-04.cfm*

possible that some progesterone or DHEA products sold without a prescription might be inferior in quality or quantity, which is why we always recommend obtaining bio-identical hormones from a compounding pharmacist.

3. Virtually *all* sex steroid hormones, bio-identical or otherwise, as well as patented "estrogens" and "progestins," are derived from wild Mexican yam (or soy) extracts that contain diosgenin. (Horse estrogens are the primary exception.) ACOG is also dead wrong when it states, "...only plants can metabolize [diosgenin] into active progesterone." In fact, diosgenin can be chemically converted – *not metabolized* – to progesterone (or any other sex steroid) *only in the*

laboratory by a process called "Marker Degradation." (*See Chapter 4.*) Neither plants nor human bodies are capable of metabolizing it. This statement by ACOG demonstrates a shocking ignorance of the manufacturing process of these hormones.

4. It's hard to know what this statement means. It seems to be suggesting that some progesterone cream products contain unprocessed diosgenin to which has been added "chemically synthesized progesterone." However, if progesterone has been "chemically synthesized," it has to have come from diosgenin; there's no other reasonable way to make it. Why a manufacturer would take "raw" diosgenin/yam cream and then add progesterone made from another batch of diosgenin is mystifying. Nevertheless, if we take the statement at face value, it's not clear why this type of preparation would be such a bad thing as long as the dose was accurate. This again indicates ACOG's profound ignorance of the hormone manufacturing process.

5. It's true that studies demonstrating the absorption and distribution of the bio-identical hormones in the body (known as *pharmacokinetic studies*) are not performed for each compounded product. Such studies would be extremely time-consuming, expensive, and impractical, given that each hormone prescription is formulated to meet the individual needs of each patient. However, if the hormone preparations are carefully formulated by a compounding pharmacist, and the doctor and patient are satisfied with the clinical results – which can be precisely and carefully monitored by 24-hour urine tests (which amounts to a basic form of pharmacokinetic analysis), as well as by the individual's personal experience – such studies are not really necessary. Moreover, if ACOG were correct, it would eliminate *all compounding*, whether of hormones or FDA-approved drugs, a result the FDA is prevented from doing by law and denies it is trying to do.

6. Again, pure nonsense. A casual review of the literature reveals *at least 14 studies*, including the well-known, NIH-sponsored PEPI study, that are published in reputable, mainstream journals and clearly demonstrate that bio-identical "progesterone creams can prevent the overstimulation of the uterine lining by estrogen or reduce the risk of endometrial cancer."[14-27] In one particularly telling study by a team

of prominent American and French researchers, postmenopausal women took doses of estradiol and progesterone daily for 5 years, during which they were carefully monitored by endometrial biopsies and hysteroscopies ("scopes" that look inside the uterus). The investigators found that no matter what dose of estradiol was used, *none of the women showed any evidence of endometrial hyperplasia* (abnormal overgrowth of the uterine lining that can lead to cancer). The researchers attributed this result to the use of a *"relatively low dose" of progesterone* with every cycle.[20] Obviously, the authors of the ACOG statement never bothered to do a 5-minute online literature search to verify this fact!

7. Another patently false statement. Please see our book, *Maximize Your Vitality and Potency*,[28] which reviews hundreds of published studies of the safety and effectiveness of bio-identical testosterone in men. In the 10 years since we wrote that book, hundreds of new studies have reinforced its major points. ACOG must have left it off their reading list. Furthermore, compounded testosterone creams, gels, and patches have been tested successfully in women in dozens of studies, but so far no bio-identical testosterone product has yet been approved for women by the FDA.[29-47]

Federal Court Rules Against FDA Harassment of Compounding Pharmacies

The FDA was re-born in 1938 when Congress passed the Federal Food, Drug, and Cosmetic (FDC) Act.* In those days, before Big Pharma had come to dominate medical practice, compounding was an essential cog in the US healthcare wheel, and the FDC Act did nothing to contradict that. For most of the intervening years, compounding pharmacies operated free of FDA interference, filling a niche that patented, off-the-shelf, one-size-fits-all, mass-produced drugs could not. In 1997, the Food and

---

*   The agency now known as the FDA originated in 1906 as the "Bureau of Chemistry." Its first Director was Harvey W. Wiley, MD. Like all other regulatory agencies, the FDA was quickly "captured" by the industries it regulated, the patent medicine and food-manufacturing industries, and the well-intentioned Dr. Wiley was forced to resign. The title of his tell-all book speaks for itself: *The History of a Crime Against the Food Law. The amazing story of the national food and drugs law intended to protect the health of the people, perverted to protect the adulteration of foods and drugs.* Harvey W. Wiley, Publisher, 506 Mills Building, Washington, DC, 1929. The entire text of this book is available online to read and download from www.soilandhealth.or g/03sov/0303critic/030305wylie/030305toc.html.

Drug Administration Modernization Act reiterated the key provisions of the FDC Act that exempted compounded medications from FDA regulation.

Nevertheless, the FDA has in recent years begun to "notice" – no doubt with lots of prodding from Wyeth and other patent medicine companies – that compounding pharmacies are apparently in violation of the law. They argue that compounding pharmacies are making "unwarranted claims" about the efficacy and safety of BHRT and may be failing to warn women of the risks involved. Not surprisingly, the agency refuses to recognize any credible scientific evidence in support of BHRT.

With increasing aggressiveness, the FDA has been applying unprecedented standards to compounding pharmacies that, if permitted, would essentially end individual compounding. The agency has been enforcing these standards via raids – *armed, knock-down-the-door, guns-drawn raids!* – on compounding pharmacies throughout the country. Since pharmacies of all kinds have long been regulated by State oversight boards, the *Federal* FDA's right to enforce its standards by raids or any other means is questionable at best.

Nonetheless, after all these years, the FDA now argues that *every* compounded medication is (and apparently always has been*)* a *new, "unapproved"* drug, thus bringing it under FDA oversight, with all the regulation that entails, including FDA-approved labeling and proof of efficacy and safety in long-term, prospective, double-blind clinical trials, costing hundreds of millions of dollars – *for every compounded prescription!*[48]

Absurd? Of course, but that hasn't stopped the FDA from claiming that compounding should be construed as a form of *drug manufacturing.* Given that there's no way compounded medicines could ever meet the regulatory requirements the FDA applies to patented, mass-produced drugs, the agency's transparent goal must be to drive compounding pharmacies out of business, thus eliminating BHRT as an option.

By 2004, compounding pharmacists had had about enough of the FDA's illegal harassment, and a group of 10 of them got together and brought suit against the agency. The case, called *Medical Center Pharmacy et al vs. Gonzalez et al*, was argued in a Federal district court in Texas.

On August 30, 2006, the court ruled decisively against the FDA, stating that compounded medications are "implicitly exempt" from the FDC Act's new-drug approval provisions. Wrote the judge, "If compounded drugs were required to undergo the [FDA's standard] new-drug approval process, the result would be that patients needing individually tailored prescriptions would not be able to receive the necessary medication due to the cost and time associated with obtaining approval. ... *It is in the best interest of public health to recognize an exemption for compounded drugs that are created based on a prescription written for an individual patient by a licensed practitioner.*" (Italics added.) In other words, the FDA cannot claim that pharmacy-compounded medications are "new drugs," and therefore, the FDA has no jurisdiction over their prescription.

Furthermore, the judge ruled that compounding pharmacy records were exempt from routine FDA inspections unless the agency could first demonstrate that the pharmacy was violating State laws and/or had crossed the line into actual manufacturing.

The FDA had also been trying to prohibit compounding pharmacists from using bulk ingredients to create customized veterinary medications (*Producing individualized prescriptions – often using special flavors – from bulk ingredients is the essence of compounding for animals and humans.*), making it virtually impossible for them to provide this *essential function* to vets, farmers, zoos, and animal lovers, not to mention people. Since relatively few mass-produced medications are indicated or formulated specifically for use in animals, compounding pharmacists have become indispensable for filling veterinarians' prescriptions.

The court ruled against the FDA on this point as well, stating that pharmacists' use of bulk ingredients for use in animal medications was legal. While those concerned with animals' health were understandably delighted with this decision, proponents of compounding for humans were also pleased, because, had the FDA's action against veterinary compounding been upheld, it was clear the agency's next step would have been to try to apply the same restriction to compounding of human meds.

Based on the Texas decision, compounding proponents are optimistic, feeling that the decision will hold up and liberate compounding pharmacies all over the country from FDA harassment. LD King, Executive Director of the International Academy of Compounding Pharmacists (IACP), stated, "The court's ruling is a precedent-setting victory for millions of patients, their doctors who prescribe compounded medicines for them, and the compounding pharmacists. This ruling affirms what the rest of the government and medical establishment have long held: *Compounding is vital and legal.*"[49]

However, this case is far from the last word on these issues. Technically, the judge's decision applies only in the Federal district in Texas (which covers Texas, Louisiana, and Mississippi) where the suit was brought, and the FDA says it intends to enforce its phantom regulations in all other jurisdictions and appealed the decision, so the case may well work its way up to the Supreme Court. Meanwhile, a decision on the appeal of this case only seems to have muddied the waters further, by rejecting some provisions of the FDA's case and upholding others. As things stand at the current time, it appears that further appeals, perhaps up to the Supreme Court, and legislative action in the Congress will be required before the issues are settled.

Wyeth's "Citizen Petition"

In October 2005, a team of Wyeth lawyers filed a "Citizen Petition" demanding that the FDA counter what they viewed as "flagrant violations of the law."[50] The petition asked for action, including *"seizures, injunctions, and/or warning letters,"* against compounding pharmacies that sold bio-identical hormones.

Wyeth insists that what they're really concerned about is *women's health.* "Wyeth *feels compelled* to advise FDA of the following activities and the *potential* risks to which American women may be exposed due to insufficient information about BHRT compounding pharmacies provide on the risks that accompany their products," states the "Citizen Petition."

Funny how Wyeth is suddenly so concerned about women's health and safety, when their HRT products have been reported in mainstream journals for decades to cause problems, such as heart disease, strokes, cancer, senility, and gall bladder disease. Only now that BHRT has become a serious threat to their bottom line have they become righteously indignant that their demonstrably dangerous "hormone replacement" products have to carry a "Black Box" warning label,* but bio-identical hormones, which are not FDA-regulated (and incidentally, have never been associated with any significant risks in published studies or otherwise), do not.

In support of its case, the Wyeth petition trots out the FDA's unscientific, misleading, and debunked survey of 12 compounding pharmacies described above, not to mention most of the same FDA complaints that had recently been shot down in Federal district court in Texas. They also argued that estriol, one of the three major natural estrogens produced by the human body, should be banned in its bio-identical form, because it is an "unapproved drug," even though estriol has been approved by the United States Pharmacopoeia (USP)† for 40 years and Wyeth itself was until recently selling estriol in Europe for the treatment of symptoms of menopause and advertising it as an "ideal treatment"!

One familiar grievance concerns the nature of compounding. Is it manufacturing or not? Isn't each compounded prescription, in fact, an unapproved, untested, unregulated *new* drug? asked Wyeth. By law the FDA regulates drug manufacturing but not drug compounding. But, just as the FDA argued – and lost – in Federal court, Wyeth's petition contends that compounding pharmacists are really *manufacturing a new drug every time they fill a prescription,* a new drug that – absent the thorough testing that all manufactured drugs must undergo – is of questionable quality, potency, and safety, and thus, may be putting its user at risk. Their conclusion: Like all patent medicines, bio-identical hormones should be regulated by the FDA, which would, in effect, end pharmacy compounding forever.

---

* The official label of Premarin® and every other FDA-approved "estrogen" product must warn about horse estrogens' nasty tendency to cause endometrial and breast cancer. The label also includes a summary of the WHI findings showing conventional HRT to be even less useful and more dangerous than previously thought.

† USP is the official drug standard setting authority for the United States.

For Wyeth, it's vital to win this point, because it represents a foot in the door for all further FDA regulation of BHRT. Without it, the FDA's jurisdiction essentially ends at the pharmacy's door (except in special instances), as it always has.

BHRT proponents have fought back vigorously, organizing those with a stake in BHRT – primarily doctors, patients, and pharmacists – to make their voices heard. Soon after the "Citizen Petition" was filed with the FDA, emails and letters began flooding into the agency. So great was the response that the FDA had to extend the standard 6-month comment period to accommodate the huge number of respondents. As of April 2007, a year and a half after the petition was filed, the FDA had received more than 70,000 individual comments, the vast majority reporting success with compounded BHRT hormones and pleading with the agency to reject Wyeth's petition and keep this vital resource available.[51] (Also in 2007, the FDA made it harder to submit such comments, by no longer accepting comments on any topic via email, but only in "snail-mailed" letters or faxes – another coincidence, no doubt.)

As the usually pro-Wyeth *BusinessWeek Online* observed, "While Wyeth clearly expected to improve its position in the multibillion-dollar market for women's hormonal products, the episode thus far shows signs of having the opposite effect. ... The huge corporation has stirred up a hornet's nest of opposition from women and doctors around the country, who see it as a classic case of Big Pharma throwing its weight around against small businesses and seeking to remove an important element of choice for suffering patients."[52]

Among the key comments to the petition was a devastating, point-by-point repudiation from the IACP, exposing each erroneous and misleading statement.[53] For example, the IACP argues, "The Citizen Petition portrays compounding pharmacies as if they were selling BHRT to hapless patients. Indeed, Wyeth states that compounding pharmacies 'are simply trying to dupe an unsuspecting patient population.' ... However, the 36-page Citizen Petition never once acknowledges that compounding pharmacies operate within the physician/patient/pharmacy triad, and that no prescription is compounded and provided to patients without receipt of a prescription from the patient's physician."

Soon after Wyeth filed its petition – in an effort that seems to have been clearly coordinated by Wyeth – several "independent" nonprofit medical professional and advocacy organizations cosigned a single letter to the FDA in support of Wyeth. These included the North American Menopause Society (NAMS), the National Association of Nurse Practitioners in Women's Health, the American Medical Women's Association, the Society for Women's Health Research, the American Society of Reproductive Medicine, the National Black Women's Health Project, the Association of Reproductive Health Professionals, the Endocrine Society, and others.[54]

Impressive as this apparently orchestrated show of support may seem on its face, it's important to realize that underlying each of these endorsements – like the SWHR connection described earlier in this chapter – lies a major conflict of interest. Wyeth has been "investing" in these organizations for years, so the upwelling of support really represents a form of payback as well as a sign that the organizations would like to keep the cash flowing in the future. As the IACP pointed out in its comment, "Each of these organizations is, to varying degrees, financially linked to Wyeth and, as a result, their comments should not be viewed as independent."[53] A prime example is NAMS, one of Wyeth's most prominent endorsers, which has received hundreds of thousands of dollars to fund research, awards, annual meetings, lectureships, educational programs, and other activities, as well as advertising in its journals and at its conventions.[55] (*See Appendix 1 for a summary of Wyeth's financial support for these supposedly "independent" advocacy and women's groups.*)

Wyeth's fingerprints can also be found all over a November 2006 resolution passed by the American Medical Association (AMA) calling for increased Federal regulation of compounded hormones, while failing to recognize the roles that State pharmacy boards, the Pharmacy Compounding Accreditation Board (PCAB), and the USP all play in regulating and setting standards for compounding pharmacies. Although the resolution does not specifically mention Wyeth's petition, its release could not help but influence the FDA's deliberations.

In the past, the AMA had evidenced a more measured approach to compounding, reflecting its consultation with the pharmacy profession. Wyeth's money may not have obviously influenced the AMA this time, but the resolution was introduced by three organizations – The Endocrine Society, the American Association of Clinical Endocrinologists, and the American Society for Reproductive Medicine – all of which receive significant funding from Wyeth (*See Appendix 1.*), financial ties that were not revealed to the AMA's House of Delegates when it approved the resolution.[56]

Surprise! The FDA Sides with Wyeth, Bans Estriol

After more than 2 years of "deliberating" and supposedly weighing the health needs and desires of 70,000 patients, doctors, and pharmacists (and the millions of others they represented) vs. the financial needs of its "client" Wyeth, the FDA finally acted on January 9, 2008. To hardly anyone's surprise, they came down on the side of Wyeth, essentially banning estriol, which just happens to compete with Wyeth's patented and dangerous "hormone" products.

The FDA's first action was to send letters warning seven compounding pharmacies that they were making false claims about bio-identical hormone replacement therapy. They also stated that estriol is not "approved" and unless pharmacies have a valid investigational new drug (IND) application *for each prescription* from the prescribing physician – a virtually impossible task – pharmacy operators may not sell compounds containing estriol.

To give you an idea of what an IND means, consider this: The IND application form alone is about 40 pages long. Each and every IND must be supervised by an institutional review board (IRB), a possibly necessary bureaucratic arrangement for usually-toxic patent medicines, but totally unnecessary for a hormone which the FDA itself admits has *never* had an adverse effect report filed despite decades of use. The delay before approval of an IND is a minimum of 30 days.

The FDA's actions against estriol are unprecedented. It is the first time the FDA had ever withdrawn from circulation a therapeutic component that had a USP monograph demonstrating its safety! It was done despite the fact that no adverse effects associated with estriol use have ever been reported by a doctor or hospital (which are obligated to report such events).

This is the FDA's most serious attack on BHRT yet, and if successful, would eliminate BHRT and make patented "HRT" regimens the only legal option available. In no uncertain terms, the battle has been joined. If they can do this with estriol, BHRT will be illegal and no other hormone, herb, or nutritional supplement that competes with a patent medicine will be safe.

Only one good thing has come out of this FDA attack on bio-identical hormone replacement therapy: it has helped mobilize the health freedom community's outrage against FDA actions. And if bio-identical hormone replacement is going to survive, it is going to take heavy doses of that outrage – focused on Congress and the courts – to save it.

(See Appendix 1 for numerous ways you, your doctor, and your pharmacist can contact the FDA and members of Congress to urge them to reverse the FDA's ban of estriol.)

Congress Gets into the Act

In May 2008, in response to the FDA's anti-BHRT actions, similar resolutions were introduced into the US House of Representatives (House Concurrent Resolution 342) and Senate (Senate Concurrent Resolution 88) urging the FDA to halt its actions against estriol and BHRT. The wording of the resolutions included the following:

Concurrent Resolution...

Expressing the sense of Congress that the Food and Drug Administration's (FDA) new policy restricting women's access to medications containing estriol does not serve the public interest...

Resolved by the House of Representatives (the Senate concurring), that it is the sense of the Congress that:

1. Physicians are in the best position to determine which medications are most appropriate for their patients;

2. The Food and Drug Administration (FDA) should respect the physician-patient relationship; and

3. The FDA should reverse its policy that aims to eliminate patients' access to compounded medications containing estriol that their physicians prescribe for them.

Initially, H. Con Res. 342 had 52 cosponsors and had been referred to the Subcommittee on Health; S. Con Res 88 had two cosponsors and had been referred to the Committee on Health, Education, Labor, and Pensions. Since no further action was taken, the resolutions will have to be re-introduced in the new Congress that started in January 2009.

The Safe Drug Compounding Act (SDCA)

Even before the FDA acted on the Wyeth petition, with its arguments defeated in Federal courts, BHRT opponents began to lean on Congress to change the law to allow the FDA to regulate pharmacy compounding. Certain members of Congress, of course, have been only too happy to oblige – in the interests of "improved patient safety," of course. In spring 2007, draft legislation – the Safe Drug Compounding Act (SDCA) of 2007 – was circulated by Senators Edward Kennedy (D-Mass), Richard Burr (R-NC), and Pat Roberts (R-Kan).

Designed to broaden the FDA's authority over compounding, the SDCA would have given the FDA undisputed power to inspect all retail pharmacies that make or dispense compounded medications and to determine whether compounded medications were medically necessary or were "essentially copies" of existing FDA-approved medications. Moreover, the act would have thrown roadblocks in the way of compounded medication distribution beyond State lines, requiring pharmacies to provide detailed documentation on all interstate orders, and to ask State pharmacy boards to "discourage the distribution of inordinate amounts of compounded drug products in interstate commerce."

Opponents of the legislation argued that the law would not only duplicate functions already performed by State pharmacy boards, the new PCAB, and the USP, but also that it would insert FDA bureaucrats between doctors and their patients by forcing prescribing doctors to prove that *each* *compounded prescription* was medically necessary. The act would also have granted the FDA broad authority to determine when compounded medications were needed and when they were not. Critics pointed out that giving the FDA these regulatory powers, dangerous and distasteful as they are, would also have put the agency on a slippery slope toward regulation or even complete prohibition of "off-label" prescribing, a practice that is jealously guarded by doctors and patent medicine companies alike, but has been selectively frowned upon by the FDA.*

The proposed law's restrictions on interstate distribution of compounded medications would have hindered patients who used pharmacies that might be located nearby but happened to be just across State borders; "snowbird" patients who continued to use their hometown pharmacies while they traveled south during the winter or north during the summer; and patients living in rural communities whose nearest compounding pharmacy might have been hundreds of miles away.

"State boards of pharmacy have done a great job to write compounding standards," said LD King of the IACP, adding that, "The PCAB just started. Our emphasis should be on these institutions, not moving power to the FDA. There's no way the FDA will be equipped to handle this."[57]
In a letter to Senators Kennedy, Burr, and Roberts, urging them to reconsider the legislation, representatives of nine different pharmacy advocacy organizations argued that the law "… would negatively impact patient care by placing undue and counterproductive restrictions on licensed prescribers and pharmacists, while doing nothing to stop the rogue compounding practices that exist."

The SDCA was originally intended to be an amendment to a larger FDA drug safety bill. However, fortunately, it did not make the final cut, due in large part to an overwhelming outpouring of grassroots opposition. According to one source, members of Congress received *more than 100,000 letters and calls* voicing concerns and opposition to the proposed law.[58] When 400 compounding pharmacists and other stakeholders descended on Capitol Hill in July 2007, the overwhelming majority of the members of Congress they met with said they had heard from members of Patients and Professionals for Customized Care (P2C2, an arm of the

---

* Once a drug is approved by the FDA for a specific indication (treating a specific disease or illness), physicians are free to prescribe it for any use they feel is appropriate, a practice that is termed "off-label" use.

International Academy of Compounding Pharmacists) – some receiving *thousands of letters* – arguing in favor of compounding. These letters did much to counteract the extensive anti-compounding lobbying by agents of Big Pharma.

What Can We Do?

Court appeals are ongoing; the FDA has nonsensically declared estriol "a new and unapproved drug" with safety and efficacy "unknown." (Your authors believe that with your help and that of hundreds of thousands of concerned women, the FDA's effort to eliminate estriol from BHRT will fail, but just in case, see Appendix 2 to read about how you and the vast majority of women can raise your own levels of estriol internally)

The forces allied against bio-identical hormones are formidable. Wyeth is a huge, powerful corporation with annual revenues approaching $19 billion dollars, financial ties to a dozen or more influential medical professional and advocacy groups and to unknown numbers of medical schools, physicians, and researchers. Of course, we can add to these a potent and well-connected DC lobbying operation, including plenty of "friends" in the Congress, FDA, and the health care bureaucracy; not to mention millions of dollars lavished each year on advertising and public relations. And Wyeth is just one company, albeit the 800-pound gorilla of conventional "hormone replacement."

What BHRT advocates lack in wealth, power, and connections, they make up in numbers and a passion bred of first-hand experience with BHRT and possibly with conventional HRT, too. Women experienced with BHRT know how well bio-identical hormones work and how good they feel when they use them. They know there's plenty of scientific evidence – not to mention common sense – to support BHRT's safety and effectiveness.

They also understand that "official" pronouncements and "news" features by TV and other media doctors regarding the alleged risks of BHRT and the "proven" benefits of HRT might well be working off Wyeth press releases. They see through the deception concealing the revolving door and the flagrant conflicts of interest among Big Pharma, the FDA, Congress, mainstream medical "experts," and the media.

The possibility that bio-identical hormones might be taken away by misguided or corrupt bureaucrats and politicians has been enough to elicit "howls" of protest to the tune of 70,000+ written comments on the "Citizen Petition" and 100,000+ phone calls, emails, and letters to Congressional offices in protest of the SDCA.

These responses have been more than mere complaints; most have included personal testimony about the benefits of bio-identical hormones to counter the misinformation, distortion, and outright lies about bio-identical hormones that characterize the conventional medical wisdom. This is information that the FDA and the Congress are not accustomed to receiving. Politicians often go where the money is, but if there's anything else they respect, it's votes; 100,000 or more unhappy women, doctors, and pharmacists translates into millions of motivated voters at the next election.

Wyeth is a past master of political manipulation and has shown it will do almost anything to keep its HRT franchise alive. Fortunately, organizations like the International Academy of Compounding Pharmacists, Patients and Professionals for Customized Care (P2C2), the American Association for Health Freedom, American Pharmacists Association, National Community Pharmacists Association, American Society of Consultant Pharmacists, American College of Apothecaries, National Association of State Pharmacies, various State pharmacists' associations, the American College for the Advancement of Medicine, the International College of Integrative Medicine, the American Academy of Environmental Medicine, the American Holistic Medical Association, and others have all been very active in opposing the powerful agents that are trying to make compounded bio-identical hormones difficult or impossible to get or even to make them illegal. These organizations need your financial *and* political support. (*See Appendix for an up-to-date list with contact information for these organizations.*)

They have raised alarms (*See ads and other articles in Appendix 1.*), argued in court, and lobbied Congress, but their efforts would be for naught if not for the enormous grassroots/netroots response from ordinary people who know first-hand the value of bio-identical hormones and refuse to relinquish their freedom to choose the best healthcare for themselves. If we are going to save BHRT, we need to keep up the pressure: stay informed, keep writing letters and emails, making phone calls, signing petitions, and providing financial support to these nonprofit organizations that can't begin to match Wyeth's resources. As P2C2 states, "Our strength is in our numbers. The more patients, physicians, pharmacists, pet owners or veterinarians we have fighting for compounded medicines, the more successful we'll be."

References

1. Weintraub A. Homegrown hormone therapy: How safe? . *BusinessWeek Online*. June 19, 2006; http://www.businessweek.com/magazine/content/06_26/ b3990070.htm?campaign_id=search: Accessed June 22, 2006.

2. Moskowitz D. A comprehensive review of the safety and efficacy of bioidentical hormones for the management of menopause and related health risks. *Altern Med Rev*. 2006;11:208-223.

3. Head KA. Estriol: safety and efficacy. *Altern Med Rev*. 1998;3:101-113.

4. Holtorf K. The bioidentical hormone debate: are bioidentical hormones (estradiol, estriol, and progesterone) safer or more efficacious than commonly used synthetic versions in hormone replacement therapy? *Postgrad Med*. 2009;121:73-85.

5. Ismail M. Spending on lobbying thrives. *Center for Public Integrity*. 2007; http://www.publicintegrity.org/rx/report.aspx?aid=823: Accessed June 10, 2007.

6. Center for Public Integrity. Lobby Watch: Wyeth. 2007; http://www. publicintegrity.org/ lobby/profile.aspx?act=clients&year=2003&cl=L003242:Ac cessed June 10, 2007.

7. Mundy A. Hot flash, cold cash. *Washington Monthly*. January/February 2003; http://www.washingtonmonthly.com/features/2001/0301.mundy.html:Accessed June 23, 2007.

8. Pipex Pharmaceuticals. TRIMESTA® (oral estriol). *http://pipexpharma.com/ pipeline trimesta.html*. 2007;Accessed November 2, 2007.

9. Barrett S. Quackwatch. *http://www.quackwatch.org/index.html*. 2007; Accessed July 4, 2007.

10. Barrett S. Steer clear of "bioidentical" hormone therapy. *Pharmwatch*. 2005; http://www.pharmwatch.org/strategy/bioidentical.shtml: Accessed July 11, 2007.

11. Center for Drug Evaluation and Research. Report: Limited FDA Survey of Compounded Drug Products. *FDA*. January 28, 2003; http://www.fda.gov/cder/ pharmcomp/survey.htm: Accessed June 26, 2007.

12. US Senate Health E, Labor and Pensions Committee,. Hearing on Pharmacy Compounding. October 23, 2003.

13. The American College of Obstetricians and Gynecologists (ACOG). No Scientific Evidence Supporting Effectiveness or Safety of Compounded Bioidentical Hormone Therapy. October 31, 2005; http://www.acog.org/from_ home/publications/press_releases/nr10-31-05-1.cfm: Accessed June 30, 2007.

14. Casanas-Roux F, Nisolle M, Marbaix E, Smets M, Bassil S, Donnez J. Morphometric, immunohistological and three-dimensional evaluation of the endometrium of menopausal women treated by oestrogen and Crinone, a new slow-release vaginal progesterone. *Hum Reprod*. 1996;11:357-363.

15. Dai D, Wolf DM, Litman ES, White MJ, Leslie KK. Progesterone inhibits human endometrial cancer cell growth and invasiveness: down-regulation of cellular adhesion molecules through progesterone B receptors. *Cancer Res.* 2002;62:881-886.

16. Leonetti HB, Anasti JN, Litman ES. Topical progesterone cream: an alternative progestin in hormone replacement therapy. *Obstet & Gynecol.* 2003;101 (4 Suppl):85.

17. Leonetti HB, Landes J, Steinberg D, Anasti JN. Transdermal progesterone cream as an alternative progestin in hormone therapy. *Altern Ther Health Med.* 2005;11:36-38.

18. Leonetti HB, Wilson KJ, Anasti JN. Topical progesterone cream has an antiproliferative effect on estrogen-stimulated endometrium. *Fertil Steril.* 2003;79:221-222.

19. Montz FJ, Bristow RE, Bovicelli A, Tomacruz R, Kurman RJ. Intrauterine progesterone treatment of early endometrial cancer. *Am J Obstet Gynecol.* 2002;186:651-657.

20. Moyer DL, de Lignieres B, Driguez P, Pez JP. Prevention of endometrial hyperplasia by progesterone during long-term estradiol replacement: influence of bleeding pattern and secretory changes. *Fertil Steril.* 1993;59:992-997.

21. Moyer DL, Felix JC. The effects of progesterone and progestins on endometrial proliferation. *Contraception.* 1998;57:399-403.

22. Moyer DL, Felix JC, Kurman RJ, Cuffie CA. Micronized progesterone regulation of the endometrial glandular cycling pool. *Int J Gynecol Pathol.* 2001;20:374-379.

23. Nisolle M, Donnez J. Progesterone receptors (PR) in ectopic endometrium? *Fertil Steril.* 1997;68:943-944.

24. Nisolle M, Gillerot S, Casanas-Roux F, Squifflet J, Berliere M, Donnez J. Immunohistochemical study of the proliferation index, oestrogen receptors and progesterone receptors A and B in leiomyomata and normal myometrium during the menstrual cycle and under gonadotrophin-releasing hormone agonist therapy. *Hum Reprod.* 1999;14:2844-2850.

25. Sager G, Orbo A, Jaeger R, Engstrom C. Non-genomic effects of progestins-- inhibition of cell growth and increased intracellular levels of cyclic nucleotides. *J Steroid Biochem Mol Biol.* 2003;84:1-8.

26. Whitehead MI, Fraser D, Schenkel L, Crook D, Stevenson JC. Transdermal administration of oestrogen/progestagen hormone replacement therapy. *Lancet.* 1990;335:310-312.

27. Effects of hormone replacement therapy on endometrial histology in postmenopausal women. The Postmenopausal Estrogen/Progestin Interventions (PEPI) Trial. The Writing Group for the PEPI Trial. *JAMA.* 1996;275:370-375.

28. Wright J, Lenard L. *Maximize Your Vitality & Potency*. Petaluma, CA: Smart Publications; 1999.

29. Floter A, Nathorst-Boos J, Carlstrom K, von Schoultz B. Addition of testosterone to estrogen replacement therapy in oophorectomized women: effects on sexuality and well-being. *Climacteric.* 2002;5:357-365.

30. Braunstein GD, Sundwall DA, Katz M, et al. Safety and efficacy of a testosterone patch for the treatment of hypoactive sexual desire disorder in surgically menopausal women: a randomized, placebo-controlled trial. *Arch Intern Med.* 2005;165:1582-1589.

31. Shifren JL, Braunstein GD, Simon JA, et al. Transdermal testosterone treatment in women with impaired sexual function after oophorectomy. *N Engl J Med.* 2000;343:682-688.

32. Bolour S, Braunstein G. Testosterone therapy in women: a review. *Int J Impot Res.* 2005.

33. The role of testosterone therapy in postmenopausal women: position statement of The North American Menopause Society. *Menopause.* 2005;12:497-511.

34. Singh AB, Lee ML, Sinha-Hikim I, et al. Pharmacokinetics of a testosterone gel in healthy postmenopausal women. *J Clin Endocrinol Metab.* 2005.

35. Somboonporn W, Davis SR. Testosterone effects on the breast: implications for testosterone therapy for women. *Endocr Rev.* 2004;25:374-388.

36. Nathorst-Boos J, Floter A, Jarkander-Rolff M, Carlstrom K, Schoultz B. Treatment with percutanous testosterone gel in postmenopausal women with decreased libido - effects on sexuality and psychological general well-being. *Maturitas.* 2006;53:11-18.

37. Nathorst-Boos J, Jarkander-Rolff M, Carlstrom K, Floter A, von Schoultz B. Percutaneous administration of testosterone gel in postmenopausal women--a pharmacological study. *Gynecol Endocrinol.* 2005;20:243-248.

38. Floter A, Nathorst-Boos J, Carlstrom K, Ohlsson C, Ringertz H, Schoultz B. Effects of combined estrogen/testosterone therapy on bone and body composition in oophorectomized women. *Gynecol Endocrinol.* 2005;20:155-160.

39. Simon J, Braunstein G, Nachtigall L, et al. Testosterone patch increases sexual activity and desire in surgically menopausal women with hypoactive sexual desire disorder. *J Clin Endocrinol Metab.* 2005;90:5226-5233.

40. Buster JE, Kingsberg SA, Aguirre O, et al. Testosterone patch for low sexual desire in surgically menopausal women: a randomized trial. *Obstet Gynecol.* 2005;105:944-952.

41. Shifren JL, Mazer NA. Safety profile of transdermal testosterone therapy in women. *Am J Obstet Gynecol.* 2003;189:898-899; author reply 899.

42. Mazer NA, Shifren JL. Transdermal testosterone for women: a new physiological approach for androgen therapy. *Obstet Gynecol Surv.* 2003;58:489-500.

43. Somboonporn W. Testosterone therapy for postmenopausal women: efficacy and safety. *Semin Reprod Med.* 2006;24:115-124.

44. Somboonporn W, Davis S, Seif MW, Bell R. Testosterone for peri- and postmenopausal women. *Cochrane Database Syst Rev.* 2005:CD004509.

45. Shifren JL. Is testosterone or estradiol the hormone of desire? A novel study of the effects of testosterone treatment and aromatase inhibition in postmenopausal women. *Menopause.* 2006;13:8-9.

46. Davis SR. The use of testosterone after menopause. *J Br Menopause Soc.* 2004;10:65-69.

47. Davis A, Gilbert K, Misiowiec P, Riegel B. Perceived effects of testosterone replacement therapy in perimenopausal and postmenopausal women: an internet pilot study. *Health Care Women Int.* 2003;24:831-848.

48. Compoundingfacts.org. Pharmacy compounding subject to FDA approval? The facts just don't fit. . *http://www.compoundingfacts.org/info.cfm?News_ID=84.* 2007:Accessed July 7, 2007.

49. Henderson D. Ruling hurts FDA push on compounds. Judge: Practice doesn't create new drugs so isn't under agency's purview. *Boston Globe.* September 1, 2006;http://www.boston.com/business/ globe/articles/2006/09/01/ruling_hurts_ fda_push_on_compounds/: Accessed July 7, 2007.

50. Wyeth Pharmaceuticals. Citizen Petition Seeking FDA Actions to Counter Flagrant Violations of the Law by Pharmacies Compounding Bio-Identical Hormone Replacement Therapy Drugs that Endanger Public Health. October 6, 2005; http://www.fda.gov/ohrms/dockets/dockets/ 05p0411/05p-0411-cp00001-01-vol1.pdf: Accessed July 12, 2007.

51. Galson S. Bio-Identical Hormones: Sound Science or Bad Medicine. *Statement before the US Senate Special Committee on Aging.* April 19, 2007; http://www. fda.gov/ola/2007/ hormone041907.html: Accessed July 12, 2007.

52. Gumpert D. Hormone Battle: Big Pharma vs. Small Biz. *BusinessWeek Online.* April 13, 2006; http://www.businessweek.com/smallbiz/content/apr2006/ sb20060413_667219.htm?campaign_id=search: Accessed July 14, 2007.

53. International Academy of Compounding Pharmacists. Comments to Citizen Petition Filed on Behalf of Wyeth. December 15, 2005; http://www.fda.gov/ ohrms/dockets/dockets/05p0411/05p-0411-c000009-vol1.pdf: Accessed July 12, 2007.

54. Food and Drug Administration. Dockets Management. 2007; http://www.fda. gov/ohrms/dockets/ dockets/05p0411/05p0411.htm: Accessed July 12, 2007.

55. Compoundingfacts.org. North American Menopause Society's Ties to Wyeth Pharmaceuticals 2007; http://www.compoundingfacts.org/info.cfm?News_ID=90: Accessed July 14, 2007.

56. International Academy of Compounding Pharmacists. Physicians, patients, Pharmacists Express Disappointment with AMA Resolution. December 18, 2006; http://www.iacprx.org/site/ PageServer?pagename=Press_Releases#111506: Accessed July 14, 2007.

57. Paul R. New bill on pharmacy compounding stirs concern. *Drug Topics.* April 2, 2007; http://www.drugtopics.com/drugtopics/article/articleDetail.jsp?id=414436: Accessed July 15, 2007.

58. Women's International Pharmacy. An update on the proposed legislation regarding BHRT/compounded medications. 2007; http://www.womensinternational.com/ legislation.html: Accessed July 15, 2007.

APPENDICES

Appendix 1: A Call to Action

"The price of freedom is eternal vigilance"
– usually attributed to Thomas Jefferson

As you're reading this, the battle for and against BHRT (*See Chapter 12.*) may still be raging, or it may be behind us, but for as long as *los Federales* as well as State and other governments exist, there will be attacks on your freedom of choice in health care. So please join us to help restore and maintain a basic American freedom enjoyed by most Americans since the 18th and 19th centuries!

To stay in touch with the latest developments in health care freedom, visit www.healthfreedom.net, the website of the American Association for Health Freedom (AAHF), 1350 Connecticut Ave, 5th Floor, Washington, DC 20036, which can also be reached at 800-230-2762. AAHF has made it possible to relay your opinion to your Senators and members of Congress with a few simple "clicks" on their website.

Also, please write, call, fax, or email your Congressional Representatives and Senators *now* (and continue to send them frequent reminders) regarding current legislation related to BHRT (and other issues related to freedom of health choice). The fight for American freedom right here at home is just as important as freedom for others abroad – for yourself, your children, and your grandchildren.

Another way to find the names, addresses, and telephone numbers of your Congressional Representatives is to visit the United States House of Representatives website – www.house.gov. To locate contact information for your State's senators, visit the Senate website – www.senate.gov. For a one-stop resource for locating and writing to your representatives, visit www.congress.org, a website run by a group called Capitol Advantage. If you don't have access to a computer, you can easily find out the contact information for your State's members of Congress and Senators by calling the United States Capitol switchboard at (202) 224-3121.

The following pages show a few of the ads BHRT supporters have been running to counter the Wyeth/FDA onslaught against BHRT and estriol in particular.

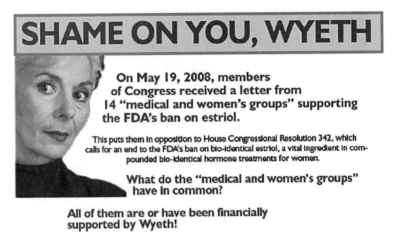

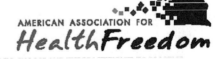

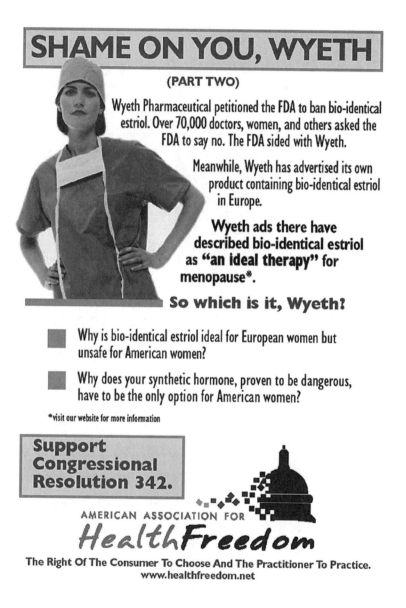

Full page ad that appeared in the *New York Times, USA Today, Wall Street Journal, Seattle Times,* and *Roll Call* on February 4, 2008

Ad sponsored by *HOME* (*Hands Off My Estrogens*), www.homecoalition.org

FDA Bans Hormone Produced by Human Body as "Unapproved" Drug

The FDA has told women and their doctors: stop using bio-identical hormones. Your choice and your doctor's prescription don't matter. Heart and cancer questions raised in 2002 about FDA "approved" synthetic women's hormones don't matter. Act now to defend your right to bio-identical hormones!

Countless women currently rely on replacement hormones that are prescribed by their doctors and compounded in local pharmacies. These compounded hormones are biologically identical to the ones produced in the human body. The formulas include bio-identical, naturally occurring estrogen hormones such as estriol.

Nevertheless, on January 9, the U.S. Food and Drug Administration ordered pharmacies to stop providing bio-identical estriol. Even though 80% of bio-identical hormone replacement therapy prescriptions use it, and estriol is manufactured by the human body, the FDA makes the outrageous and nonsensical claim that estriol is "a new and unapproved drug" and that "the safety and effectiveness of estriol is unknown."

Bio-Identical Estriol is Safe

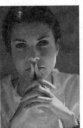

In a press conference, the FDA admitted that no adverse event involving compounded bio-identical estriol has ever been reported. Research involving 15,000 women funded by the Department of Defense and conducted at Kaiser-Permanente Oakland found that women who produced the most estriol during their first pregnancy had 58% less breast cancer over the next forty years.

Every woman who has ever had a menstrual cycle or been pregnant knows that natural estriol is both safe and effective. Estriol is a major estrogen throughout a woman's reproductive years, and soars to enormous levels (up to a thousand times) during pregnancy.

How can bio-identical estriol, identical to every woman's natural estriol, be unsafe or ineffective? And how can the FDA claim that a substance present in our bodies from the dawn of humanity is a "new and unapproved drug"?

Speaking the Truth is Not a "False Claim"

The FDA is also ordering pharmacies to stop using the terms "bio-identical hormone replacement therapy" and "BHRT" on the grounds that these terms represent "false claims."

False claims do exist in any field and should not be allowed. But describing these hormones accurately is not a false claim.

What's Going on Here?

For decades the FDA has called any claim about a natural substance, no matter how accurate, a "false claim" if it is not specifically FDA "approved." But there's a big "Catch-22": It costs up to a billion dollars to achieve FDA approval. As a general rule, companies cannot afford to spend these huge sums unless their drug is patent-protected. And again, as a general rule, natural substances such as bio-identical hormones cannot be patent-protected. As a result, the FDA has "approved" only a very small handful of natural substances, sometimes only after being sued and ordered to do so by a judge.

Bottom line: The FDA says that natural substances must be "approved" to make any claims about them, but knows full well that, under the current FDA system, there is no way to get most natural substances "approved."

Why is the FDA So Hostile to "Natural" Medicine?

"Alternative," "natural," and "integrative" medicine is booming today. A growing number of doctors and patients believe that natural substances are often safer and more effective than synthetic, hyper-expensive but "approved" patent medicines (drugs). So why is the FDA so hostile?

A possible explanation: the FDA is worried that natural substances will eat into the sales and profits of its clients, the big drug companies. Fees from the big drug companies pay for a sizeable share of the FDA's budget and staff. There are many other financial ties as well.

In October 2005, Wyeth, a large patent medicine (drug) company, filed a "citizens' petition" demanding that the FDA ban bio-identical hormones that compete with Wyeth's synthetic hormones. Sales of Wyeth's hormones had plummeted as more and more women and their doctors turned to bio-identical hormones. (Recently Wyeth has faced layoffs and facility closings for this and other reasons.)

Over 70,000 women, pharmacists, and doctors wrote to the FDA, the overwhelming majority asking the Agency to reject Wyeth's attempt to shut down the competition and preserve access to bio-identical hormones. The FDA sided against the women and with Wyeth.

Are the FDA "Approved" Drugs Safe?

And what do we know about the "approved" patent medicines (drugs) from Wyeth and others that the FDA wants you and your doctor to use for hormone replacement? These once-bestselling drugs come from horses or are imprecise versions of natural human hormones. Why would any woman prefer horse hormones or imprecise-yet-patentable copies of human hormone molecules to ones precisely identical to those found naturally in her body?

Studies have also raised questions about possible heart and cancer risks from these hormones. (See the *Journal of the American Medical Association* 288 [3], pp. 321-333; [7], pp. 872-884). This is why these drugs currently have Black Box Warnings on them.

Why Shouldn't Women and Their Doctors Have a Choice?

It's time to take action again!

We are the HOME (HANDS OFF MY ESTROGENS) Coalition, a coalition of licensed doctors and concerned citizens. *Please contact your congressional representative, senators, and the White House Immediately.* For sample letters and e-mails, and a simple interactive form for sending your messages, visit the HOME Coalition website:

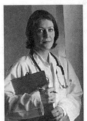

www.homecoalition.org

Or contact your elected officials directly. You can use these numbers to obtain an address or to leave your comments:

The U.S. Senate and the House of Representatives:
(202) 224-3121 (switchboard)

The White House:
(202) 456-1414 (switchboard);
(202) 456-1111 (comments)

Please do it NOW, or your access to bio-identical hormones will disappear!

—*Jonathan V. Wright, MD*
Tahoma Clinic, Renton, Washington
A.B., Harvard University (1965)
M.D., University of Michigan (1969)
First North American prescriber of bio-identical
hormones for clinical use, 1983

For the HOME Coalition:
American Academy for Advancement in Medicine (ACAM)
American Academy of Environmental Medicine (AAEM)
International College of Integrative Medicine (ICIM)
The Bio-identical Hormone Initiative (BHI)

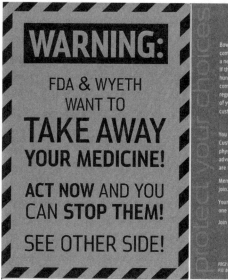

What BHRT Supporters Are Saying About the Wyeth/FDA Campaign to Ban Estriol

---

American Academy of Environmental Medicine
6505 E Central, Ste 296, Wichita, KS 67206
Tel: (316) 684-5500; Fax: (316) 684-5709
Internet: www.aaemonline.org

"The American Academy of Environmental Medicine believes that physicians are in the best position to determine which medications are most appropriate for their patients and that the FDA should never stand between a medical decision made by a patient and their chosen physician. If FDA's action is allowed to stand, it would force hundreds of thousands of women off of medications that their doctors have prescribed for them – and for no scientific or medical reason."

American Board of Clinical Metal Toxicology
4889 Smith Road, West
Chester, Ohio 45069
Phone 1.800.356.2228 or 513.863.6277
Fax 513.942.3934
Email secretary@abcmt.org

"The attempt by the FDA to suppress custom compounding of safe, natural, bioidentical hormones is a broad overreach, a thinly-veiled effort to increase the profits of major manufacturers at the expense of the health, comfort, and happiness of the 100 million adult women in America. This far exceeds the federal authority, creating new problems for helpless but hopeful individuals rather than protecting their rights to a better life. One company "leading the charge" hides behind a double-standard: Wyeth includes estriol in at least one of its drug combinations marketed in Europe … but wants the very same hormone to be outlawed here!"

American College for the Advancement of Medicine
24411 Ridge Route, Ste 115
Laguna Hills, CA 92653
Phone: 949.309.3520
Fax: 949.309.3538
Internet: www.acamnet.org

"ACAM believes women have a right to treatment options that are best suited for their health and well-being as prescribed under the auspices of a licensed physician. We find the FDA's attempt to ban estriol overly restrictive. Additionally, the FDA has failed to show a compelling federal interest in banning estriol as no serious or adverse effects have been reported with the use of compounded bio-identical estriol."

Association of American Physicians and Surgeons
1601 N. Tucson Blvd., Suite 9
Tucson, AZ 85716
Phone: (800) 635-1196
Fax: (520) 325-4230
Internet: www.aapsonline.org/

"Doctors are in the better position to determine which medications are appropriate for their patients, and the FDA needs to respect the doctor-patient relationship and reverse its misguided and harmful policy that seeks to eliminate patients' access to compounded medications in general and medications containing estriol in particular."

Citizens for Health
26828 Maple Valley Highway, #242
Maple Valley, WA 98038
Email: info@citizens.org
Internet: www.citizens.org/

"CFH believes that a patient's health care provider is in the best position to determine which medications or treatments are most appropriate for him/her – the FDA should never stand between a medical decision made by a patient and his/her chosen health care provider. [House Concurrent] Resolution 342 emphasizes this, and it is one of the reasons CFH supports the resolution.

"If the FDA is allowed to maintain its position regarding bio-identical hormones containing estriol, it would result in hundreds of thousands of women losing access to medications that their health care providers have prescribed for them. Is it right that millions of American women who rely on this safe, proven and effective healthcare option will have it denied them when the FDA has never before taken action against a USP-monographed drug in the absence of any adverse events?

"The FDA should refrain from interfering with state regulations and stick to its intended mission. It would better utilize its time, energy and resources by standardizing bio-identical hormones, making them more available and accessible rather than restricting them."

Integrated Healthcare Policy Consortium
240 Maple Street
Burlington, VT 05401
Phone: (802) 658-8525
Internet: www.ihpc.info/

"In January of this year, the U.S. Food and Drug Administration (FDA) initiated steps to restrict the provision of prescriptions containing bio-identical estriol by compounding pharmacies to post-menopausal women. We find this action to be an unwarranted invasion of the physician-patient relationship, and an unjustifiable restriction of a woman's individual right to choose from among treatment options sharing similar risks and therapeutic benefits ... Compounding pharmacists and healthcare practitioners should be allowed to perform to the limits of their licensed scope of practice, and patients should have access to the medications and remedies prescribed and deemed safe by their doctors. Estriol should not be taken off the market; rather factual information should be made available to the public in support of informed decision-making."

International College of Integrative Medicine
122 Thurman St. Box 271
Bluffton, OH 45817
E mail: wendy@icimed.com
Phone: (866) 464-5226, (419) 358-0273
Internet: www.icimed.com/

"Estriol is an essential compounded substance for the safe, effective treatment of [women with debilitating hormone imbalance]. Estriol has been available for this use through the US Pharmacopeia for 50 years. No significant safety concerns have been reported to the FDA or observed by our physicians. There is not a rational reason for the FDA to restrict the use of estriol. The only apparent reasons I can see are a petition by a competitor (Wyeth, maker of Premarin® and Prempro®) and the desire of the FDA to restrict compounding pharmacies from doing their job of preparing prescriptions for physicians to treat patients. These should not be the role of the FDA."

Life Extension Foundation
1100 W. Commercial Blvd.
Fort Lauderdale, FL 33309
Phone: 954-766-8433 or 800-544-4440
Internet: www.lef.org/

"Unlike Premarin® and Prempro® that have been demonstrated to increase cancer and vascular disease risk, we have accumulated a significant amount of evidence that estriol (especially when combined with natural progesterone) may protect against common female cancers.

"The FDA has admitted that it is taking enforcement action against estriol on behalf of drug companies that stand to economically benefit if estriol is banned from the marketplace. The fact that an agency of the federal government charged with protecting the public's health is instead being used by vested financial interests to deny American women a safe form of estrogen (estriol) is a mockery of the system.

"Please know that in the 14 years that we have been recommending estriol drugs, there has never been a report of serious adverse events reported by our members. In fact, the FDA itself acknowledges that it has received no reports of adverse reactions. All of this points to the obvious, ie, the FDA is acting to protect the financial interests of drug companies who continue to sell forms of estrogen that are proven to increase risk of lethal disease."

The North Carolina Integrative Medical Society
PO Box 6472
Raleigh, NC 27628
Internet: www.ncims.com/

"NCIMS supports the ability of a patient to access individualized medication, which can only be created by a Compounding Pharmacy... It is criminal for the FDA, whose purpose is to protect the health and lives of Americans, to attempt to deny the basic right to freedom of healthcare. The FDA itself admits no adverse events caused by the use of Estriol, which has been listed in the US Pharmacopeia for 50 years.

Is the FDA actually motivated to promote the interests of the pharmaceutical industry? The FDA should not pursue a short-sighted plan to promote pharmaceutical profit. The FDA should refocus on its mission to protect the health and lives of Americans. They should be wary of the motives of large pharmaceutical companies, which seek a "one-pill-fits-all" mass-produced monoculture of health. This may work well with car manufacturing, but when applied to living organisms, results in tragic disaster."

Organic Consumers Association
6771 S. Silver Hill Drive
Finland, MN 55603
Phone: 218-226-4164
Fax: 218-353-7652
Email: ronnie@organicconsumers.org
Internet: www.organicconsumers.org/

"The FDA has never before taken action against a USP monographed drug where there have not been any adverse events. …Congress should ask the FDA to focus on its mission of protecting consumers from real harms, avoid unnecessary interference with state regulations, and refrain from creating problems where there are none."

Semmelweis Society International
80 12th Street, Suite #307
Wheeling, WV 26003
Phone: 724-678-2648
Internet: www.semmelweis.org/

"The resolution [H Con Res 342] … calls on the FDA to respect the physician-patient relationship and recognizes that doctors, not the FDA, are in the best position to determine which medications are appropriate for their patients. It highlights the FDA's own acknowledgment that it is unaware of any adverse events associated with the use of estriol over the past three decades."

The Bioidentical Hormone Initiative
5821 W. Maple Rd. Ste 192
West Bloomfield, MI 48323
Internet: www.bioidenticalhormoneinitiative.org/

"The FDA needs to act in the best interests of the public. The banning of the natural hormone estriol does not serve this purpose. Estriol has been listed in the U.S. Pharmacopeia for over 50 years. There have been no adverse events associated with estriol and studies demonstrate that it is both safe and effective. FDA has acknowledged no adverse events.

Since the FDA has never taken action against a USP monographed drug where there have been no adverse events, why is FDA taking action against estriol? When indicated, we have successfully used estriol in our practices. It is an extremely safe and effective bioidentical, natural hormone. We have not heard any complaints about estriol from our patients. There is no reason for FDA to actively move against estriol.

"We urge Congress to ask FDA to not interfere with state regulations and create problems where none exist. FDA is not acting in the interest of the public. It is time for Congress to act and redirect FDA to properly do its job."

Women in Balance
Post Office Box 12004
Overland Park, KS 66282
E-Mail: information@womeninbalance.org
Internet: www.womeninbalance.org/

"The FDA claims that there is no safety and patient response data for Estriol, yet there is a body of literature about this, as Estriol is a fundamental element of female biology. In addition, Estriol has been used in Europe and Japan for years with no reported ill effects. And this ingredient is used in several drugs manufactured by Wyeth in Europe, Cyclo-Menorette® and Estriolsalbe®. We hear from thousands of women who have been helped with physician prescribed bioidentical hormone therapy. Please allow the continued availability of compounded bioidentical hormones like Estriol that women need for quality of life."

International Academy of Compounding Pharmacists
4638 Riverstone Blvd.
Missouri City, TX 77459
Phone: 281-933-8400
Fax: (281) 495-0602
www.iacprx.org

"Estriol medications compete directly with Wyeth's synthetic products that have been linked by the Women's Health Initiative to heart disease, cancer and [fill in the blank]. Women want a choice, and the FDA and Wyeth are essentially seeking to deny their doctors the right to prescribe many of the treatments that compete with Wyeth's products. ...Wyeth provides funding to these organizations. We understand that the very letter they sent you was coordinated by a Wyeth lobbyist. Because Wyeth is a major manufacturer of patented, horse-derived hormones, it is waging a fierce lobbying campaign to restrict a woman's access to alternatives to its own products – alternatives like compounded hormones that contain estriol."

WYETH'S "INDEPENDENT" SUPPORT?

When Wyeth first filed its "Citizen Petition" in October 2005, and again in May 2008, as the FDA/Wyeth attack on estriol was being debated in Congress, the "independent" advocacy and women's groups listed below cosigned a single letter urging "support" of the Wyeth/FDA position. As compiled by the *American Association for Health Freedom (AAHF)*, here is a summary of Wyeth's "generosity" to these organizations over the last few years. How independent are these organizations? ***Judge for yourself.***

American College of Obstetricians and Gynecologists	Wyeth funds several annual awards for the American College of Obstetricians and Gynecologists (ACOG), totaling approximately $29,000 per year. Wyeth is also a Friends of ACOG Participant, where Friends donate $3,000 per annum; is a frequent exhibitor at ACOG's Annual Clinical Meetings; and sponsors ACOG's annual "Resident Reporter" Program.
American Medical Women's Association	On its web site, the American Medical Women's Association (AMWA) lists Wyeth as one of 12 members of its Corporate Partners Program, which it "thank[s] for their generous support." Wyeth is also listed as a member of AMWA's Elizabeth Blackwell Diamond Circle of Honor, which recognizes donations of $10,000 and above.
American Society for Reproductive Medicine	Wyeth is a member of The American Society for Reproductive Medicine's 2007 Corporate Council. The Society received at least $75,000 from Wyeth last year, which placed it in the top echelon of sponsors of its annual meeting.
Association of Reproductive Health Professionals	Wyeth is a founding member of the Association's Corporate Advisory Board, and its dues benefit the Fund for the Future of Reproductive Health. In 2005, they gave an award called "Wyeth Pharmaceuticals New Leaders Award." Wyeth was a Gold sponsor at their 2007 conference at a cost of at least $15,000.
Black Women's Health Imperative	Wyeth was an underwriting sponsor of "Celebration of Activism for Black Women's Health and Lives in 2004."
Center for Women Policy Studies	Wyeth is listed as one of the Center's funders from 1972 until 1997.

The Endocrine Society	Wyeth Pharmaceuticals is a Corporate Liaison Board member of The Endocrine Society as well as a frequent exhibitor at the Society's Annual Meetings. The Society recognized Wyeth as a Leadership Donor in 2002, honoring those donors who have contributed at least $100,000 to the Society in the previous year.
National Association of Nurse Practitioners in Women's Health	Wyeth is a Gold Corporate Sponsor for the National Association of Nurse Practitioners in Women's Health. The Association's President and CEO, Susan Wysocki, serves on both Wyeth's advisory board and speaker's bureau.
National Black Nurses Association	In 2000, Wyeth provided funds to help support the NBNA Women's Health Research Agenda. In 2002, Wyeth contributed funding for the NBNA Women's Health Grant Program.
National Consumers League	According to the Center for Science in the Public Interest, Wyeth was the largest single corporate contributor to the National Consumers League for the period 2001 and 2002, with total contributions of $337,500. In 2003, Wyeth began funding an NCL campaign called MenoPAUSE: Take Time to Talk about Your Symptoms. According to an NCL press release, [MenoPAUSE] … "is made possible by an unrestricted educational grant from Wyeth." Wyeth has also sponsored various NCL surveys and reports going at least as far back as 1999.
National Partnership for Women and Families	Wyeth was a sponsor of their 2007 Annual Luncheon – at the Leadership Circle (2nd highest level) with a donation of at least $10,000.
National Women's Law Center	According to the National Women's Law Center's 2005-2006 Annual Report, Wyeth was listed as a sponsor ($25,000-$49,999).
North American Meno- pause Society	Wyeth endows a $200,000 lectureship fund named for NAMS President Dr. Wulf Utian and was named a "Partner in Menopause Education" (requiring a contribution of at least $8,000) for the NAMS' 2007 Annual Meeting. Additionally, half of NAMS's Board of Trustees for 2007-2008, including Dr. Utian, receives "consulting fees" or "research support" from Wyeth.
Society for Women's Health Research	Wyeth serves on the Society for Women's Health Research's Corporate Advisory Council and served as one of the corporate dinner chairs of the Society's 2007 Annual Gala Dinner. SWHR also received a $250,000 donation in 2002 at Wyeth's 60th anniversary celebration of Premarin®, one of the company's HRT drugs. (See Chapter 12)

This article is excerpted from Dr. Jonathan V. Wright's Nutrition & Healing *monthly newsletter, available by subscription and online at www.wrightnews-letter.com.*

DON'T BE FOOLED BY BIG PHARMA'S MOVE INTO BIO-IDENTICAL HORMONE REPLACEMENT THERAPY

Big Pharma is threatened by the increasing popularity of bio-identical hormones, and with good reason: They're safer, they're cheaper, and they actually work. So it wasn't too surprising when the patent medicine company Wyeth wrote a citizen's petition to severely restrict − if not eliminate − individually compounded bio-identical hormones.

Thanks to hundreds of thousands of women and men (thanks to you too, if you were one of them) who wrote, faxed, emailed, and called the FDA and their congressional representatives in opposition to the petition. (My favorite letter was by a woman who threatened to "…have PMS at FDA headquarters every month if my individually compounded bio-identical hormones are taken away.") In response to the unexpectedly large volume of protest, the FDA took from October 6, 2005 until January 8, 2008 to even start the process of trying to ban estriol and severely restrict pharmacy compounding.

In August 2006, Federal District Judge Robert Junell decided for compounding pharmacies and against the FDA in Medical Center Pharmacy, et al v. Gonzales, et al, writing: "The Court finds that the compounding of ingredients to create a drug pursuant to valid prescription from a health care provider does not create a new drug." Judge Junell's order became final a month or two later, and it appeared as if bio-identical hormones were safe from the FDA and the patent medicine companies.

Unfortunately, those were just the opening salvos in what looks to be a long, drawn out struggle. (There has been other "court action" since which did nothing to clarify the issue.) There's big, big, money in bio-identical hormones − for patent medicine companies, for FDA approval, and, of course, yet another potentially big increase in power and control for the FDA. So if patent medicine companies and the FDA can't win by one route, they'll just try another.

Their New Strategy? If You Can't Beat 'em, Join 'em.

Patent medication companies are now latching onto these bio-identical hormones and are renaming them, getting FDA approval, and jacking up the price. The end result would be increased FDA regulation, bio-identical hormones at 5 times the cost, and less freedom for your doctor to individualize your hormone treatment. But as bad as those things are, they're still only scratching the surface of just how damaging this could ultimately be for the unrestricted use of relatively inexpensive bio-identical hormones.

Bio-Identical Hormones in Disguise

Estriol is an estrogen that's produced in substantial quantities in nonpregnant, cycling women, but it's especially high in pregnant women. In 2002, UCLA researchers reported that, in women with multiple sclerosis, pregnancy-high doses of estriol significantly improved symptoms, MRI scans, and many tests of immune function.

For those of you who are technically inclined, I've included what the researchers wrote about the results of the study (if you're not in this category, you can skip to the following paragraph): "As compared with pretreatment baseline, relapsing remitting [multiple sclerosis] patients treated with oral estriol (8 mg/day) demonstrated significant decreases in delayed type hypersensitivity responses to tetanus, interferon-gamma levels in peripheral blood mononuclear cells, and gadolinium-enhancing lesion numbers and volumes on monthly cerebral magnetic resonance images. When estriol treatment was stopped, enhancing lesions increased to pretreatment levels. When estriol treatment was reinstituted, enhancing lesions again were significantly decreased."

Since that study was published in the *Annals of Neurology* in 2002, I've prescribed estriol (as well as other individually specific remedies) for a few women with multiple sclerosis and other autoimmune diseases, including lupus, rheumatoid arthritis, and type 1 diabetes. And in nearly every single case, the women involved could tell that estriol made a significant difference in the way they felt.

But even though this is "old news" in the world of alternative medicine, a certain patent medicine company is trying to reinvent the wheel. Apparently, Pipex Therapeutics hasn't heard about the extensive use of estriol as a bio-identical hormone here in these United States. As stated in a press release: "Pipex is also developing Trimesta® (oral estriol) for the treatment of relapse-remitting multiple sclerosis (MS). Estriol, an estrogenic molecule approved and marketed in Europe and Asia for the treatment of postmenopausal hot flashes for over 40 years but never introduced to the US, is a pregnancy hormone that is believed to be responsible for the high rates of spontaneous remission experienced by female MS patients during pregnancy."

Never introduced to the US? Pipex researchers seem to be blissfully (or perhaps for corporate reasons, purposefully) unaware of bio-identical hormone replacement here in these United States. I wrote the first prescription for Tri-Est (an 80% estriol prescription filled by compounding pharmacist Ed Thorpe of Kripps Pharmacy in Vancouver, BC, Canada) in the 1980s for just one woman suffering with symptoms of menopause. And now, Tri-Est and its close cousin Bi-Est (also 80% estriol) are prescribed by thousands of physicians through thousands of compounding pharmacies to millions of women in the US. Estriol alone is a fairly frequent prescription for some women, such as those with a prior history of cancer. Remember: Trimesta® is just estriol repackaged!

The same is also true of DHEA and 2-methoxyestradiol, two naturally occurring hormones in the body. I'm sure you've heard of DHEA, but did you know it's been renamed Prestara®? Under that name, it's already approved by the FDA for the prevention of loss of bone mineral density in patients with systemic lupus erythematosus.

The hormone 2-methoxyestradiol is another estrogen metabolite produced naturally in women's bodies. Although this hormone isn't available yet, it's still been found to have major anti-tumor effects against a range of cancers, including (but not limited to) breast, cervical, prostate, pancreatic, endometrial, myeloma, leukemia, and osteosarcoma. As described above, under nearly everyone's radar screen, EntreMed corporation has morphed entirely natural 2-methoxyestradiol into Panzem®.

Misuse and Abuse of Bio-Identical Hormones

Renaming bio-identical hormones to turn a quick profit is certainly bad enough. But as I said earlier, that's just the start of the disaster that's sure to follow.

Any physician skilled and knowledgeable in the use of bio-identical hormones knows that natural steroids, such as estriol, DHEA, and 2-methoxyestradiol, should NOT be taken orally. According to one study, taking only 1 to 2 mg orally of low-potency estrogen formulations increased the relative risk of developing endometrial cancer.

So which route of administration has been chosen by the company pushing for estriol (aka Trimesta®) approval? *Oral.* And when the inevitable findings of excessive endometrial cancer are ultimately disclosed, you can bet the blame will fall on the bio-identical hormone itself − and not on the oral route of administration, which is known to be more risky.

The patent medicine company that recently received approval for DHEA (aka Prestara®) isn't doing any better. In addition to using oral doses instead of the more physiologic transdermal route, the quantities given − 200 milligrams daily for women − are well known to physicians skilled and knowledgeable in the use of bio-identical hormones to be enormous overdoses. But when the inevitable side effects come rolling in, you can be sure it'll be the DHEA itself − not it's abuse and misuse − that gets the blame.

It's been 50 years now since bio-identical cortisol went down this same path of destruction. Doctors prescribed much larger than physiologic doses of cortisone for months to years, and now the public is blaming cortisone for causing hypertension, diabetes, osteoporosis, peptic ulcers, and the occasional cortisone psychosis − rather than blaming themselves for cortisone abuse and misuse!

If Trimesta®, Prestara®, and Panzem® are all approved, misused, and abused as patented cortisone was, the entire field of physiologic-dose bio-identical hormone replacement will be condemned by organized medicine and the FDA, and we could very well lose our individually compounded bio-identical hormones due to "bio-identical hormone abuse" encouraged by patent medicine companies and abetted by mainstream medicine!

Goliath Joins the Battle

Can you guess which side the American Medical Association is on? It's certainly not yours! The AMA is obligingly helping out patent medication companies and the FDA, and is renewing the call to remove compounded bio-identical hormones from the market altogether – or at least to regulate them into uselessness.

According to a recent press release: "The American Medical Association's (AMA) House of Delegates unanimously and enthusiastically passed a resolution introduced by the Wyeth-funded Endocrine Society and other "concerned" organizations urging the US Food and Drug Administration (FDA) to increase its oversight and regulation of so-called bio-identical hormones." Apparently, the AMA has no respect for the long tradition of individual state regulation of pharmacy compounding, but just wants to give yet more power to *los Federales*.

How can we hope to win a battle against the AMA, multibillion dollar patent medicine companies, and the FDA? The following three steps should go a long way toward advancing our cause:

- The first step is renewed, overwhelming protest – like last year when we battled against Wyeth's citizen petition. Start by becoming more informed about the stealth movement to have natural products renamed and sold at enormous mark-ups. Use the examples in the box below to predict to your state and local representatives what will happen to the price of Prestara® (DHEA), Trimesta® (estriol), Panzem® (2-methoxyestradiol), and any other bio-identical hormones and other natural products if they become FDA-"approved."

- Contact your insurance company. Inform them about the present cost of your bio-identical hormones (which they frequently won't pay because they're not "approved") compared with the enormously inflated cost of the FDA brand name version of the product.

- Stay alert for the next big campaign push against your individually compounded bio-identical hormones. It's coming as surely as patent medicine companies love big money, and *los Federales* love power!

Price Comparison for Natural Products and Their FDA-"Approved" Counterparts

		Number of capsules	Dosage per serving	Cost per bottle
Natural name	DHA-EPA fish oil	120	1,200 mg	$14
Patented name	Lovaaza®	120	1,000 mg	$150
Natural name	L-carnitine	90	500 mg	$25.40
Patented name	Carnitor®	90	330 mg	$81.89

The prices for the patented, brand name drugs can be found at www. drugstore.com. The natural products can be found at www.vitacost. com.

International Hormone Society
Statement on Bio-identical Hormones
December 05, 2006

After a literature review and discussions with physicians from all over the world who are well versed in treating patients with endocrine abnormalities, we, the members of the International Hormone Society, think the time is right to release a statement on the use and delivery of bio-identical hormones.

A "bio-identical hormone" has exactly the same chemical structure as a hormone produced by the human body. The term "bio-identical" is generally used for preparations containing sex hormones such as estradiol, estrone, estriol, progesterone and testosterone. The alternatives are non-bio-identical hormone preparations such as those widely commercialized in most birth-control pills and in post-menopausal hormone treatments. The prevailing concept is that bio-identical hormones may be safer to use than non-bio-identical hormones because they fit the body, in particular when a safer route of administration is used such as transdermal delivery.

The members of the International Hormone Society were concerned about product safety long before the publication of studies such as Women's Health Initiative (WHI) in 2002 and the British One Million Women study in 2003 that found an increase in the incidence of breast cancer in postmenopausal women using non-bio-identical hormones as compared to placebo or nonusers. In the WHI study, the use of non-bio-identical female hormones was also associated with an increased risk of cardiovascular and cerebrovascular diseases.

In accordance with the recommendations of a growing number of medical societies, the International Hormone Society, in a consensus on "Estrogen and Progesterone Treatment of Pre- and Postmenopausal Women" issued on December 11, 2005, did not and still does not recommend the use of non-bio-identical estrogens and progestogens for the treatment of ovarian deficiencies. However, the use of synthetically modified female hormones used for birth control may be considered for a limited time if no other contraceptive alternative exists. The consensus is based on an extensive review of the literature on the use of bio-identical and non-bio-identical estrogens and progestogens. Greater potential toxicity and risks were found in the non-bio-identical compounds.

On the other hand, the International Hormone Society did and still does recommend in the consensus the use of bio-identical estrogens, in particular estradiol and estriol, and also bio-identical progesterone, for the correction of ovarian deficiencies. In contrast with the recent Endocrine Society's position (October 2006) and the American Medical Association's resolution (November 2006) that state that little or no scientific and medical evidence exists to support the claims that bio-identical hormones may be safer, a review of the literature contradicts this statement. There currently is sufficient evidence confirming the greater safety of bio-identical sex hormones compared to the non-bio-identical ones, in particular when the transdermal, nasal or intramuscular routes are used instead of the oral route.

Critics object to bio-identical hormones sold by compounding pharmacies due to the lack of oversight by the Food and Drug Administration (FDA), and assume that there is no guarantee of dosage, purity, efficacy and safety. We share with the American Medical Association, the Endocrine Society, the American College of Obstetricians and Gynecologists, and the American Academy of Family Practitioners the concern that patients should be offered the best products at all times, and that all products must be as consistent as possible in dosage, and as pure, efficient and safe as possible.

The physicians of the International Hormone Society think they can provide a valuable, decisive opinion in this debate for two reasons. First, many of them have broad experience in the use of bio-identical hormones compounded by compounding pharmacies, experience which does not seem to be shared by the writers of the various positions and resolutions of the aforementioned societies. Second, the opinion of the International Hormone Society members is independent of any pressure from advertisers, sponsoring pharmaceutical firms, or compounding pharmacies.

The physicians of the International Hormone Society wish to stress the following points:

- *Control of compounding pharmacies:* The production of bio-identical hormone preparations by compounding pharmacies is under control of the pharmacy state board in each state. This control has sufficiently warranted high quality products, in dosage, purity, efficacy and safety, to satisfy physicians. Better control may be acceptable as long as it does not restrict physicians from exercising their therapeutic freedom to prescribe compounded preparations for the full benefit of patients.

- *Major advantage of compounded preparations:* Compounded preparations of bio-identical hormones offer a major, indispensable advantage over standardized preparations, namely that the dosage and formulation of the product can be tailored to each patient. Concentration and composition, including solvents or fillers, can be individualized to what the patient needs or is able to tolerate. We think personalized treatments such as those offered by compounding pharmacies offer the best prospect for optimal health care.

- *Production and distribution of bio-identical hormones is not limited to compounding pharmacies:* The FDA approval of "bio-identical" hormones already exists in the form of patches and mass-produced estrogen gel and cream. Compounding pharmacies are merely making a cream or gel that better suits the individual patient.

- *Conjugated estrogens, an example of widely sold non-bio-identical hormones:* The form of estrogen, conjugated estrogen, which initiated this entire debate, is actually an estrogen waste product found in the urine of pregnant mares. Many of the estrogens in horse urine cannot be considered "bio-identical" to the human body because they are structured differently than human estrogens. Although some of the estrogens are equivalent to human estrogen, they have been altered biochemically by conjugation. Conjugation takes place in the liver of horses and humans in order to excrete unwanted estrogen. Therefore, conjugated estrogen medications are not bio-identical because they are waste product forms of estrogen marked for removal by a horse liver.

- *Use of the term "bio-identical" hormones.* The AMA's request to the Food and Drug Administration to prohibit use of the commonly employed term "bio-identical hormones," unless the preparation has been approved by the FDA, contradicts the first amendment rights of the Constitution of the United States, denying the freedom of speech ensured by the amendment, and unacceptably interferes with the rights of medical doctors currently prescribing compounded preparations of bio-identical hormones. Section 503A of the FDA Modernization Act of 1997 attempted to restrict the first amendment rights of compounding pharmacies, stipulating "that they refrain from advertising or promoting particular compounded drugs". However, the Supreme Court, in a 2002 decision, found that restriction unconstitutional. In the words of the FDA itself: "The Supreme Court affirmed the 9th Circuit Court of Appeals decision that found section 503A of the Act invalid in its entirety because it contained unconstitutional restrictions on commercial speech." This Supreme Court decision should firmly establish for all parties that first amendment speech applies to compounding pharmacies as to all Americans, and that first amendment speech does not require approval from anyone, including the FDA.

- *Testing*: Most physicians who work with bio-identical hormones from compounding pharmacies use traditional blood tests, not saliva tests, as incorrectly stated by the American Medical Association (resolution of November 2006) and the Endocrine Society (position statement of October 2006).

- *Safety*: As previously stated, there is currently sufficient evidence confirming the greater safety of bio-identical sex hormones as compared to non-bio-identical ones, particularly when administered transdermally, nasally or intramuscularly instead of orally.

- *Research*: We recommend future research in this area, and, in particular, we support independent research on the potential risks and benefits of bio-identical and non-bio-identical hormones.

In conclusion, we urgently advise the American Medical Association to revise its position and the Food and Drug Administration to take all points of the International Hormone Society's statement into consideration and to preserve physician's rights to prescribe the best possible products for their patients, including compounded preparations of bio-identical hormones.

APPENDIX 2:
BHRT – UP CLOSE AND PERSONAL

- Contact your insurance company. Inform them about the present cost of your bio-identical hormones (which they frequently won't pay because they're not "approved") compared with the enormously inflated cost of the FDA brand name version of the product.

- Stay alert for the next big campaign push against your individually compounded bio-identical hormones. It's coming as surely as patent medicine companies love big money, and *los Federales* love power!

Price Comparison for Natural Products and Their FDA-"Approved" Counterparts

WOULD YOU LIKE TO HELP MAKE MEDICAL HISTORY?

Although Big Pharma is not about to run any comparative head-to-head clinical trials between conventional HRT and BHRT, one small, *independent FDA-approved* trial is currently underway, the first of its kind, anywhere.

Funded privately through the University of Kansas (*ClinicalTrials.gov Identifier: NCT00302731*), the trial is a 12-month, randomized, double-blind, placebo-controlled study ("gold-standard" design) comparing the safety and efficacy of the "standard of care" (low-dose Prempro™) with that of placebo and three different combinations of estradiol and/or estriol combined with progesterone. Participants (40 healthy women aged 40 to 65 and within 7 years after menopause) are randomly and blindly assigned to each arm of the study.

Safety evaluations include measurements of lipid (cholesterol) levels and electrocardiograms (ECGs) at the start of the trial (baseline) and again after 6 and 12 months; and mammograms, ultrasound exams of the uterus, and bone scans, at baseline and 12 months. Hormone levels are measured by 24-hour urine samples. (All at no cost to participants.)

The trial's principal investigator is Jeanne A. Drisko, MD, of the University of Kansas Medical Center, Kansas City, Kansas, and current president of the American College of the Advancement of Medicine (ACAM). Dr. Drisko and her colleagues expect that the data gathered from this pilot study, in addition to providing validation of BHRT's efficacy and safety, will open the door to larger, more definitive studies in the future.

If you would like to make history and participate in this groundbreaking trial, and you live within a reasonable driving distance of Kansas City, please contact Dr. Drisko at 913-588-6208 or jdrisko@kumc.edu.

The following articles are all adapted from Dr. Jonathan V. Wright's Nutrition & Healing *monthly newsletter, which is published by Healthier News, LLC, 702 Cathedral Street, Baltimore, MD 21201. The newsletter is available by subscription and online at www. wrightnewsletter.com.*

TAKING THE FEAR OUT OF BIO-IDENTICAL HORMONE REPLACEMENT THERAPY – ONE URINE TEST AT A TIME

If you're a woman, your average life expectancy is about 80 years. That means you're going to spend more than one-third of your life in a post-menopausal state, facing all the adverse health effects associated with reduced levels of the hormones your body made internally before meno-pause (estrogens, progesterone, DHEA, testosterone, thyroid hormones, melatonin, and others). These effects range from mild but annoying – things like increased fatigue and decreased libido – to serious threats to your ability to lead a normal daily life – osteoporosis, muscle weakness, atherosclerosis, loss of cognitive function, and many more.

And those of you men reading this aren't out of the woods either. Although your hormones decline more gradually, men face very similar challenges.

But there is a way to effectively prevent many of these problems, "diseases of aging" as they've come to be known, and promote longevity in both women and men during the later stages of your lives. The only problem is, many of us are afraid to use it.

As we discuss throughout this book, concerns about the risks associated with "hormone replacement therapy" have been a hot topic of discussion, especially over the last few years, since the results of the "Women's Health Initiative" (WHI) were released.

Although its results were released only 7 years ago, a recent survey conducted by researchers at Stanford University found that fewer than 30% of women remember this pivotal study. What does seem to have made a lasting impression are the dangers that were uncovered by that trial, namely increased risks of heart attack, stroke, and cancer.

But the HRT in the WHI study used horse estrogens and a "space alien" progestin (not natural progesterone), neither of which have any business being in your body. So it's critical to make the distinction between HRT using "hormones" that are completely foreign to human bodies and the kind used in BHRT, which exactly mimic what your body produces (or produced) naturally all on its own before menopause or andropause set in. Unfortunately, the mainstream media – even articles by "leading science writers" – very rarely makes that distinction. As a result, I get lots of questions about BHRT safety every day, from *Nutrition & Healing* readers and Tahoma Clinic patients.

Today I'll do my best to answer them all in one comprehensive article. So let's start with the question that is typically forefront on everyone's mind: ***How do you know for sure that BHRT is safe?***

Know Where Your Safety Stands

Even though I wrote the first prescriptions for bio-identical HRT in the early 1980s, and in that time (as far as has been reported to me) only one individual out of several thousand has developed a cancer that could possibly be related to hormones, I'm the first to admit that my experiences are not "controlled research."

As we document throughout this book, many aspects of BHRT safety have fortunately been researched in depth. Numerous studies have found that BHRT has many advantages over conventional "horse and alien molecule" HRT, but two of the most striking are that, unlike the "other" form, BHRT decreases cardiovascular risk, as well as estrogen-related cancer risk.

But BHRT research still has some gaps. There's not been time for long-term controlled studies. Also, very few studies are done on a cellular level because the hormones used in BHRT – estradiol, estriol, sometimes estrone, progesterone, testosterone, DHEA, and others – are not always used by your cells in exactly these molecular forms. Instead, they get "metabolized" by your body into other molecules (which we'll get into in just a bit). Research so far has found some of these metabolized

How Pre-Menopausal Women Can Predict
– and Reduce – Breast Cancer Risk

Low estriol isn't usually something that most BHRT users need to worry about, since estriol is already in their prescriptions. But premenopausal women with a family history of breast cancer should also consider getting all of their estrogen metabolites checked with a 24-hour urine test, since low levels of estriol can help predict breast cancer risk. The good news is, if your estriol levels are low, the problem is easily corrected with *iodine* or *iodide*.

In the 1970s, when using John Myers' iodine treatment for fibrocystic breast disease, I observed that iodine and iodide both could increase a woman's own secretion of estriol while lowering her estrone and estradiol. It's also well known in the epidemiologic community that high-iodine diets (such as Japanese diets that include lots of high-iodine seafood and seaweed) are associated with the lowest cancer risks, and the effect of iodine increasing estriol may be at least part of the reason.

There's also a 15-year "prospective" study of over 15,000 women that demonstrated that those in the upper quarter of estriol secretion during their pregnancies (which is predictive of relative estriol secretion throughout a woman's "cycling" years) had a 58% lower risk of breast cancer over the next 15 years than women in the lowest quartile.

But since iodine and iodide in larger quantities taken for longer periods of time can suppress thyroid function, if you find you have relatively low estriol, it's best to work with a practitioner skilled and knowledgeable in nutritional and natural medicine to "normalize" this ratio.

hormones to be procarcinogenic, others anticarcinogenic, and the status of others is still uncertain. "Ratios" between some of these hormones are also important.

But even though at present, these metabolites can't be monitored at the cellular level, they can be at a "whole body" level, which is how we maximize BHRT safety.

The most comprehensive and accurate way to monitor hormone metabolites is with a 24-hour urine test. Many of the people I work with are surprised that I don't recommend blood testing to measure hormone levels, but there are a few factors that explain why blood testing isn't the best choice.

When your body produces hormones internally, they're secreted in "pulses," (bursts and pauses), and when you use BHRT, you supplement with the hormones once or twice a day. This way they're not continuously circulating throughout your body at steady levels, which makes obtaining an accurate measurement from a blood sample extremely difficult. Blood levels of any hormone can be quite variable, depending on the time of day the sample is drawn. Urine testing, on the other hand, determines the entire amount produced − or supplemented − in a 24-hour period.

Also, except with testosterone, blood tests don't distinguish between the "free" and "bound" forms of hormones. And, according to researchers, the "bound" forms are inactive. Thus, nearly all of the estrogens and progesterone measured in blood are the inactive "bound" form. The "free" forms − the active forms − are actually not measured at all. On the other hand, urine testing measures the sum of free and "conjugated" hormonal steroids. (Conjugated steroids are ones that have combined with other simple molecules.) The "free" form of any hormone is the most active form, but the "conjugated" form can be active, too, so it's beneficial to know how much of these types of hormones are in your body, as opposed to a measurement that includes forms that researchers have found to be inactive.

One other quirk of blood testing is that estriol − one of the most important protective estrogens − is practically unmeasurable in blood samples by most labs. By contrast, estriol is found in urine in greater quantities than nearly any other single estrogen. While they aren't absolutely certain why, experts think this may occur, because even though considerable estriol is secreted every day, it's "cleared" from the blood very rapidly.

On top of these drawbacks, blood testing just isn't presently available for many of the steroid metabolites that are important for ensuring BHRT safety.

In addition to estriol, at present, blood tests for 2-methoxyestradiol (a "good" estrogen), 4-hydroxyestrone (considered the "worst" estrogen), androstanediol (a "good" testosterone), and others are not available.

What about saliva testing? Well, it's true that saliva testing is convenient, noninvasive, and somewhat accurate for younger individuals not using BHRT. Its main drawback for practitioners is that salivary levels of

Why Your Bones Don't Want Your 2/16 Ratio Too High

Believe it or not, there is one caution about the "2/16" ratio being too high. Back in 1997, one research group found that a very high ratio (perhaps higher than 4:1 to 6:1) may predict a higher risk for osteoporosis.

steroid hormones for individuals using BHRT are "sky-high," and usually bear no resemblance to normal physiologic ranges. Also, even though saliva testing is said to measure the "free" form of steroid hormones, studies have shown that steroid binding proteins do appear in saliva, so it's possible that these measurements include some "bound" (or inactive) hormone, too. And, like blood testing, saliva testing is not available for many of the metabolites necessary to monitor for safety.

So urine testing is really the "gold standard" for monitoring BHRT safety. This test keeps tabs on literally dozens of steroid hormones and their metabolites. It does this by testing each urine specimen with something called gas chromatography (GC). According to nearly all experts, GC is unsurpassed in its potential for determining a multitude of steroid metabolites simultaneously in a single specimen. The GC is also coupled with "mass spectrometry" (MS), which literally identifies the "molecular fingerprint" of each individual steroid molecule.

Not All Estrogens Are Created Equal: Which Ones Should You REALLY Be Concerned About?

Now that we've covered the testing you'll need to undergo to keep BHRT safe, let's move on to the actual hormones involved, starting with estrogen, and talk about which ones can be cause for concern and why.

What Else Can You Learn From Your Urine?

24-hour urinary steroid tests aren't just useful for checking and adjusting quantities of hormones to ensure BHRT safety. The GC/MS urine-testing technique can also monitor many other natural steroids and metabolites, too, including cortisol, cortisone, and their metabolites, and aldosterone.

These measurements can help you and your doctor identify any unusual stress (indicated by high cortisol and cortisone levels), weak adrenal function (indicated by low levels of cortisol, cortisone, and several of their metabolites), or even extra risk for age-related hearing loss (indicated by aldosterone levels).

If you already have age-related hearing loss and your aldosterone is low, supplementing bio-identical aldosterone can actually improve your hearing significantly. (See *Nutrition & Healing* for May 2006, or check the on-line archives.)

There are more than 20 circulating estrogens in the body. Estrone, estradiol, and estriol are frequently thought of as the main players, although researchers have found that 2-hydroxyestrone is also present in large quantities. Estrone and estradiol are potent estrogens, generally thought to be procarcinogenic – when they're acting alone, that is. But when you add the right amount of estriol to the mix (as Mother Nature intended), it neutralizes those effects by acting as an anticarcinogen. Before menopause, most women's bodies secrete more estriol than estrone and estradiol, so BHRT generally contains more estriol, too.

Next there are the hydroxyestrogens. Like estriol, 2-hydroxyestrone (and other 2-hydroxyestrogens) are considered to be "weak" but anticarcinogenic estrogens. $16\text{-}\alpha$-hydroxyestrone (and other $16\text{-}\alpha$-hydroxyestrogens), on the other hand, are procarcinogenic. This is where the "2/16 ratio" (*See Chapter 7.*) comes into play, and allows BHRT users to get the benefits of these estrogen metabolites without putting themselves at risk.

Considerable research shows that the ratio of 2-hydroxyestrogens to $16\text{-}\alpha$-hydroxyestrogens can predict breast cancer risk for premenopausal women. Higher 2/16 ratios indicate lower breast cancer risk, and low 2/16 ratios (particularly those less than 1.0) indicate higher risk. While this ratio doesn't appear to be helpful for predicting breast cancer risk in postmenopausal women who aren't using BHRT, it's been my experience (although no actual research data exists), that it is indeed predictive for postmenopausal women who are using BHRT.

And before you men tune out, those 2-hydroxyestrogen and 16-α-hydroxyestrogen measurements are important for you too: Research has found men in the highest third of 16-α-hydroxyestrogen had the highest risk of prostate cancer, while men in the highest third of 2-hydroxyestrogen had the lowest risk.

If your 24-hour urine test shows that your 2/16 ratio is low, there are two simple ways to boost it back into the "safe" zone. Start by adding more "cruciferous" vegetables (broccoli, cauliflower, bok choy, cabbage, Brussels sprouts), flaxseed, and soy (but not too much soy for men) to your diet. These foods can all help raise your 2-hydroxyestrogen levels, which, in turn, will help move your 2/16 ratios in a favorable direction.

You can also take supplements of the active compound in the cruciferous vegetables, a substance called di-indolylmethane (or DIM). Usually 100 milligrams 2 to 3 times daily can bring a low 2/16 ratio back up to a safe range. (One thing to keep in mind: Many practitioners still recommend supplements of the precursor molecule to DIM, called indole-3-carbinol, or I3C. But I3C only becomes active after it's transformed into DIM by stomach acid. Since so many individuals are low in stomach acid, I've found that it's more effective just to use DIM itself.)

While 16-hydroxyestrogens are considered pro-carcinogenic, the estrogen metabolites that appear to pose the biggest threat to your health are the ones with the number "4" in front of them – 4-hydroxyestrone and other 4-hydroxyestrogens. These are the ones considered to be the most carcinogenic of all estrogens, stimulating the growth of both breast and prostate cancer. At present, only the 24-hour urine test using GC-MS can measure your levels of these metabolites (so you see, again, why urine testing is such an important part of BHRT safety).

If your levels of any 4-hydroxyestrogens are higher than normal, you should also increase your intake of cruciferous vegetables and/or start taking DIM. One research report found that I3C supplements could lower 4-hydroxyestrogens, so cruciferous vegetables and DIM can very likely do the same thing.

Unlike patent medicine versions of HRT, the human body is all about balance when it comes to hormones. Since we naturally produce some procarcinogenic estrogens, Mother Nature also made sure we produce anticarcinogenic ones as well. One of these anticarcinogenic estrogen metabolites is 2-methoxyestradiol. It's actually only found in very small quantities in the body. But this is one of those situations where a little goes a long way. Small quantities or not, 2-methoxyestradiol is a very potent anti-carcinogen. So potent, in fact, that one patent medicine company has recently "renamed" it "Panzem®" and is trying to get the FDA to "approve" it as a patented "drug." (Unfortunately, the clinical trials on Panzem® are using enormous and entirely unnatural quantities of 2-methoxyestradiol introduced into the body in an entirely unnatural way: by swallowing it. Estrogens and other steroid hormones simply don't − and shouldn't − enter the body through our GI tracts!)

One group of researchers has also found that even very tiny quantities of 2-methoxyestradiol (less than 1 micromole, for the technically inclined) are effective against uterine fibroid (leiomyoma) cells. Others are finding that 2-methoxyestradiol may be a very important factor in protecting against the artery damage that leads to atherosclerosis.

Since 2-methoxyestradiol plays such important roles in the body, it's important to keep your own levels in a normal range so that this powerful metabolite can offer the maximum amount of protection possible. 2-methoxyestradiol is something known as a "methylated" estrogen, so nutrients that induce the process of "methylation" may help increase its levels. Folate and vitamin B12 both help stimulate methylation, so if your 24-hour urine test shows low 2-methoxyestradiol, work with a practitioner skilled and knowledgeable in nutritional and natural medicine to determine the best doses of these and other nutrients to help increase your levels.

Taking on Testosterone – Safely and Naturally

When you're talking about estrogen, you can bet that testosterone isn't far behind. The good news is, things are a little simpler when it comes to monitoring this hormone for safety (which, I suppose proves that men who claim that women are "complicated" are at least partially correct!). Although there are testosterone metabolites that you do need to keep track of, there aren't as many as there are with estrogen.

The first testosterone metabolite on the list is one you've probably already heard of, since there are patent medicines designed to lower it: DHT (di-hydrotestosterone). But using one of those patent medications or too much alpha-linolenic acid (ALA), zinc, or saw palmetto can lower DHT levels too far. This does lower over-all prostate cancer risk, but, as strange as it sounds, it actually increases the risk of developing a more aggressive form of the disease. Although research isn't definitive on this point, it appears that this could occur because low levels of DHT can lessen the formation of an anticancerous testosterone metabolite called androstanediol, which is actually made from DHT. In fact, it's likely that the ratio between DHT and androstanediol is even more important than the level of either one on its own.

Another aspect of BHRT safety that men need to keep tabs on is "excess aromatization," a technical term used to describe the entirely natural but quite unhealthful process – for men – of metabolizing testosterone into too much estrogen. Aromatization itself is normal: Even the most masculine men need some estrogen for their bodies to operate at peak performance. But when overactivity of that process transforms testosterone into too much estrogen, problems – like prostate enlargement and even prostate cancer – can occur.

Excess aromatization becomes more common with increasing age, but it's even more common in men with insulin resistance. Type 2 diabetics always have insulin resistance, but if you haven't been diagnosed with diabetes, that doesn't necessarily mean you don't need to worry about excess aromatization: Insulin resistance usually occurs years – even decades – before type 2 diabetes is ever diagnosed.

If you have type 2 diabetes or an increased risk of insulin resistance (which you do if type 2 diabetes runs in your family), check with a physician skilled and knowledgeable in bio-identical hormone use to see if your 24-hour urine test shows excess aromatization. (For a more detailed explanation of insulin resistance and how to test for it, see *Nutrition & Healing* for July and August 2001. You can download these issues for free from the on-line archives.)

Fortunately, there are two very effective ways to slow aromatization to a normal rate. One is a combination formula of Chinese botanicals called "Myo-min" (from Chi Enterprises). I've observed that 2 or 3 tablets twice daily will almost always return excess estrogen to normal. The other male "excess estrogen normalizer" is the flavonoid chrysin, derived from passion flower. One important caveat, though: It's typically not very effective in capsule or tablet form. The best delivery system of chrysin is the liposomal spray form, (from LipoLab) which I have found to be effective for most men. Two sprays twice daily usually does the job. Both Myo-min and liposomal spray chrysin are available through natural food stores, compounding pharmacies, and the Tahoma Clinic Dispensary.

Researchers have also found that melatonin can inhibit aromatization. Sometimes it can take rather large doses – up to 20 milligrams a day – to do the job, though. While this amount is free of serious side effects, it can make you more drowsy or groggy than you would typically be in the morning, so it may not be useful for everyone.

Putting BHRT Safety into Practice

As technical as all the preceding information has been, it truly does make an impact on your daily functioning. The following examples might do a better job of showing you how the 24-hour urine test can help make sense of hormone levels and the symptoms that imbalances can cause.

Frank was 72 when he came in to the office complaining of muscle weakness, lack of stamina, and erectile dysfunction. Among various other supplements, he was taking 100 milligrams of pregnenolone daily. Pregnenolone is sometimes called the "mother of all steroids," as it is at the top of the hormone metabolism tree, and may be converted to any other steroid metabolite at all: cortisol, estrogen, testosterone, DHEA, aldosterone – any of them.

24-hour urine testing using GC/MS determined his testosterone levels to be on the very low end of normal. His estrone was 3 times higher than his testosterone, actually at the same level as most premenopausal women!

Frank stopped taking the pregnenolone and started taking testosterone instead. Three months later, Frank returned with improved stamina, muscle strength, and erectile function. His follow-up urine test confirmed a decrease in estrone to normal male levels, as well as an increase in testosterone values.

Barbara was in her late 30s, the last of 9 sisters. All 8 older sisters had had breast cancer, and Barbara wanted to do everything she could to avoid getting it herself. She was actually working at the Tahoma Clinic at the time and had heard about the 2/16 ratio test from employees at nearby Meridian Valley Labs. Although these estrogen metabolites had been researched for years, Meridian Valley Labs was the first lab to introduce the test for practitioners – and Barbara was the first woman to get the test done.

Her test showed 2-hydroxyestrogens to be very low, and her 16-hydroxyestrogens high – her "2/16" ratio was just 0.5, which definitely indicated that she was at higher risk for breast cancer. Barbara's first step was the same one I recommended to you earlier: She added more broccoli, cauliflower, cabbage, ground flaxseed, and soy to her diet. But her next test disclosed a 2/16 ratio of 0.6 – not a significant improvement. So she added di-indolylmethane (DIM) supplements (60 milligrams 3 times a day) to her extra cruciferous vegetable intake. Several weeks later her 2/16 test was up a bit – but only to 0.8. Barbara continued eating as many cruciferous vegetables as she could and increased her DIM dose to 120 milligrams 3 times a day, and finally boosted her 2/16 ratio up over 1.0.

Michael was 51 when he came to the Tahoma Clinic. In his mid-40s he'd started having symptoms of prostate enlargement (BPH) – getting up more than once at night to urinate, decreased force of his urine stream, and a bit more difficulty getting urination started. He read about and started taking a standardized preparation of saw palmetto, 160 milligrams 3 times daily. Over 3 to 4 months, his symptoms faded to the point that they were "almost unnoticeable," and stayed that way for several years.

But when he came in for his appointment, I was concerned about the amount of saw palmetto he was taking, and also that he wasn't using any supplemental zinc or essential fatty acids such as ALA or GLA (gamma-linolenic acid, which is actually more effective for BPH than ALA). So I recommended he take a 24-hour urine test.

Michael's test showed that his 5-α-reductase was severely overinhibited. I explained (as you read earlier) that while reducing levels of this enzyme along with DHT may lower his overall risk of prostate cancer, it could actually increase his risk of developing a more aggressive form of prostate cancer. I also explained that zinc and essential fatty acids such as GLA and ALA are essential nutrients, and saw palmetto isn't, so these essential nutrients should be the first line of defense for reducing over-active 5-α-reductase. He eliminated the saw palmetto, and over several months was able to find quantities of zinc and GLA that worked for him, both for symptom control and for normalizing his enzyme activity as seen on the 24-hour urine test.

These are just a handful of examples of people who have benefited from bio-identical hormone replacement therapy along with careful monitoring of not only the hormones themselves, but also their equally important metabolites. Of course, BHRT continues to evolve. While there's no longer any doubt that BHRT is safer than horse hormones and patented "space alien" progestins, BHRT is not and can never be perfectly safe. After all, our own internally produced hormones aren't perfectly safe either: Research shows that even younger people whose own bodies produce higher levels of sex hormones have a somewhat higher hormone-related cancer risk.

But unlike those versions of HRT the patent medicine companies continue to try to force on you, keeping BHRT as safe as possible is often as simple as taking a regular urine test and working with your doctor to adjust any imbalances naturally.

Thanks to Christa Hinchcliffe ND, and Wendy Ellis ND, for their contributions to this article.

The "Unimportant" Molecule That's Curing Cancer

Do-It-Yourself Tips for Boosting Your Levels – Without Big Pharma's Help

Earlier, you read about Panzem®, one of "Big Pharma's" aggressive moves into bio-identical hormones. But for decades before the pharmaceutical industry changed its name and spent hundreds of millions of dollars trying for FDA "approval" Panzem®, was actually known by its *real* name, 2-methoxyestradiol.

For much of that time, no one really knew the function of 2-methoxyestradiol, and since there are such tiny quantities of it in our bodies, it was dismissed (as scientists so often do when they don't yet know what one of Nature's "minor" molecules is for) as "unimportant."

But now the gold rush of research is on for 2-methoxyestradiol, because it appears that it may be able to actually cure – or at least significantly slow – many types of cancer, including some of the most commonly feared forms, including prostate, breast, and ovarian.

An "Inactive" Hormone Shows Its True Cancer-Fighting Potential

As usual with patent medicine research, the emphasis (and the rush) is on the "gold" that can be produced by selling an "approved" form of this entirely natural molecule (at an unnaturally high price), rather than learning how to work with Nature as closely as possible, which would offer the most benefit at the least possible cost to patients everywhere. But that's just one of many "fatal flaws" of the current "health care" system here in these United States. And even though that's unlikely to change anytime soon, we still may be able to salvage something from this situation.

Before turning the spotlight on 2-methoxyestradiol itself, it's always important to have a little bit of general background on how these things work in the body. Estrogens and androgens are steroid hormones (Nature's own original steroids, not the "extraterrestrial-molecule," pumped-up-to-be-patentable, pseudosteroids currently scandalizing athletics). These natural steroids are produced by the ovaries or testes, adrenal cortices, and other body tissues of both men and women.

But, too much estrogen, especially too much of the "wrong kind" of estrogen increases the risk of new cancers and promotes the development of any tumors that are already present. This occurs primarily when two of the "major" forms of estrogen – estradiol and estrone – follow a pathway that metabolizes them into estrogen compounds that promote tumor formation. Other pathways produce estrogen metabolites that protect against tumors.

As it turns out, 2-methoxyestradiol isn't inactive, as the "experts" once assumed. In fact, it's one of the most potent anti-carcinogenic estrogen metabolites. This metabolite is formed from the hydroxylation of 17β-estradiol followed by O-methylation in the liver. (I know that's highly technical, but remember the word "*methylation*" for later.)

Some recent studies have shown that, 2-methoxyestradiol inhibits the growth of prostate cancer cells by inducing apoptosis (cell "suicide") and preventing tumor growth in rapidly growing cells. It showed similar benefits for both breast and prostate cancer when it was used in combination with other chemotherapeutic therapies. And speaking of its role among chemotherapy drugs, not only does 2-methoxyestradiol have potent effects against pancreatic and gastric cancers that have become resistant to other chemotherapeutic drugs, but it also reduced the amount of other chemotherapeutic drugs needed in cases of ovarian cancer by enhancing their anti-tumor effects.

Researchers have seen similar results using 2-methoxyestradiol in many other kinds of cancer, including osteosarcoma, leukemia, and chondrosarcoma, a type of cancer affecting the cartilage.

In addition to promoting apoptosis in cancer cells and working with chemotherapy drugs to boost their effects with lower doses (which, hopefully, will help minimize the harsh side effects of these drugs), 2-methoxyestradiol also works against cancers by inhibiting angiogenesis, the formation of new blood vessels, which is how many cancers nourish themselves. To top off this roster of benefits,

2-methoxyestradiol has also shown the ability to inhibit the spread of cancer through metastasis.

All of these various approaches to fighting cancer (and likely some that haven't even been discovered yet), make 2-methoxyestradiol an extremely promising tool for treating the disease at many different stages.

Giving Nature the Cancer-Curing Credit It's Due

The study results I listed above are really just the tip of the proverbial iceberg when it comes to the clinical trials being done on 2-methoxyestradiol. As a matter of fact, just as I was sitting down to write this article, yet another "2-methoxyestradiol might cure cancer" study was released – and made quite a splash in the media (probably because it was done at one of the most mainstream of mainstream institutions, the Mayo Clinic). The press report started:

> "A new study of an estrogen-derived drug shows promise as a treatment for breast cancer and breast cancer metastases to bone. A drug that has shown promise in treating sarcoma, lung, and brain cancers, demonstrates that the drug may also be effective in treating breast cancer, in particular the spread of breast cancer."

I'm sure you've noticed the typical patent medicine company language "spin" right away. *2-methoxyestradiol is a natural estrogen, not a "drug,"* but the word "drug" is used three times in the first two sentences. And the spin didn't stop there.

> "[Mayo Clinic researchers] studied the effect of 2-methoxyestradiol on the bone…In breast cancer, the cancer commonly lodges in the bone, destroying it in a debilitating painful process called osteolysis. Osteolysis can lead to bone fractures and causes patients to feel tired, or even to lose consciousness.

> "According to one of the researchers, 2-methoxyestradiol is potentially very important in the treatment of breast cancer metastatic to bone, because it has few of the unpleasant side effects of most chemotherapy drugs and targets both bone resorption and the cancerous tumor cells. According to another researcher,

> "We were expecting the 'drug' (quotation marks added) to have an effect, but we were not expecting to have as big of an effect as it did."

I suppose getting the mainstream to give credit to Nature instead of "drugs" is too much to hope for. But at least they haven't tried twisting all-natural 2-methoxyestradiol into a patentable, "space-alien" version – yet.

And these researchers did make one other bit of progress: They appear to be among the first to notice that swallowing steroids is not Nature's preferred route of administration. Of course, that should have been obvious from the start to any MD, PhD, or intelligent student of the human body. But, obvious or not, nearly all other researchers have had their volunteers swallow 2-methoxyestradiol, which may be one of the reasons such enormous doses have been required in the research to-date. According to the news report on the Mayo Clinic study:

> "Clinical trials of 2-methoxyestradiol (2ME2) for breast cancer patients are in progress. These trials are based on an oral version of 2ME2 to treat primary tumors, but this method has limitations, as the oral version of 2ME2 is poorly suited to getting into the blood system and reaching tumors. Researchers resolved this problem by delivering 2ME2 by injection and found it was much more effective."

To put it simply, the Mayo Clinic study found that 2-methoxyestradiol can:
- Effectively target breast cancer cells
- Prevent the spread of breast cancer cells to bone
- Protect bone from osteolysis, a type of bone metastasis in which the bone is eaten away by cancer cells.
- Is much more effective in smaller quantities when *not* swallowed, but (in this case) injected.

Safety in Numbers – and Larger-Than-Normal Doses

The Mayo Clinic study may be the most recent – and accurately conducted – research on 2-methoxyestradiol so far, but there are lots of other studies on this estrogen metabolite as well that show just as much promise, even with some wrinkles in the methodology.

In a Phase I clinical trial of 2-methoxyestradiol in 15 women with metastatic breast cancer, 10 patients stabilized in their disease progression and two reported reductions in bone pain and the use of painkillers. And there were no adverse effects from daily *oral* doses of 200, 400, 600 or 800 milligrams, although at 1,000 mg per day, all 15 patients in the study reported hot flashes.

Another Phase I study of 2-methoxyestradiol examined its effects when combined with the cancer drug, docetaxel, in 15 patients with metastatic breast cancer. This time, no adverse effects were observed when oral 2-methoxyestradiol was administered in concentrations between 200 and 1,000 mg per day for 28 days following 4 to 6 weeks of docetaxel therapy.

The next clinical trial on 2-methoxyestradiol's résumé involved 11 men and 9 women, who were given oral doses of the estrogen metabolite to find the maximum-tolerated dose and determine any level of toxicity. To be enrolled in the study, patients had to have malignant, metastatic, inoperable solid tumors and to have exhausted standard treatment options. Prostate and ovarian cancers were the most commonly represented tumors in the study group. Patients were initially given a specific oral dose of 2-methoxyestradiol over the course of 28 days. When a treatment cycle was completed without adverse effects or progression of disease, doses were escalated to the next highest dose. Results of the study determined that 2-methoxyestradiol was well tolerated *orally* at dose levels ranging from 400 mg to 3,000 mg, although side effects, such as hot flashes and thrombosis, did occur in some participants.

As the previous study indicated, 2-methyoxyestradiol may be as beneficial for men as it is for women. In one randomized, placebo-controlled study specifically on PSA levels and prostate cancer, 33 patients were given either 400 or 1,200 milligrams per day of oral 2-methoxyestradiol over the course of 16 weeks. PSA numbers either stabilized or declined by as much as 40 percent in many of the patients receiving the 1,200-milligram dose. Several patients developed abnormalities in liver function that resolved when 2-methoxyestradiol was discontinued, but other than those few instances, it was well tolerated in the study participants.

Once again, no matter how the media – or the patent medicine industry – tries to spin it, *2-methoxyestradiol is a naturally occurring estrogen metabolite, not a "drug."* And this natural substance has enormous potential as an anticancer agent for a wide variety of cancers, particularly when it's administered properly (into the bloodstream first, before the liver gets a chance to change it and destroy it, which is actually the liver's job with steroid hormones.) But even the studies that used the wrong method of administration demonstrated that 2-methoxyestradiol has few adverse effects and little toxicity.

The Good News and Bad News About This Revolutionary Cancer Therapy

The good news we can take away from the 2-methoxyestradiol research to date is that a much safer and effective form of cancer treatment is coming. Now for the bad news: Given the "approval" process, it's still years away. And, unfortunately, like all other newly introduced "approved drugs," it will be enormously expensive (although more likely to be covered by insurance than non-"approved" natural treatments).

But by now you might be wondering why you need to wait around for approval at all. Since 2-methoxyestradiol is a naturally occurring estrogen, doctors, especially ones skilled and knowledgeable in the safe and effective use of bio-identical hormones, should be able to order it through their compounding pharmacies, and prescribe it for you just like the other estrogens used in an overall BHRT program. Not to mention the fact that, even though they've been proven safe, it's also very likely that you wouldn't need doses as large as the ones used in the research studies: There's every reason to believe that much lower doses of 2-methoxyestradiol will be just as effective if they're used as part of an overall, natural anti-cancer approach, in combination with excellent diet, detoxification, immune support and stimulation, and many other safe and natural anti-cancer compounds. So why not just talk to your doctor about adding this safe and all-natural hormone to your current BHRT regimen now?

Well, unfortunately, it's not that easy – and, believe me, I've tried. One compounding pharmacist told me that chemical supply sources advertising 2-methoxyestradiol for sale "on-line" refused to sell to compounding pharmacies, giving various excuses. Another compounding pharmacist actually was able to purchase a very small amount, which arrived in a package emblazoned with a skull and crossbones, accompanied by a "safety sheet" that cautioned about potentially toxic effects of 2-methoxyestradiol! Either these sources don't have a clue what they're selling, or the fix is in (but most likely it's a mixture of both).

Since 2-methoxyestradiol is, in fact, a relatively harmless natural metabolite with great potential for good, I'm hoping it becomes available through the same sources as other bio-identical hormones at a reasonable price sometime in the near future. Otherwise, it'll be the same ol' story: If you develop cancer, don't call your doctor, call your travel agent!

In the meantime, though, there are some things you can do to increase your body's own 2-methoxyestradiol levels.

Stockpiling Your Own Internal Reserves

2-methoxyestradiol is one of the metabolites monitored in the 24-hour urine evaluation. (*See Chapter 9.*) Even though it's present in very tiny quantities, don't be fooled by the research studies using huge doses by unnatural means (oral administration). As I mentioned above, even tiny quantities can be pivotal as "signaling molecules" when they occur naturally in your body.

For example, one research study found that an exceptionally tiny quantity –1 "micromole" – has "antiproliferative, antiangiogenic, and apoptotic effects" on uterine fibroid cells. Although there's no concrete proof, it's very likely that one function of the very tiny quantities of 2-methoxyestradiol in our bodies is to prevent both benign hormone-related tumors, such as fibroids, as well as hormone-related cancers before they get started.

So how can you increase your own level of 2-methoxyestradiol? Remember the term *"methylation"* from the beginning of this article? It's the process that produces 2-methoxyestradiol from other forms of estrogen. Methylation relies on certain enzymes and molecules called "methyl donors" to function properly. Making sure you're supplying your body with enough of these methyl donor molecules is key to raising your 2-methoxyestradiol levels.

The list of foods that contain the necessary methyl donor molecules will probably look familiar: green leafy vegetables, legumes, citrus, berries, and nuts. Although in this particular case, it's very important that the foods have been processed as little as possible before you eat them – and that includes heating and freezing. Keeping these foods as fresh and "raw" as possible helps preserve the methyl donor molecules they contain.

There are also a few supplements that supply methyl groups, including particularly S-adenosylmethionine (SAMe), followed by methylsulfonylmethane (MSM), betaine (including the betaine from betaine hydrochloride), 5-methyltetrahydrofolate (a "new-in-the-stores" and more natural form of folic acid), and methylcobalamin (a form of vitamin B12).

If your 24-hour urine test reveals that your levels of 2-methoxyestradiol are low, increase your consumption of the foods listed above, and check with your physician skilled and knowledgeable in bio-identical hormone replacement therapy about which and how much of these supplements to take.

And on a non-supplemental note: stress, especially prolonged stress, reduces methylation of estrogens since the required "methyl groups" get used by the body to make adrenaline instead. Meditation, biofeedback, and other stress and "adrenaline-reducing" techniques can make more methyl groups available to make 2-methoxyestradiol, and reduce your risk of cancer at the same time.

Thanks to Lauren Russel, ND, for her organization and summary of the data collected for this article.

The Lung Health Secret Every Woman Needs To Know

Protect Yourself from Emphysema and COPD – and Even Reverse Damage That's Already Been Done

Aside from the fact that, as free citizens of these United States, we should have the right to choose any type of medical treatment we feel is best suited to keeping us healthy, the ongoing threat of *los Federales* taking away access to bio-identical hormone replacement therapy (BHRT) puts women at a significant disadvantage in many other ways too. If you're a long-time reader of *Nutrition & Healing*, you already know that, as part of BHRT, estrogen replacement can lower a woman's risk of Alzheimer's disease and cognitive malfunction, protect her against cardiovascular disease, strengthen her bones, and slow down skin aging. But one of the other important benefits of BHRT is something you've probably never heard about.

A series of research reports from the respected Lung Biology Laboratory at Georgetown University School of Medicine (led by Drs. Donald Massaro and Gloria DeCarlo Massaro) dating back to 1994 have established that estrogen is extremely important to lung health, too, especially for women. Unfortunately, most people have no idea about estrogen's role in lung health, since reporting about these studies has been minimal to nonexistent in newspapers, television, radio, and major internet webpages, all of which appear to prefer reprinting financially-driven news releases from patent medicine companies, instead of doing their own investigative research and reporting.

But despite the lack of media coverage, these studies made some groundbreaking discoveries. Although chronic obstructive pulmonary disease (COPD) and emphysema are obvious and well-known results of smoking, nonsmokers sometimes develop COPD and emphysema, too. And instances of both conditions are much higher in nonsmoking women than they are in men. These studies help explain why – and show just how simple it can be not only to protect your lungs, but also to repair any damage that's already been done.

Why Women "Outbreathe" Men

The first research report in this series was published in 1995. Working with female rats, the researchers discovered that oxygen uptake almost doubled during pregnancy and nursing, even though the structure and surface area of the lungs remained the same as before (total surface area of the lungs directly correlates with the degree of oxygen-carbon dioxide exchange). They suspected that the hormonal increases of pregnancy were responsible for the increased oxygen uptake.

But even though the female rats' lung surface area didn't change during pregnancy, the research team also found that mature female rats naturally have a higher total lung surface area for oxygen-carbon dioxide exchange than male rats of the same age. The females also had significantly smaller alveoli (the billions of tiny oxygen-carbon dioxide exchanging "sacs" that comprise the lungs' spongy tissue). And the smaller the alveoli in the lungs, the more there are, which accounts for the greater gas-exchange surface area.

A year after they made these initial discoveries, the same research team proved in two ways that estrogen is directly responsible for the difference between the lungs of female and male rats. First, they removed the ovaries from immature female rats and found that when they had fully matured, these females had larger alveoli and a smaller gas-exchange surface area than female rats of the same age that hadn't had their ovaries removed. In the second phase of the study, the researchers gave a group of immature female rats extra estrogen and found that these females developed smaller, more numerous alveoli (resulting in greater gas-exchange surface area) than immature rats not given estrogen.

To rule out the possibility that hormones in general are responsible for lung development, the researchers gave androgens (testosterone and testosterone-related hormones) to a group of newborn female rats. But the extra androgens made no difference to the ultimate size or total oxygen-exchange surface area of their lungs. They also discovered that male newborn rats that had been genetically engineered to be deficient in androgen receptors (so that their own testosterone would be less effective) had the same lung development as newborn male rats with normal androgen receptors.

With all of the information they'd compiled, the researchers concluded that estrogen is primarily responsible for lung function in females. From there, they moved on to test the effects of estrogen loss – and replacement – on lung health.

Reversing Lung Damage with Estrogen

First they found that removing the ovaries (a procedure technically known as "ovariectomy") of adult female mice resulted in both loss of alveoli and of lung surface area. Loss of surface area reduces oxygen-carbon dioxide exchange (in other words, it negatively affects the ability to breathe easily).

But when the researchers gave the rats that had had their ovaries removed estrogen replacement, not only did they regain some of the alveoli they'd lost, but the ones that were damaged actually got better.

They concluded in part that "estrogen is required for maintenance of already formed alveoli and induces alveolar regeneration after their loss in adult ovariectomized mice, and [this research] offers the possibility that estrogen can slow alveolar loss and induce alveolar regeneration in women with COPD."

In 2006, the research team finished their series of studies with a review article of their own work as well as research of others. The review pointed out that normal aging already results in loss of lung alveoli, and that menopause further accelerates the loss of lung surface area, which, in turn, reduces oxygen-carbon dioxide exchange and makes breathing more difficult. In other words, since estrogen is critical to long-term protection of women's lungs, after menopause, there's just not enough estrogen for some women, and their lungs suffer.

They also pointed out that their work and work in other laboratories "has disproved the notion that pulmonary alveoli are incapable of regeneration," and that research indicates that the factors regulating both alveolar loss and regeneration are "conserved" (scientese for "the same") for rats, mice, and humans.

Breathe Easier with BHRT

So what do all of these study results mean for you (or at least the women in the audience)? Well, there are several implications of this research work. First, even if you're healthy, you should seriously consider BHRT if you want to maximize your lungs' ability to absorb oxygen and get rid of carbon dioxide as you get older. This is especially important if you're an athlete, and want to continue your athletic activities for as long as you can – but maintaining healthy lungs also helps make simple daily tasks like walking up and down the stairs easier.

And BHRT may be especially important for women (nonsmokers) who have emphysema and/or COPD. If your estrogen levels are low enough to have caused (or at least contributed to) these problems, chances are that you're also at a significantly higher risk for the other problems associated with low estrogen levels, such as Alzheimer's disease, heart attack and other cardiovascular disease, and osteoporosis. But BHRT can help protect you from all of these conditions while it's helping to repair the damage that has been done to your lungs.

Even if your emphysema and/or COPD can be linked to smoking, BHRT is still worth trying. It may not help as much as if you'd never smoked, but if you're past menopause, your estrogens are already low, so replacing what your body is missing certainly won't hurt.

And what about men? As the researchers pointed out, male lungs and their alveoli aren't nearly as sensitive to hormonal variation as women's. However, there is at least one potential exception: Men whose testosterone gets so low that their bodies can't make much estrogen at all. (Remember, in both sexes the body makes estrogen by converting testosterone to estrogen – a process known as "aromatization.") So if you're a man who has been diagnosed with emphysema or COPD, you might want to get your estrogens checked along with your testosterone. If it turns out that your levels are too low, BHRT (in different proportions than those given to women, of course), may very well help you too.

Whether you're a woman or a man – with or without emphysema or COPD – if you're considering having your hormones checked and possibly using BHRT, make sure to consult a physician skilled and knowledgeable not only in BHRT but in nutritional and other natural therapies as well.

Singing BHRT's Praises – Literally

Although I'm not aware of any "controlled research," this is one topic that doesn't really require any. We've all experienced what happens to our voices as we enter and go through puberty, both in ourselves, and in our children and grandchildren. Vocal change during puberty is one of the signs of an increase in hormones. So it makes sense that, as you get older and these same hormones (particularly estrogen and testosterone) decline, your voice may change again – only not for the better this time.

But just like the other negative changes that accompany declining hormone levels, BHRT can also combat the "aging" of your speaking and singing voice. In fact, I've heard from many, many women whose increasingly unreliable voices returned to their former fullness after just a few weeks of BHRT.

Research has shown that estrogen is particularly important for women's lung function, so this may be part of the reason BHRT often helps women's singing. However, this application of BHRT seems a bit more universal: I've heard the same positive feedback about "voice recovery" with BHRT from older men, too.

Once again, anytime you're considering BHRT– whether it's to maintain your singing voice or any other purpose – make sure to consult a physician skilled and knowledgeable in BHRT as well as nutritional and other natural therapies.

ELIMINATING FIBROCYSTIC BREAST DISEASE – EVERY TIME!

Fall is "convention season" in the medical community. In the fall of 2004, I spoke to approximately 400 physicians at two different conventions. Among many other topics, I asked how many were familiar with Dr. John Myers's treatment for fibrocystic breast disease. Surprisingly, less than 10% of each group raised their hands. So in addition to telling these doctors about it, I thought I'd best tell you too, so that this exceptionally effective treatment won't "get lost," as so many natural, nonpatentable treatments have.

But before we get to Dr. Myers's cure for fibrocystic breast disease, let's cover the role of caffeine in this problem.

The Caffeine-Fibrocystic Breast Disease Controversy

Fibrocystic breast disease is characterized by hard lumps and bumps of varying sizes − *cysts* − in the breasts, which are often uncomfortable and even painful. It's one of the most common female health problems, occurring in over 60% of women, usually between the ages of 30 and 50.

Two decades or so ago, researchers reported that caffeine appeared to significantly aggravate this condition. So a "controlled trial" was organized to study the subject further, enrolling women with and without fibrocystic breast disease. Some women were asked to continue caffeine use, and others were asked to completely eliminate it. After some time, comparisons were made, and the researchers concluded that the use of caffeine made no significant difference in either causing or aggravating fibrocystic breast disease.

But a careful analysis of this study disclosed that it had some fundamental problems, which made the results essentially meaningless: Some women in the "zero-caffeine" group actually had traces of caffeine in their breast cyst fluid. Since human bodies don't make their own caffeine, those "zero-caffeine" women must have been using some caffeine after all − perhaps without even realizing it. It's not hard to do, since caffeine appears in some places you might not expect, such as chocolate and some over–the-counter pain relievers (especially headache medications like Excedrin®). Even decaf coffee has trace amounts of caffeine.

But aside from the caffeine factor, it's highly probable that some women are genetically predisposed to develop fibrocystic breast disease, and some simply aren't, caffeine or no caffeine. For a more meaningful study, only women with fibrocystic breast disease (or a family history of it) should have been enrolled, and then divided into "caffeine" and "no-caffeine" groups, with better control of caffeine intake in the zero-caffeine group.

Despite the flawed study, years of observation point to a clear connection between caffeine and fibrocystic breast disease. While caffeine doesn't cause this condition (if it did, there would be a much higher incidence), it can and does aggravate it.

Physicians skilled and knowledgeable in natural medicine have observed repeatedly that caffeine elimination usually results in a degree of improvement in women with fibrocystic breast disease. I continue to recommend it.

Results You Can Feel in Just 30 Minutes

Now, back to Dr. Myers's even more effective therapy − and my own "eyewitness" introduction to it.

In 1976, Dr. Myers came to the Seattle area to teach a seminar. He had arranged with the physicians in attendance for two local volunteer women with the very worst cases of fibrocystic disease to be present so that he could demonstrate the effectiveness of his treatment.

The women were given a few minutes to explain their very similar symptoms. Both had had fibrocystic disease for more than 5 years. Both reported pain nearly all month long, with relief only during menstruation, and they experienced major discomfort even from wearing some bras or heavier clothing. Neither could sleep on her stomach, nor hug anyone, without severe pain.

The women had agreed to let the doctors attending the seminar examine them before and after Dr. Myers's treatment − truly brave and generous of them. They took turns lying on an exam table as one doctor after another checked them as gently as possible. Despite the doctors careful efforts, the examinations were obviously painful; both women clenched their teeth frequently and tried not to complain.

When my turn came, I apologized (as did all the doctors) and checked as carefully as I could. The women's breasts felt as if they contained dozens and dozens of rock-hard marbles of varying sizes and sometimes irregular shapes.

After the examinations were completed, Dr. Myers thanked the women, and then a nurse took them (one at a time) into a small treatment room. Dr. Myers went in also; they emerged in less than 10 minutes. After the second woman had her treatment, everyone sat down again to resume listening to Dr. Myers.

Thirty minutes later, Dr. Myers asked the two women how they felt. Each was obviously surprised to report that she felt better already. Dr. Myers asked if they would agree to another examination. Both said "Yes."

Like the other physicians in attendance, I was amazed. Instead of grimacing in pain, both women were smiling as they were examined. The "rock-hard marbles" weren't gone, but they were much softer, more pliable, and obviously much less painful. Even the tissue between the cysts felt softer. And it had been less than 1 hour since Dr. Myers and the nurse had done the treatments.

Even more amazingly, Dr. Myers then told us that with just 2 to 3 months of repeated treatments, neither of these women would suffer from fibrocystic breast disease at all, and that the same would be the case for any woman suffering from fibrocystic disease treated by his methods. He emphasized that in some cases small remnants of the cysts would remain, but in all cases the pain would be gone, in most cases permanently, with follow-up treatment rarely required.

The Method Behind the Miracle

Dr. Myers explained that he had used a solution of iodine,* which he swabbed into the entire vaginal area of each woman, followed within 2 minutes by an intravenous injection of magnesium sulfate. That's all there was to it, and less than 1 hour later there had been substantial improvement.

---

* Dr. Myers' treatment has changed very little over the years. For awhile, the type of iodine he preferred ("di-atomic") became unavailable, so I switched to "Lugol's iodine," which is 5% "di-atomic" and 10% SSKI (saturated solution of potassium iodide). It works just as well.

Right away, one of the seminar attendees asked why the iodine had to be swabbed into the vagina, rather than just swallowed. Dr. Myers explained how he arrived at this particular protocol by relating some of the early research he did in the dog laboratories of Johns Hopkins University Medical School using iodine for fibrocystic breast disease.

There's a type of beagle (the females, of course) that "normally" develops fibrocystic breast disease. Dr. Myers had removed both ovaries from one group of these female beagles, and performed "sham" surgery on the other group, leaving their ovaries in place and intact as a control. He'd applied his series of treatments to both groups of beagles. Those with ovaries had complete elimination of their beagle-breast-cysts; the dogs without ovaries had no improvement at all.

Dr. Myers concluded that the ovaries must combine iodine with another molecule or molecules to make an unknown (to this day) iodine-containing compound that resolves fibrocystic breast disease. He pointed out that when we swallow iodine, most of it is "trapped" by our thyroid glands, and much less is available to the ovaries, so it's only logical to apply the iodine as close to the ovaries as possible.

Also during his work with the beagles, he had found that intravenous magnesium sulfate improved the efficiency of the iodine treatment; once again, the reason for this still hasn't been discovered.

Following Dr. Myers's seminar, I started using his treatment at the Tahoma Clinic. It was just as successful as he promised. As word spread, we worked with over 100 women in the first year or 2. Some were left with much smaller but pain-free cysts; others had them disappear completely. But *every single woman treated had complete relief of pain* within a few weeks to 3 months maximum.

How I Accidentally Discovered the Effect of Iodine on the EQ (Estrogen Quotient)

In the 1970s, it was still controversial whether women with fibrocystic breast disease were at greater risk for breast cancer. Some of the women I worked with were concerned about that, so I told them about the work of Dr. Henry Lemon at the University of Nebraska, which indicated that estriol might be protective against breast cancer. (*See Chapter 7 for a review of the EQ and the work of Dr. Lemon.*) I asked each woman with fibrocystic breast disease to do the type of test Dr. Lemon had been doing, a 24-hour urine collection examined in the laboratory for relative levels of estrone, estradiol, and estriol, as I thought it might tell us about cancer risk for women with fibrocystic breast disease.

More than a few of these tests came back showing a low EQ – low levels of estriol compared with the other 2 estrogens. According to Dr. Lemon, this did indicate an elevated risk of breast cancer. But, at the time, I wasn't sure what to recommend to correct the problem, so I started researching possible solutions. In the meantime, though, I recommended that the women continue their iodine treatments.

Several of the women completed their treatments before I'd found anything useful at the library. Since their breast condition had changed dramatically, I thought that their estrogen ratio tests might have changed, too, so I recommended they repeat them. *In every case* the proportion of estriol had increased dramatically between the first test and the second one.

And that's how I learned that iodine has a remarkable effect on estrogen metabolism, normalizing the EQ nearly every time I've recommended it to a woman over the last 30+ years. Later on, I observed that iodide would do the very same job as iodine in improving women's estriol levels, both in women with and without fibrocystic breast disease. By contrast, the results aren't nearly as good for men with a low EQ, only a minority of whom have improved estriol levels and higher EQs with iodine or iodide use.

More recent research (See "Iodine Kills Breast Cancer Cells!") has found that iodine (but not iodide) might actually be a useful treatment for breast cancer. Thus, it appears that iodine may both help to prevent and to effectively treat this condition.

One of the theoretical "risks" of using high-dose iodine in the amounts needed to treat fibrocystic breast disease is hypothyroidism (weak thyroid function). However, I have never witnessed an instance of this occurring in nearly 30 years of administering this therapy. It appears that fibrocystic breasts "soak up" large amounts of iodine, leaving the thyroid gland unaffected.

Iodine Kills Breast Cancer Cells!

If someone had predicted 30 years ago that iodine would become one of the most important breast cancer treatments, I doubt many people would have believed it. And they would have been right – it isn't one of the most important cancer treatments. In fact, it's hardly used at all.

But it should be.

Iodine kills breast cancer cells without killing off normal cells in the process. In other words, it's ideal for both the treatment *and* prevention of breast cancer.

Chances are your doctor hasn't heard of this (I'll tell you why in just a minute). So if you want the treatment – and believe me, you should – it's up to you to share this information with your doctor.

Solid Research Conveniently Ignored

In the 1960s and '70s, pioneering iodine researcher Bernard Eskin, MD, reported time and again that iodine is a key element in breast health. (At one time I counted over 80 of his research papers on the topic.)

In one of his studies, Dr. Eskin demonstrated that deliberately blocking breast cells from access to iodine resulted in precancerous changes – changes that were aggravated when those same cells were exposed to either estrogens or thyroid hormone. Surprisingly, in the absence of iodine, thyroid hormone appeared to be more likely to produce abnormalities in breast cells than estrogen.

In another report, he noted that when breast tissue cells are lacking in iodine (in both humans and rodents), the cells are more likely to be abnormal, precancerous, or cancerous. He said, "Iodine-deficient breast tissues are also more susceptible to carcinogen action and promote lesions earlier and in greater profusion. Metabolically, iodine-deficient breasts show changes in RNA/DNA ratios, estrogen receptor proteins." He concluded that: "[Iodine] presents great potential for its use in research directed toward the prevention, diagnosis, and treatment of breast cancer."

Despite its obvious potential, not much has been done with this treatment over the past 30 to 40 years – at least not in the US. Since iodine isn't patentable (and is therefore unlikely to be "approved" for use to prevent or treat breast cancer), Dr. Eskin's work has been ignored. Patent medicine companies simply looked elsewhere for profits. Sadly, since most mainstream doctors are dependent on patent medicine company sales reps for much of their up-to-date information, doctors have been kept in the dark regarding this potential use for iodine.

Over the past 2 years, though, researchers in Mexico and India (where low-cost, unpatented medicine is a necessity) have begun further investigations into iodine's potential as a breast cancer treatment. So far, all of their results confirm Dr. Eskin's original research: Iodine directly kills many types of human breast cancer cells, and it doesn't kill healthy cells in the process.

Traveling Beyond the Border for Natural Cancer Cures

In 2005, researchers from the Autonomous National University in Juriquilla, Mexico, reviewed evidence showing that iodine supports breast health by slowing or preventing the spread of cancerous cells. They said, "In animal and human studies, molecular iodine [I(2)] supplementation exerts a suppressive effect on the development and size of both benign and cancer neoplasias…Iodine, in addition to its incorporation into thyroid hormones, is bound into antiproliferative iodolipids [iodinated lipids with anticancer activity] in the thyroid called iodolactones, which may also play a role in the proliferative control of mammary gland." They concluded that breast cancer patients should consider supplementing with I2 in addition to their traditional breast cancer therapy.

In June 2006, a group from the Sanjay Ghandi Institute of Medical Sciences in Lucknow, India, found that iodine is cytotoxic (kills cancer cells) to several human breast cancer cell lines, including (for the technically inclined) MCF-7, MDA-MB-231, MDA-MB-453, ZR-75-1, and T-47D. When iodine was applied to human blood cells (monocytes), it inhibited growth and proliferation, but it didn't kill the cells.

Then, in December 2006, the group in Mexico tested the effect of iodine on the MCF-7 form of human breast cancer cells. (They didn't try iodine against the other human breast cancer cell lines noted above.) They found that iodine (but not iodide), along with an iodinated fatty acid, inhibited the MCF-7 cancer cells. At the same time, the iodine neither harmed nor inhibited fibroblasts, a normal type of human connective tissue cell that helps to support breast tissue and other tissues throughout the body. Other technical details led the researchers to suggest that iodine may become active against cancer cells when it is bound to certain lipids or proteins that are normally present in the breasts.

A Safe Adjunct Treatment to Conventional Cancer Therapies

These recent research reports give new hope and an added tool for breast cancer patients. It's true that the research isn't conclusive at this point, but you don't need to wait for academic and scientific certainty – which will likely take many more years – to try out the benefits for yourself.

If you have breast cancer and you're undergoing regular treatment, adding iodine to your treatment plan will only increase your odds of a favorable outcome – and it's perfectly safe. Numerous studies have proven that iodine (and its iodide form) are among the safest of all the elements.

In one case, a 54-year-old man mistakenly drank 600 mLs (over 20 ounces) of a saturated solution of potassium iodide – 100,000 times the recommended daily allowance. The initial reaction was a bit scary: He developed swelling in his neck, mouth, and face, and he experienced transient heart rhythm abnormalities – but he recovered uneventfully.

In another instance, a researcher had 2,400 patients with asthma take 5,000 milligrams of potassium iodide daily on a cycle of 4 days on, followed by 3 days off. Only 12 of the individuals (0.5%) became hypothyroid as a result, and 4 developed swollen thyroid glands. There was no report of any adverse reaction among the rest.

Even though iodine is generally safe, some individuals are sensitive to iodine and/or iodide. There have been anecdotal reports of iodide causing autoimmune thyroiditis, hyperthyroidism, and hypothyroidism. Too much iodine in a few individuals has caused iodism, an acne-like rash accompanied by a runny nose and a bad taste, all of which go away when the dosage is reduced or eliminated.

But the possible consequences of an unchecked breast cancer are considerably more likely – and of course much worse – than experiencing a negative reaction to iodine. So if I were you, I'd give it a try.

Rub Away Your Breast Cancer?

A suggestion for you and your doctor to consider: Put the treatment right onto the problem! Mix a solution of 50% iodine/50% DMSO and rub it directly onto your breast nearest to where the cancer is (or used to be). The DMSO will ensure penetration deep into the tissue. A 70% DMSO solution is widely available, and iodine is available by prescription as Lugol's Iodine or in natural food stores and the Tahoma Clinic Dispensary as Triodide (from Scientific Botanicals). If you're worried about the breast cancer spreading, you can rub the mixture into the area under the arms rich in lymph glands (nodes) where breast cancer spreads first.

But please don't do any of this without consulting a physician skilled and knowledgeable in the use of high-dose iodine!!

You should also be sure that your physician monitors your thyroid function and gives you other nutrient suggestions while you use iodine as an adjunct in your regular breast cancer treatment.

For more information about iodine and iodide, I recommend two excellent books: Dr. David Derry's *Breast Cancer and Iodine: How to Prevent and How to Survive Breast Cancer*, and Dr. David Brownstein's *Iodine: Why You Need It, Why You Can't Live Without It.*

Forget Those Needles: Erase Your Wrinkles with a Powdered Drink Mix

Plus Two Other All-Natural Age-Fighters Your Skin Will Thank You For

A few weeks ago, our 31-year-old daughter came home for a visit. She hadn't seen her mother for several weeks, and not long after she arrived, she asked what Holly had been doing "this time" to make her skin look so good. As she put it, Holly's skin looked "healthier than ever." She commented that her skin tone was deeper and more vibrant and that some of the little wrinkles around Holly's eyes were actually gone.

Holly's always taken very good care of herself: never smoked, doesn't drink alcohol, eats as much "organic" and "free range" as possible, uses absolutely no sugar, refined food or food chemicals, and takes her vitamins, minerals, and botanicals. She's also used bio-identical hormones for over 15 years, and most of that time she's also used a skin cream containing a tiny amount of estriol (more on that a little later). Of course, I have always considered her beautiful, but she really does appear much younger than her actual age: In fact, from time to time she's asked to show her driver's license to prove that she qualifies for the "over-55" discount offered at certain places.

But she had been doing something extra "this time." I admit that I hadn't noticed a great difference, but, in my defense, it's harder to see changes in someone you're around every day (or perhaps because men just aren't as "tuned in" to those sorts of details as women are), but regardless of whether or not I'd noticed, our daughter certainly had.

Holly's improvements had come about as a result of her taking (for the second time – I'll tell you about the first time in just a bit) a combination containing collagen, hyaluronic acid, and other natural ingredients.

Why These Anti-Aging "Miracles" Aren't Always All They're Cracked up to Be

You've likely already heard of products containing collagen and hyaluronic acid (HA). They've both been touted for their skin "anti-aging" effects (especially for facial skin) for awhile. And using them is logical since collagen is the major extracellular protein responsible for the strength and flexibility of connective tissue, including the skin. In fact,

25 to 30% of bodily protein is collagen. And HA is one of the biological hallmarks of youth: Baby skin has the most hyaluronic acid and content declines with age.

But if it were as easy as it sounds in the commercials advertising products containing collagen and HA, everyone would be using them – and would have younger-looking skin with fewer wrinkles as a result. Since that isn't the case, you've probably gathered that there are a few problems with using many of these products.

"Generally accepted" opinion has been that swallowing collagen and hyaluronic acid won't do that much good, as they'd be completely digested (or nearly so) in the intestines. So emphasis has been placed on injecting them directly into the skin, especially facial skin, to replace the collagen and hyaluronic acid our own skin makes less of as we grow older.

Since all the "approved" forms of collagen and HA are injectable, they all require visits to a doctor – and they're quite costly. But even worse than these drawbacks is that the injectable forms of collagen and HA used in most cases are not exactly the same as the human forms. Collagen shots typically include cow collagen instead of human collagen, and HA injections come from rooster and bacterial sources, so the chances of unwanted "side effects" are higher. To be fair, there is at least one injectable that uses bio-identical hyaluronic acid. (For a more complete review of several of these products, see *Nutrition & Healing* for February 2004.)

But it wasn't injections of bio-identical HA that had elicited such praise from our daughter about Holly's appearance. In fact, she hadn't been using injections of anything. Even though most sources agree that taking collagen and HA orally won't help the skin, at least one study – not to mention Holly's first-hand experience – has shown that it <u>does</u>.

Say Goodbye to Sagging, Puffy, Wrinkled Eyes

In this blinded and randomized 8-week research trial, 40 women, aged 35 to 60, took 7.5 or 8.5 grams daily of a product called *Toki*®. Toki is a powdered drink mix that combines collagen, hyaluronic acid, and other natural ingredients and is sweetened with stevia. According to the researchers, the formulation "resulted in a highly statistically significant improvement in periorbital [around the eyes] wrinkling, in periorbital aging, and periorbital over-all facial aging. The investigator's mean global improvement scores of overall facial aging as compared to baseline photographs were also highly significant."

The women participating in the study also did self-evaluations. And each of them also reported significant improvement in sagging, puffiness, and wrinkling around the eyes, as well as noticeable improvement in overall facial aging – the same improvements our daughter noticed in Holly after she started taking Toki®.

This research also certainly appears to disprove the idea that injecting collagen is the only way to prevent it from being broken down during digestion: Levels of collagen in the participants' blood were 114% higher at the end of the 8 weeks than at the outset of the study. So apparently, at least some of the collagen swallowed in the Toki® formula "made it through" without being broken down in the gut.

Of course, that doesn't prove outright that the very same collagen caused the women's significant facial improvements, but there's no question that something in Toki® *did*.

Holly's Toki® regimen started with 6 grams (one packet) 3 times a day for 2 weeks. Then she tapered back to 2 doses daily for another 2 weeks. Now she's following the "maintenance" dose of 1 packet daily.

First Time's a Charm

As I mentioned earlier (and as our daughter's comment implied), this isn't the first time Holly has tried injection-less anti-aging treatments. Three or 4 years ago at yet another convention, she was given a small sample bottle of a hyaluronic acid product called Synovoderma®. Knowing that babies' skin has considerably more hyaluronic acid than adult skin, and that dermatologists and plastic surgeons were using non-bio-identical injections of hyaluronic acid to improve their patients' appearance, she decided that a natural form might be worth a try. At the very least, she knew it wouldn't hurt to swallow it, especially since the capsules contained nothing else but rice bran and beeswax (apparently fillers). So she read the label, and took 2 of the capsules twice daily.

Towards the end of the first week, she was washing her face, and asked me to come take a look. "There's all this dead skin coming off," she pointed out. "I've never had that much dead skin come off at one time, ever!" Her face cloth was definitely covered with shreds of old skin; the only time I've seen that much coming off someone at once has been the "peeling" that sometimes occurs awhile after a sunburn, and Holly definitely hadn't had that.

For the next few days, more dead skin than usual came off each time Holly washed her face, although each day it was a little less, until the exfoliation subsided to normal. She continued to use 3 capsules twice daily for 3 weeks, as the product packaging instructed, then cut back to 3 a day for several weeks. About that time, our daughter (the same one who visited recently) came by, and noticed an improvement in her mother's facial skin then too.

While it's true that *Synovoderma®* may be more expensive than many other supplements, and *Toki®* is definitely more expensive than other supplements, the difference either one can make to your complexion may be worth it. Unlike most of the facial injections, both these supplements are all natural, and very unlikely to cause significant "side effects." And if cost is an issue to you, facial injections are way, way more expensive than either *Synovoderma®* or *Toki®* − and take considerably more time and trouble. If you've been thinking at all of cosmetic facial injections, it's worth your while to try one or both first.

In addition to these, there is yet another natural anti-aging tool for your facial skin that you may want to consider.

Bio-Identical HRT: Good for You Inside *and* Out

The other skin treatment Holly has been using for years is a topical cream containing bio-identical estriol. Usually, when I mention this hormone it's in reference to its role in bio-identical hormone replacement therapy, which is typically prescribed for women dealing with the various symptoms associated with menopause (hot flashes, vaginal dryness, etc.). But over 10 years ago, I read about the results of a 1987 study in which 14 postmenopausal women were treated for 3 weeks with a topical skin application containing estriol (and compared with another 6 women who received the same topical treatment without estriol).

According to the researchers, after 3 weeks "The elastic fibers in the [skin] were thickened, better orientated and slightly increased in number in half of these patients but in none of the control patients. The epidermal thickness was slightly increased in 4 of the patients treated with estriol." And this after only 3 weeks!

I guessed that a longer period of time would have shown a greater success rate, and even better results. So I asked my compounding pharmacist friends at Key Pharmacy (www.keynutririonrx.com, 1-800-878-1322) to put estriol together with other ingredients into a skin crème.

Since the quantity of estriol in the skin crème was small, and not likely to have a systemic effect, Holly started using it. Since then, she's noticed that she's gotten considerably fewer and less noticeable wrinkles than many of her friends (and the benefits she's gotten from other products like Synovoderma® and Toki® are just "icing on the cake," so to speak).

But Holly's experiences aren't the only support for this approach to skin anti-aging. In 1996, another research group examined the effects of tiny concentrations of bio-identical estrogens applied to the skin. In this study, 59 premenopausal women with signs of skin aging applied crèmes containing either 0.01% estradiol or 0.3% estriol. The researchers also measured the women's blood levels of estradiol and two other hormones, FSH (follicle stimulating hormone, which stimulates estrogen secretion from the ovaries) and prolactin (which, among other things, stimulates milk secretion in nursing mothers). Skin biopsies were also taken for measurements of collagen in 10 of the women.

According to the researchers: "After treatment for 6 months, elasticity and firmness of the skin had markedly improved and the wrinkle depth and pore sizes had decreased by 61 to 100 percent in both groups. Furthermore, skin moisture had increased and the measurement of wrinkles…revealed significant, or even highly significant, decreases of wrinkle depth in the estradiol and the estriol groups…significant increases of Type III collagen labeling were combined with increased numbers of collagen fibers at the end of the treatment period."

The researchers also noted that only blood levels of prolactin increased significantly, while estradiol and FSH did not. They pointed out that this indicated there were no systemic effects of the use of these hormones, only the local − and desirable − skin changes.

And in 2005, another research group reported on the use of progesterone skin cream in 40 women during and after menopause. The study measured skin elasticity, epidermal hydration (skin water content) and skin surface lipids, along with measurement of blood levels of estrogen, progesterone, FSH, and LH (luteinizing hormone), which is known to stimulate progesterone secretion.

According to these researchers: "The 2% progesterone cream yielded consistent superiority over [placebo] in counteracting different signs of aging in the skin of peri- and postmenopausal women. Clinical monitoring showed a greater reduction in wrinkle counts (29.10% vs. 16.50%) and wrinkle depth (9.72% vs. 7.35%)… and a significantly higher…increase in skin firmness (23.61% vs. 13.24%) in the treatment group…No serious side-effects of the treatment were observed."

Ladies, it's never too late to consider using topical BHRT. It's safe, and can be monitored for any systemic effects (and adjusted accordingly in the unlikely event that one should occur). If you're interested in trying this "anti-aging" tool, contact a physician skilled and knowledgeable in BHRT!

But before you do, there is just one small note of caution: Two percent of a hormone (progesterone, in the case of the last study mentioned above) in a skin crème doesn't sound like much. However, it did produce a small but significant increase in blood progesterone in the women who used it. On the other hand, the 0.01% estradiol and 0.3% estriol crèmes used in the other studies didn't increase blood levels of these hormones significantly.

Although your body isn't likely to absorb each of these hormones at the same exact rate, it's probably close, so even though they are applied topically and haven't been shown to affect blood levels significantly, you should still undergo regular interval monitoring for systemic absorption of any topical hormones (and their potential metabolites) you decide to take (just as you do during "regular" BHRT). It's also likely best to keep the concentrations of any topical hormones at no more, and possibly less, than the concentrations mentioned in the research articles.

****

Readers of *Nutrition & Healing* know that while I work with clients at Tahoma Clinic, I'm also consultant to Meridian Valley Labs (www.meridianvalleylab.com, 425-271-8689). Ever since I was the first to prescribe bio-identical estrogens along with progesterone, testosterone, and DHEA in the early 1980s, I've been working with Meridian Valley Labs to continually develop safety monitoring testing for what's come to be known as BHRT. The 24-hour urine test is by far the best test for this purpose, and Meridian Valley Labs has far and away the best of these tests at the best price, with peer-to-peer consultation for practicing physicians included in the price of the test. See the website listed above for further details.

****

Take
our
FREE

hormone assessment online at:

www.smart-publications.com/

hormone-self-assessment

INDEX

D

I